AF564413

Recent Advances in Poultry Nutrition

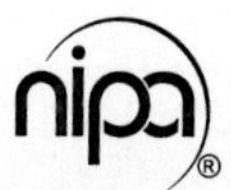

NIPA® GENX ELECTRONIC RESOURCES & SOLUTIONS P. LTD.
New Delhi-110 034

Recent Advances in Poultry Nutrition

M.T. Banday
Dean
Faculty of Veterinary Sciences and Animal Husbandry
Shre-e- Kashmir University of Agricultural Sciences and Technology, Kashmir
Jammu & Kashmir, India

Sheikh Adil
Assistant Professor
Department of Livestock Production and Management
Faculty of Veterinary Sciences and Animal Husbandry
Shre-e- Kashmir University of Agricultural Sciences and Technology, Kashmir
Jammu and Kashmir, India

Manzoor A. Wani
Lecturer
Department of Livestock Production and Management
Faculty of Veterinary Sciences and Animal Husbandry
Shre-e- Kashmir University of Agricultural Sciences and Technology, Kashmir
Jammu and Kashmir, India

NIPA® GENX ELECTRONIC RESOURCES & SOLUTIONS P. LTD.
New Delhi-110 034

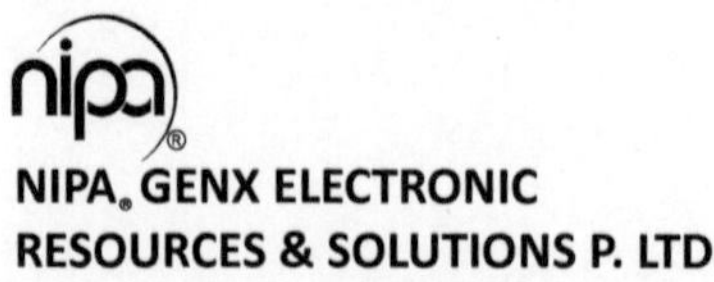

NIPA® GENX ELECTRONIC RESOURCES & SOLUTIONS P. LTD.

101,103, Vikas Surya Plaza, CU Block
L.S.C.Market, Pitam Pura, New Delhi-110 034
Ph : +91 11 27341616, 27341717, 27341718
E-mail: newindiapublishingagency@gmail.com
www: www.nipabooks.com

For customer assistance, please contact
Phone: + 91-11-27 34 17 17
Fax: + 91-11- 27 34 16 16
E-Mail: feedbacks@nipabooks.com

ISBN: 978-81-19103-79-9

Composed and Designed by NIPA.

ABOUT THE EDITORS

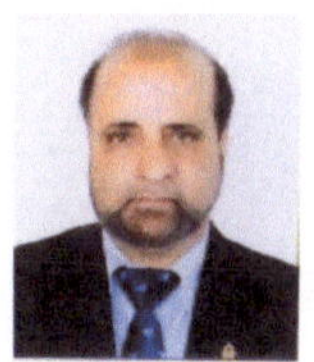

Dr. M.T. Banday is currently Dean, FVSc & AH, Shuham, SKUAST-Kahmir. He is recipient of Fellow National from Animal Production Management Society of India. He received SK Ranjhan Award from Animal Nutrition Society of India for his doctoral Programme. He has published about 250 research papers/abstracts/popular scientific articles, 3 books, 2 book chapters, 5 technical bulletins, one monograph, four practical manuals and edited learning material on Poultry Production for National Institute of open School, New Delhi. He is associated with a number of internal and external research projects. He is in the editorial board of two Poultry magazines. He has guided 5 students for Ph.D programme and 13 students for MVSc programme He has been a life member of a number of professional/scientific bodies. He is Vice President of ISAPM. He can be contacted at drbandayade@gmail.com.

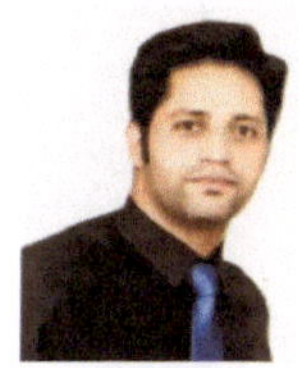

Dr. Sheikh Adil is currently working as an Assistant Professor in the Department of Livestock Production and Management, F.V.Sc. & A.H., SKUAST-Kashmir. He has a vast experience in teaching, research and extension activities. He got third rank in B.V.Sc. and first rank in M.V.Sc. His area of interest is poultry nutrition. He is recipient of various awards. He has guided a number of students at UG and Postgraduate level. He has published a number of research and technical papers in various national and impact factor international journals. Besides he has number of book chapters, manuals, monographs, pamphlets etc to his credit. He is an Editorial board member in various reputed national and international journals. He is a life member of number of professional/scientific bodies. He is associated with many internally & externally funded projects. He can be contacted at drsheikhadil@skuastkashmir.ac.in.

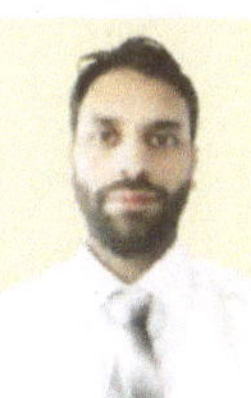

Dr. Manzoor A. Wani is working as a lecturer in the Department of Livestock Production and Management, F.V.Sc. & A.H., SKUAST-Kashmir. He has graduated from SKUAST-K. He secured JRF for his Master's degree programme and Institute fellowship of ICAR-IVRI for his doctoral programme. He has published research papers in national and international reputed journals. He has been awarded with best PhD thesis, Young scientist award and a number of best presentation awards. He is a life member of number of professional/scientific bodies. He has been a part of various internally & externally funded projects. He can be contacted at manzoorwani5193@gmail.com.

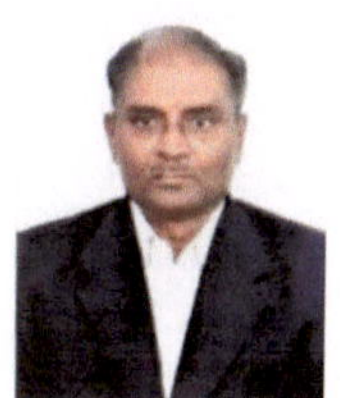

V Ramasubba Reddy
Retired Professor
Agricultural University, Hyderabad

Foreword

There is a marked improvement in the Animal Husbandry sector and in particular in the Poultry Sector in India as it is emerging as an important activity for enhancing nutrition and providing employment as the broiler production has grown in importance. According to industry sources, the animal output of broilers has multiplied six-fold in the current decade with annual rate of growth amounted to 20 percent for broilers and ten percent for eggs.

Today, India ranks as the world's third largest egg producing country and fifth largest poultry meat producer. Today a network of over 500 commercial hatcheries and breeding farms, 100 commercial feed mills, Veterinary pharmaceuticals and equipment manufacturers has made poultry farming a dynamic agri-business, duly supported by research and development.

Given the tightening supply and ever increasing cost of raw materials, there will be more pressure to extract every unit of energy and nutrients from feed ingredients. In this context, a number of feed additives are expected to play an increasingly significant role. Among these additives, enzymes, crystalline amino acids, and phytogenics will have a profound effect on future sustainability of poultry industry. Thus, future nutritional research needs to focus on identifying the barriers to effective digestion and utilization of nutrients to achieve the positive effect.

This book would be of great use to undergraduate, post-graduate students, teachers and scientist's affiliated to poultry science. An attempt has been made to compile most of the scientific interventions made, in order to enlighten and update the knowledge of students, teachers, research scholars, and industrialists in the field of poultry nutrition. It is a first edition of the book and we hope it will be very useful to all the target groups and end-users.

V Ramasubba Reddy
Retired Professor
Agricultural University
Hyderabad

Preface

Poultry sector has witnessed many ups and downs as a result of lack of information on nutrient requirements and feeding programmes for chicken. However, compared to other types of livestock sectors, poultry industry has advanced in terms of technologies, improved productivity and consistent improvements in nutrition. Poultry nutrition and other management practices have improved through education expansion, trainings, and competition and survival instincts.

The small improvement in feed efficiency is economically important as feed alone accounts 60-70% of total production cost. Nutrition plays a vital role in economic production and maintenance of proper poultry health. Major objective of poultry nutrition is to improve the performance, efficiency of gain and quality of products (meat & eggs). Therefore, there is an urgent need to update the nutrient requirements of high yielding and fast growing chicken; evaluate and utilize alternate feed resources, explore the possibility of using new feed additives to optimize production and overall health of birds while excluding antimicrobial feed additives. Key advances in poultry nutrition are discussed and future directions which can be expected are highlighted in this book.

Nutritional advances as discussed in the various chapters in this book embrace historical perspectives as well as futuristic perspectives. Indeed we must have a clear understanding of the past to identify advances that will mold the future of poultry nutrition. Generally in the past, poultry nutrition has focussed on increasing the production efficiency of meat and eggs to meet the ever achieving demand of animal protein globally. However, futuristic demand in poultry is driven not only by the need to maximize biological and economic performance of birds, but also by societal issues (environmental, welfare, antibiotic growth promoters, traceability and use of genetically modified ingredients).

We are thankful to all the Professors, Scientists and teachers for providing the up to date information of their respective chapters in the area of poultry nutrition. We owe our special thanks to publisher NIPA Genx Electronic Resources & Solutions Pvt. Ltd. for publishing the book in most presentable form.

We sincerely hope that the present form of book will be found useful by all the concerned. Let this book set the path for future research work to be carried out in the area of poultry nutrition. Comments and suggestions for further improvement of this book are solicited.

Editors

Contents

1

Nutritional Requirements of Chicken An Overview

S.V.S. Verma[1], S.K. Bhanja[2] and M.T. Banday[3]

[1]Retired Principal Scientist & Head NT, ICAR-Central Avian Research Institute, Izatnagar, Uttar Pradesh, Uttar Pradesh

[2]Principal Scientist, ICAR-Central Avian Research Institute, Izatnagar, Uttar Pradesh Uttar Pradesh

[3]Dean, Faculty of Veterinary Sciences and Animal Husbandry, Shre-e- Kashmir University of Agricultural Sciences and Technology, Kashmir.

Introduction

Until the 1960's poultry in India remained largely a backyard dual purpose activity for eggs and meat. People from low social order and economically weaker sections in villages and suburbs generally took to poultry keeping primarily to supplement their diet with more nutritious eggs and meet, and secondly to enrich their livelihood. Despite on a small scale, the activity attracted sizeable proportion of population contributing immensely to the egg and meat supply. The Indian society, though largely vegetarian, gradually accepted eggs and meat in their diet. As demand for poultry products increased, small units transformed into larger well organized farms paving way for a poultry products supply network throughout the country.

By 1980's Indian poultry emerged a fastest growing segment of the Indian Agriculture. Scientific inputs in terms of poultry science education, training and extension provided a much needed boost to modernize Indian poultry on scientific lines to establish it well on the world's poultry map. Genetic selection and breeding helped evolve potential egg laying strains (300 + eggs in a year) and fast growing broiler chicks capable of attaining 2 kg body weight by 6 weeks of age (Table 1, 2) with a satisfactory feed conversion efficiency (FCE). Befitting nutritional management, housing and health care measures revolutionized poultry operations further. Realization of the fact that cocks were not necessary to enable hens lay eggs, came a big surprise for the common people. Germ-free eggs, so obtained (came to be known by farm eggs), stormed into the market, helping in promotion of egg consumption greatly. This attracted fresh investments in the form of ancillary industries providing all-round support to poultry network building up within and around India.

Table 1: Certain performance indices typical to egg laying stocks in India

Age (weeks)		Egg Production	Egg weight	Feed Intake
Range	No.	Range (%)	(g/egg)	(g/b/d)
19-20	02	05-15	30-40	60-75
21-24	04	40-80	38-42	90-100
25-52	28	92-97	45-48	100-110
53-73	21	89-80	48-52	110-113
74-84	11	79-60	51-55	100-110

Table 2: Certain performance indices typical to commercial broiler chickens in India

Age	**Live Weight (g/b)**			**Feed Intake (g/b)**			**Cumu-lative Feed Intake (g/b)**	**Feed Conver-sion (Feed/ live wt.)**
(weeks)	**Male**	**Female**	**Average**	**Male**	**Female**	**Average**		
1	150	140	145	132	130	131	131	0.90
2	370	340	355	286	276	281	412	1.16
3	672	615	644	484	440	462	874	1.36
4	1078	964	1021	696	638	667	1541	1.51
5	1570	1340	1455	942	728	835	2376	1.63
6	2082	1738	1910	1112	992	1052	3428	1.79
7	2580	2130	2355	1270	1062	1166	4594	1.95

The road to poultry development was however never smooth, it always had its own pitfalls. Widespread drought and resultant general food, feed and fodder scarcity during the 1980s gripped the nation to its fold. Poultry, being largely dependent on cereal grains and their by-products for its food, was hit the most. Prices of essential commodities went up unabated attracting malpractice of the trade. The industry crippled and many farmers closed down operations due to prohibitive costs and poor feed quality throwing an open challenge to the nutritionists. Accordingly, the poultry nutritionists rose to the occasion and evolved production-oriented, nutritionally-sufficient, economically-viable feed formulae through utilizing alternate unconventional feed resources, saving the Indian poultry industry in crisis.

Significant alterations in the productive capacity of the egg and meat lines of chickens have become a prominent supportive development to the Indian poultry during the past few decades. Improved germplasm supported with befitting nutritional management, comforting environment with proper healthcare made such achievements a reality. We now understand nutritional management of chickens better than those of the other farm livestock. However, in view of the ever-changing ecological impacts, gaps in the knowledge of nutrient requirements are, indeed, a natural phenomenon and updation of such aspects through search and research is a continuous process.

Nutrition-the base of life

The study of nutrition involves a combined effort of the knowledge of chemistry, biochemistry, microbiology, toxicology and processing technologies all applied to understand nutrients in various feedstuffs, their nutritive quality and bioavailability on ingestion as part of diet. An ideal poultry diet consists of energy-rich cereal grains (bajra, barley, jowar, maize, rice kani, wheat), grain by-products (ricebran, ricepolish, wheatbran), proteinous oilseed meals (groundnut meal, rapeseed meal, soybean meal, sunflower meal), animal protein sources (fish meal, meat-cum-bone meal, meat meal), calcarious limestone, oystershell grit, micronutrient premixes (trace elements, vitamins) and any medicaments. Conventional poultry rations so formulated are coarsely milled and mixed into a uniform blend. Suggested levels of certain nutrients in diets for layer and broiler chickens are given in Table 3 and 4.

While dealing with poultry nutrition many words (basal, diet, feed, mash, pellets, premixes, ration, supplements) have invariably been in vogue and with specific meanings too. The terms allowance and requirement are of special significance, when formulating diets for chickens raised for specific purposes. Feed and nutrient requirements refer to the amount of composite diet or any specific nutrient needed by birds of a particular age group reared for any specific purpose. It is the amount that has been so determined through experimentations, and is actually needed for body maintenance, tissue growth, wellbeing, production and for reproductive purposes. On the other hand, an allowance is the amount a little more than the actual requirement so as to take care in any exigency.

The publications (ARC, 1977; NRC, 1994; BIS, 2007) hold excerpt of the enormous data based on extensive reviews of published reports (bioassays, growth experiments, egg laying and reproductive performance, egg and meat quality, physiological responses, eggshell quality, survivability and the like) globally thereby suggesting requirement figures for most nutrients as needed by different categories of chickens to perform optimally. Such recommendations may generally hold good for most poultry stocks raised for various purposes and reared under the usual climatic conditions. Even though, certain degree of safety margin in the nutrient requirement figures is warranted keeping in view various situations and factors affecting them.

Table 3: Suggested levels of certain nutrients in diets for layer chickens

Constituent	Commercial Layer Feed				Layer Breeder Feed			
	Chick Starter (1-7 wk)	Grower (8-18 wk)	Layer Ph-I (19-52 wk)	Layer Ph-II (52 wk on wards)	Chick (1-7 wk)	Grower (8-18 wk)	Female (>19 wk)	Male (>19 wk)
Nutrient (%)								
Moisture	10.00	10.00	10.00	10.00	10.00	10.00	10.00	10.00
Protein (Nx6.25)	20.00	16.00	18.00	16.00	20.00	16.00	17.00	16.00
Eather Extract	3.00	2.50	2.50	2.50	3.00	2.50	2.50	2.50
Fibre	7.00	9.00	9.00	10.00	7.00	9.00	9.00	10.00
Acid-insoluble ash	4.00	4.00	4.50	5.00	4.00	4.00	4.50	5.00
Linoleic acid	1.00	1.00	1.00	1.00	1.00	1.00	1.00	1.00
Amino acid(g/kg Diet)								
Arginine	10.00	8.50	6.70	5.10	7.00	6.00	5.00	4.50
Glycine + Serine	12.00	9.50	6.00	4.50	11.00	8.50	5.00	4.50
Histidine	5.00	3.30	2.10	1.60	1.60	1.50	1.60	1.20
Isoleucine	9.00	6.00	4.50	5.50	9.00	5.00	5.30	5.00
Leucine	14.00	9.90	8.40	6.60	12.00	6.80	6.80	6.00
Lysine	10.00	7.00	7.00	6.50	9.50	7.00	7.00	8.00
Methionine	4.00	3.50	3.50	3.00	4.00	4.00	4.00	4.00
Methionine + Cystine	7.00	6.00	6.00	5.50	7.00	6.00	6.00	6.00
Phenylalanine or	8.00	6.50	4.90	3.90	4.50	4.00	4.10	4.00
Phenylalanine + Tyrosine	15.00	10.00	8.00	7.00	10.00	7.00	7.70	7.00
Threonine	7.00	5.00	4.20	3.50	5.00	4.00	3.50	3.00
Tryptophan	2.00	1.50	1.20	1.20	1.50	1.20	1.40	1.00
Valine	9.00	6.60	5.30	5.10	6.50	5.00	5.30	4.50
Metabolizable energy (Kcal/ kg)	2800	2500	2600	2400	2800	2600	2600	2600
Aflatoxin-B_1 max. (ppm)	20.00	20.00	20.00	20.00	20.00	20.00	20.00	20.00
Calorie: Protein Ratio	140	150	145	150	140	163	153	163

Table 4: Suggested levels of certain nutrients in diets for broiler chickens

Constituents	Commercial Broiler Feed			Broiler Breeder Feed			
	Pre Starter (1-7d)	Starter (8-21d)	Finisher (22-Finish)	Chick	Grower	Female	Male
Nutrient (%)							
Moisture	10.00	10.00	10.00	10.00	10.00	10.00	10.00
Protein (N x 6.25)	23.00	22.00	20.00	20.00	16.00	16.00	15.00
Ether Extractives	3.00	3.50	4.00	2.50	2.50	2.50	2.50
Fibre	5.00	5.00	5.00	7.00	9.00	9.00	9.00
Acid-insoluble ash	2.50	2.50	2.50	4.00	4.00	4.00	4.00
Linoleic acid	1.10	1.10	1.10	1.10	1.10	1.10	1.10
Amino acid (g/kg Diet)							
Arginine	12.50	11.50	10.00	10.00	9.00	9.00	8.50
Glycine + Serine	9.00	7.00	6.00	6.00	4.50	4.50	4.00
Histidine	4.80	4.50	4.00	4.00	3.20	3.20	3.00
Isoleucine	8.60	7.60	7.20	7.20	6.00	6.00	5.80
Leucine	15.00	13.00	12.00	10.00	8.50	8.50	8.00
Lysine	13.00	12.00	10.00	10.00	8.00	8.50	8.00
Methionine or	5.00	5.00	4.50	4.50	4.00	4.50	4.00
Methionine + Cystine	9.00	9.00	8.50	7.00	7.00	7.00	7.00
Phenylalanine or	8.00	7.00	6.40	6.40	5.00	5.00	4.80
Phenylalanine + Tyrosine	15.00	14.00	11.60	11.50	8.00	8.00	8.00
Threonine	7.40	7.00	6.30	6.30	5.20	5.20	5.00
Tryptophan	2.10	2.00	1.90	1.50	1.00	1.00	1.00
Valine	10.00	9.00	8.30	8.30	7.10	7.10	7.00
Metabolizable energy (Kcal/kg)	3000	3100	3200	2800	2750	2800	2750
Aflatoxin-B_1, max(ppm)	20.00	20.00	20.00	20.00	20.00	20.00	20.00
Calorie: Protein Ratio	130	141	160	140	172	175	183

Nutrients

A nutrient is a substance needed by all organisms for survival, growth and wellbeing. Chickens require 40 odd different nutrients for normal growth, sound health, optimum productivity and reproductive efficiency, and all of which need to be furnished through the diet in specified amounts and relative proportions to each other. The nutrients are classified into seven major heads:

1. **Carbohydrates:** A major portion of dietary energy for chickens is derived from carbohydrates which plentifully occur in cereal grains and their by-products primarily in the form of starch that is readily digested, converted into soluble sugars and made use of by the simple-stomach creatures like poultry. Other carbohydrates occur in form of polysaccharides (cellulose, hemicelluloses, pentosans), oligosaccharides (stachyose, raffinose), and all of which are poorly digested by poultry hence have no nutritional worth. On the contrary, such carbohydrate sources exert adverse effects on the digestive processes in the alimentary tract unless appropriate enzymes have been supplemented to degrade these into simpler units.

2. **Proteins and Amino Acids:** Proteins are the main reservoir of amino acids (AAs), the building blocks to synthesise body tissue particularly the musculature, protective tissues (skin, feathers, bone matrix, ligaments), and the soft tissues including vital organs. Body proteins are composed of 22 AAs, all being physiologically essential. Of these, 12 are dietary essential, as the chickens cannot synthesise in their body, or not in amounts needed. Out of these, cystine, lysine, methionine and tryptophan are critical in practical diets. Dietary requirement of protein is in fact that of the essential amino acids (EAAs) contained therein, and which serve variety of metabolic functions. Body proteins, therefore, stay in a dynamic state with degradation and synthesis occurring continually to maintain an adequate supply of AAs. Any shortfall will result in cessation of growth and production accompanied by withdrawal of protein from less vital body tissues to maintain vital functions.

3. **Fats and Oils:** These are concentrated sources of energy and often incorporated in diets for broiler chickens to enhance growth and feed conversion efficiency (FCE). Feed-grade fats and oils may originate from many sources (rendering of animals, refuse from vegetable-oil refining) and besides providing energy, these serve also as chief sources of essential fatty acids (EFAs)-linoleic and linolenic, which are not synthesized by chickens but are metabolically essentials. Linoleic acid is essentially needed to maintain cell membrane integrity, an issue very much important to strengthen immunity against diseases. It is also necessary to ensure optimum egg weight in laying hens. Fats and oils in diet extend extra-

calorific value, help bind fine feed particles for ease of apprehension, and add sheen to the diet all of which promote feed intake of birds.

4. **Minerals:** Inorganic chemicals free of carbon molecules are required by chickens (Table 5, 6) for normal growth, construction and providing rigidity to the skeleton, maintenance of sound bodily health, performance of various physiological and metabolic functions, and as integral part of body cells and fluids. Calcium (Ca) and phosphorous (P) are the major minerals needed to construct bony skeleton, and also form essential part of body fluids. Manganese (Mn) and zinc (Zn) together with vitamin B_2 are needed to prevent the development of perosis, a condition characterized by curled toe. Cobalt (Co), copper (Cu) and iron (Fe) are essentially needed in traces for the formation of haemoglobin. Sodium chloride (NaCl), the common salt, is an essential part of body fluids helping perform biochemical functions including nutrient uptake and maintenance of acid-base balance. Information on typical mineral resources together with their elemental composition commonly employed in poultry feed manufacturing has been presented in Table 7, whereas salient features of their deficiency in poultry diets are presented in Table 8.
5. **Vitamins:** A collective name given to certain organic compounds required in minute quantities to accomplish vital functions in the body. These micronutrients are indispensable to all living beings and found naturally in feeds and feedstuffs in varying amounts and degree of stability.

Upto 14 vitamins are known to be required (Table 5, 6) to support various physio-metabolic functions enabling chickens grow fast, produce more and perform efficiently. Of these, four (Vitamins A, D_3, E and K) are fat-soluble, whereas those of the B-complex group and the vitamin C are soluble in water. Some water-soluble preparations of vitamin K are now available. Chickens are able to synthesise vitamin C (ascorbic acid) in their body but not in amounts actually needed, hence supplemented liberally to enable them tide over inclement weather conditions not uncommon to the Indian sub-continent.

Wide variability existed in the bioavailability of various naturally occurring vitamins; biotin in maize is 100% bioavailable, but only about 10% in barley and wheat. Synthetic forms of vitamins with well-established potency are now available commercially, and employed in poultry feed formulations ignoring the amounts present naturally in feedstuffs.

The requirement figures for most vitamins in diet for chickens are expressed in terms of mg/kg except for vitamins A, D_3 and E which are given in Units. Vitamin D exists in several forms but for poultry form D_3 is preferred. It is found naturally in the fish liver oil or synthesized through irradiation of animal sterol. One unit of vitamin D_3 (ICU, IU or USP) is defined as the activity of 0.025 mg cholecalciferol.

Table 5: Suggested levels of minerals and vitamins in diets for layer chicken

Substance	Commercial Layer				Layer Breeder			
	Chick	Grower	Layer Phase-I	Layer Phase-II	Chick	Grower	Female	Male
Minerals (%)								
Calcium	1.00	1.00	3.00	3.50	1.00	1.00	3.50	1.00
Phosphorus, Total	0.70	0.65	0.65	0.65	0.65	0.60	0.60	0.60
Phosphorus, Available	0.45	0.40	0.40	0.40	0.45	0.40	0.40	0.40
Sodium Chloride	0.50	0.50	0.50	0.50	0.50	0.50	0.50	0.50
Potassium	0.20	0.20	0.20	0.20	0.20	0.20	0.20	0.20
Magnesium	0.05	0.05	0.05	0.05	0.05	0.05	0.05	0.05
Micro-minerals (mg/kg)								
Copper	12.00	9.00	9.00	9.00	12.00	12.00	12.00	12.00
Iodine	1.00	1.00	1.00	1.00	1.50	1.50	1.50	1.50
Iron	70.00	60.00	60.00	60.00	80.00	80.00	80.00	80.00
Manganese	70.00	60.00	60.00	60.00	100.00	100.00	100.00	100.00
Zinc	60.00	60.00	60.00	60.00	80.00	80.00	80.00	80.00
Selenium	0.15	0.15	0.15	0.15	0.15	0.15	0.20	0.15
Vitamins (I.U./kg)								
Vitamin A	9000.00	8000.00	8000.00	8000.00	12000.00	12000.00	15000.00	12000.00
Vitamin D_3	1800.00	1600.00	1600.00	1600.00	2500.00	2500.00	3000.00	2500.00
Vitamin E	15.00	10.00	10.00	10.00	20.00	20.00	50.00	25.00

Vitamins (mg/kg)								
Vitamin K	1.50	1.50	1.50	1.50	2.00	2.00	3.00	2.00
Thiamine B_1	2.00	1.50	1.00	1.00	2.00	2.00	3.00	2.00
Riboflavin B_2	6.00	5.00	5.00	5.00	5.00	5.00	6.00	5.00
Nicotinic Acid	40.00	20.00	20.00	20.00	40.00	40.00	50.00	40.00
Pantothenic Acid	10.00	9.00	7.00	7.00	15.00	15.00	25.00	15.00
Pyridoxine B_6	3.00	3.00	3.00	3.00	5.00	5.00	6.00	5.00
Biotin	0.10	0.10	0.10	0.10	0.20	0.20	0.20	0.20
Folic Acid	1.00	0.50	0.50	0.50	3.00	3.00	4.00	3.00
Choline	500.00	200.00	400.00	400.00	800.00	800.00	600.00	800.00
Vitamin B_{12} μg/Kg	10.00	8.00	8.00	8.00	20.00	20.00	30.00	20.00

As opposed to backyard poultry, chicken in organized farming systems are raised indoors with practically no access to sunlight. Requirements for all vitamins for poultry, therefore, are furnished through the diet only observing all precautions and considering the potency, adequacy to save birds of possible vitamin deficiencies and consequential health problems (Table 9).

Table 6: Suggested levels of minerals and vitamins in diets for broiler chicken

Substance	Commercial Broiler Chick			Breeding Stock			
	Pre Starter	Starter	Finisher	Chick	Grower	Layer	Male
Mineral (%)							
Calcium	1.00	1.00	1.00	1.00	1.00	3.50	1.00
Phosphorus, Total	0.70	0.70	0.70	0.70	0.70	0.70	0.70
Phosphorus, Available	0.45	0.45	0.45	0.45	0.45	0.40	0.40
Sodium Chloride	0.50	0.50	0.50	0.50	0.50	0.50	0.50
Potassium	0.20	0.20	0.20	0.20	0.20	0.20	0.20
Magnesium	0.05	0.05	0.05	0.05	0.05	0.05	0.05
Micro-minerals (mg/Kg)							
Copper	12.00	12.00	12.00	12.00	12.00	12.00	12.00
Iodine	1.20	1.20	1.20	1.50	1.50	1.50	1.50
Iron	80.00	80.00	80.00	80.00	80.00	80.00	80.00
Manganese	100.00	100.00	100.00	100.00	100.00	100.00	100.00
Zinc	80.00	80.00	80.00	80.00	80.00	80.00	80.00
Selenium	0.15	0.15	0.15	0.15	0.15	0.20	0.15
Vitamins (I.U./Kg)							
Vitamin A	11000.00	11000.00	10000.00	12000.00	12000.00	15000.00	12000.00
Vitamin D_3	3000.00	3000.00	3000.00	2500.00	2500.00	3000.00	2500.00
Vitamin E	30.00	30.00	30.00	20.00	20.00	50.00	20.00

Vitamins (mg/Kg)							
Vitamin K	1.50	1.50	1.50	2.00	2.00	3.00	2.00
Thiamine B_1	1.00	1.00	1.00	2.00	2.00	2.00	2.00
Riboflavin B_2	4.00	2.00	2.00	4.00	4.00	4.00	4.00
Nicotinic Acid	40.00	40.00	40.00	40.00	40.00	50.00	40.00
Pantothenic Acid	15.00	15.00	15.00	15.00	15.00	25.00	15.00
Pyridoxine B_6	2.00	2.00	2.00	2.00	2.00	2.00	2.00
Biotin	0.10	0.10	0.10	0.10	0.10	0.10	0.10
Folic Acid	0.50	0.50	0.50	0.50	0.50	0.50	0.50
Choline	1300.00	1300.00	1300.00	1200.00	1000.00	1200.00	1000.00
VitaminB_{12} (µg/Kg)	10.00	10.00	10.00	15.00	15.00	15.00	15.00

Table 7: Mineral resources for use in poultry feeding

Source	Chemical Formula	Elements (%)	
Calcium and Phosphorus			
Bone meal		Ca 30.00;	P 15.00
Calcium carbonate	$CaCO_3$	Ca 40.05;	CO_3 59.95
Dicalcium Phosphate, dihydrate	$CaHPO_4.2H_2O$	Ca 23.29;	P 18.01,
Limestone grit		Ca 38.00	
Oystershell grit		Ca 37.00	
Cobalt			
Cobaltous Chloride, Pentahydrate	$CoCl_2.\ 5H_2O$	Co 26.80;	Cl 38.28
Copper			
Cupric sulphate	$CuSO_4$	Cu 39.81;	$SO_4$60.19
Cupric sulphate Pentahydrate	$CuSO_4.\ 5H_2O$	Cu 25.46;	$SO_4$38.49
Cupric Chloride	$CuCl_2$	Cu 47.27;	Cl 52.73
Iodine			
Potassium Iodide	KI	I 76.45;	K 23.55
Potassium Iodate	KIO_3	I 59.31;	K 18.27
Calcium Iodate	$Ca(IO_3)_2$	I 65.09;	Ca10.28
Sodium Iodate	NaI	I 84.68;	Na15.32
Iron			
Ferrous sulphate heptahydrate	$FeSO_4.\ 7H_2O$	Fe 20.09;	SO_4 34.59
Magnesium			
Magnesium carbonate	$MgCO_3$	Mg 28.84;	CO_3 71.16
Magnesium sulphate	$Mg\ SO_4$	Mg 20.19;	SO_4 79.81
Magnesium sulphate heptahydrate	$Mg\ SO_4.\ 7H_2O$	Mg 09.87;	SO_4 39.01
Manganese			
Manganese dioxide	MnO_2	Mn 63.19	
Manganese carbonate	$MnCO_3$	Mn 47.79;	CO_3 52.21
Manganese chloride tetrahydrate	$MnCl_2.\ 4H_2O$	Mn 27.76;	Cl35.86
Manganese sulphate	$Mn\ SO_4$	Mn 36.36;	$SO_4$63.64
Manganese sulphate tetrahydrate	$Mn\ SO_4.\ 4H_2O$	Mn 24.63;	$SO_4$43.10
Potassium			
Potassium chloride	KCl	K 52.44;	Cl 47.56
Potassium carbonate	K_2CO_3	K 56.58;	$CO_3$43.42
Potassium bicarbonate	$KHCO_3$	K 39.05;	HCO 60.95
Potassium sulphate	$K_2\ SO_4$	K 44.87;	SO_4 55.13
Sodium			
Sodium chloride	NaCl	Na 39.35;	Cl 60.65
Sodium bicarbonate	$NaHCO_3$	Na 27.38;	HCO_3 72.62
Sodium sulphate	Na_2SO_4	Na 32.39;	$SO_4$67.61

Zinc			
Zinc carbonate	$ZnCO_3$	Zn 52.14;	CO_2 47.86
Zinc chloride	$ZnCl_2$	Zn 47.97;	Cl 52.03
Zinc oxide	ZnO	Zn 80.35;	
Zinc sulphate	$Zn\ SO_4$	Zn 40.47;	SO_4 59.33
Zinc sulphate, hydrate	$Zn\ SO_4.\ H_2O$	Zn 36.42;	SO_4 53.55

Table 8: Salient deficiency features of mineral elements in chickens

Minerals	Deficiency Symptoms
Calcium	Rickets; young – osteomalacia, Poor eggshell quatlity, osteomalacia, low hatchability
Copper	Anemia
Iron	Anemia
Iodine	Goiter
Magnesium	Convulsions, Sudden death
Manganese	Perosis, poor hatchability of eggs
Phosphorus	Rickets, poor eggshell quality, low hatchability of eggs
Selenium	Accumulation of fluid under the skin
Zinc	Poor feathering, stunted growth, short bones

Table 9: Response of chickens to vitamin inadequacies in diet

Vitamin	Salient Observations
Vitamin A	Poor growth, debility, Atexia, Xerophthalmia, Egg production decreased, Poor Immune response, Nutritional Roup.
Vitamin D_3 (Cholecalciferol)	Growth retardation, Rickets, Osteomalacia, Thin shelled eggs, Egg production and hatchability lowered.
Vitamin E (α–Tocopherol)	Encephalomalacia (Crazy-Chick Disease), Muscular dystrophy, Enlarged Hock joint.
Vitamin K_3 (Menadione Sod.)	Blood-clotting time prolonged, intra- muscular bleeding.
Vitamin B_1 (Thiamine)	Anorexia, Polyneuritis, convulsions, Star-gazing posture, Increased mortality.
Vitamin B_2 (Riboflavin)	Poor growth, dermatitis, Curled-toe paralysis, reduced egg production and hatchability.
Vitamin B_3 (Niacin)	Stunted growth, Hock enlargement, Black Tongue and mouth Cavity.
Vitamin B_5 (Pantothenic acid)	Poor growth, Dermatitis, Scaby lessons on feet, corners of mouth and eyes.

Vitamin B_6 (Pyridoxine HCl)	Involved in protein metabolism, Deficiency may lead to poor N-retention. Retarded growth, dermatitis, anemia, gizzard erosion in chicks. In adult birds: loss of appetite, reduced egg production and hatchability.
Vitamin B_7 or H (Biotin)	Retarded growth, brittle feathers, dermatitis around the eyes, beak and on the feet, reduced hatchability, perosis, parrot-beak embryos, chondrodystrophy, involved in fatty Liver Kidney Syndrome (FLKS)in broiler chicks.
Vitamin B_9 (Folic acid / Folate)	Poor growth and feathering, anaemia, reduced egg production and hatchability, comb becomes a waxy-white colour.
Vitamin B_{12} (Cyanocobalamin)	Slow growth, Pernicious anaemia, embryonic mortality.
Vitamin C (Ascorbic acid)	Not always a dietary essential for being synthesised in the body. Helps birds sustain through to the extreme weather conditions. Being an antioxidant, helps promote healthy tissue.
Choline	Though not regarded a vitamin, choline is considered one and discussed along with, Retarded growth and development of perosis in young chickens, prevention of Fatty liver and Kidney Syndrome (FLKS) in broiler chicks.

6. **Fiber:** Dietary carbohydrates are, invariably, accompanied with a cellulosic fibrous fraction which the birds scarcely digest. Being associated with lignin and silica, the fiber has no nutritional value as such, and excreted. The fiber, however, helps cleanup the intestinal lumen of the noxious substances clinging thereon. A small amount of dietary fiber, therefore, has its own advantages too.

7. **Water:** A simple yet most essential of all nutrients, the water is, indeed, synonymous to life. Water is the medium to dissolve and transport nutrients all over the body, helps regulate body temperature and saves poultry from heat stress as well as dehydration. Any slackness in drinking water supply to chickens will prove disastrous. Clean fresh water (~ 20°C) must be made available to chickens at all times. Water from borewell is usually clean, odourless and free of microbes. Frequent checks for the salt contents, total dissolved solids (TDS) and turbidity indicating microbial population must be carried out, and guidelines followed to safeguarding health of the flock (Table 10).

   Excessive intake of high-salt water may be problematic for birds of any kind or age leading to wet droppings and insanitation in the poultry house. Downs, feet and feathers all get soiled with the excrement giving a shabby look and causing downgrading of the stock. Tentative daily water intake by chickens at ambient temperature ~20°C has been shown in Table 11. Chickens normally drink twice as much as the amount of feed they consume. The egg laying flock needs nearly twice as much as water than the non-layers. Young fast- growing chicks consume twice as much water as the slow growers. All kinds of stock during the dry hot periods require twice as much water as in cool pleasant weather conditions. A simple rule of thumb has been to provision 3 to 4 times more water than the tentative feed requirement. Also, the water containers must be cleaned and sanitized prior to refilling.

Table 10: Suitability of water for poultry in relation to total dissolved solids (TDS)

Total Dissolved Solids (PPM)	Salient Observations
Less than 1000	Generally suitable for any class of poultry.
1001-3000	Normally satisfactory yet may tend to cause wet droppings.
3001-5000	Poor quality water adversely affects flock performance through in-house insanitation and morbidity.
5001-7000	Intake of such water by poultry certainly creates digestive disorders leading to drastically poor performance and increased mortality. Not acceptable for poultry.
Over 7001	Just unfit water for use by any kinds of poultry flock.

Table 11: Tentative daily water intake by chickens with advancement of age at ambient temperature-20^{0}C

Age of the bird (week)	Water intake per bird (ml/d)	
	White Leghorn	White Rock Broilers
1	30	32
2	42	65
3	55	110
4	70	140
5	85	180
6	100	215
8	105	225
10	110	250
20	120	272
50	220	300
70	250	300

1. Energy nutrition

Energy nutrition of farm livestock has been an area of interest for researchers ever since. Primarily driven by the need to design diets for controlled experimentations on large animals, poultry were generally kept out of its perview. Main responses to dietary energy level in poultry feeding have come due to intake and the choice of a practical level depended merely on economic considerations.

Several terms have been in use for expressing dietary energy content. Gross Energy (GE) is the total calorific value when a particular feed/feedstuff is completely combusted in a Bomb calorimeter. The value can also be calculated from the chemical composition of a feedstuff by applying the GE value for carbohydrate (4.1 Kcal/g), protein (5.4 Kcal/g), and fat (9.3 Kcal/g) to the amounts of such nutrients. GE in the digested components of diet is referred to as digestible energy (DE) which, on further correction for the energy excreted in form of urine, is term metabolisable energy (ME), apparent ME (AME) or the Classical ME. Unlike the other farm livestock, poultry voids undigested food and metabolic rejects in form of feces and urine as a single excrement called droppings. Owing to this feature, estimates of digestibility in poultry are not available, instead a more precise term metabolisability of dietary nutrients or the diet dry matter (DM) is practiced. Metabolisable energy is the net energy available after the fecal and urinary energy losses have been accounted for and presents for body maintenance, growth and reproduction.

Nitrogen deposition in the body tissues and excretion in case of tissue breakdown is a normal phenomenon, wherein energy in the nitrogen component associated with gain or loss of AME is termed N-corrected ME (AMEn). Additional correction for the metabolic fecal and endogenous urinary losses defined as excretory energy (EE) of non-dietary origin is referred as the true metabolisable energy (TME). Correction of TME to zero nitrogen balance (TMEn) reduces variation and provides energy estimates independent of feed intake.

Metabolisable energy has widely been accepted and used to describe energy values of poultry feeds/feedstuffs, and the energy requirements customarily expressed in these units (NRC, 1994). It is a common practice to correct ME for the energy component trapped along per unit of N retained to bring all data to N-equilibrium enabling meaningful comparisons between values for feeds and the birds of different genetic makeup. Energy data on certain poultry feedstuffs has been presented (Table 12), as a reference guide.

Table 12: Salient nutrients in feedstuffs commonly employed in poultry feed formulations

Feedstuff (DM~90%)	Protein (NX6.25) (%)	Amino acid (g/Kg)					Ether Extract (%)	Crude fiber (%)	Linoleic acid (%)	Mineral Elements (%)		Energy AME (Kcal/Kg)
		Cys	LYS	MET	THR	TRP				Ca	P_{total}	
Energy - Rich												
Bajra	12.5	0.14	0.43	0.24	0.44	0.18	4.8	2.2	-	0.13	0.71	2640
Barley	11.5	0.24	0.44	0.18	0.52	0.12	1.7	5.6	1.0	0.03	0.36	2650
Jowar, White	9.8	0.20	0.25	0.16	0.31	0.10	3.0	4.1	1.1	0.04	0.28	3050
Maize	9.1	0.20	0.27	0.18	0.30	0.08	3.6	2.8	0.6	0.25	0.40	3300
Maize-gluten feed	20.0	2.6	0.8	1.8	1.1	0.20	2.0	7.0	-	0.20	0.28	2600
Ragi grains	12.8	0.2	0.08	0.14	0.32	0.32	1.8	2.8	-	0.10	0.12	2950
Rice bran	16.0	0.33	0.68	0.31	0.54	0.17	1.0	12.0	-	0.18	0.16	1800
Rice Kanni	7.9	0.17	0.28	0.20	0.26	0.09	1.7	1.5	0.6	0.40	0.20	3010
Rice Polish	13.0	0.26	0.60	0.24	0.40	0.14	18.0	6.9	4.0	0.05	1.20	3050
Sal seed extractions	9.0	0.20	0.32	0.36	0.30	0.10	1.0	3.0	0.3	0.22	0.18	2600
Tapioca	2.0	-	-	-	-	-	0.70	12.8	-	0.58	0.12	3300
Wheat	13.0	0.25	0.48	0.25	0.38	0.15	3.0	2.8	2.0	0.18	0.42	3160
Protein-Rich												
Fish meal	40.6	0.27	2.5	0.88	1.40	0.70	6.60	1.50	-	10.90	4.75	2460
Groundnut Extractions	44.0	0.47	1.77	0.42	1.44	0.50	1.0	6.0	0.1	0.16	0.64	2690
Guar meal	41.0	0.46	1.68	0.48	4.90	0.68	4.2	6.8	-	0.80	0.82	2200
Maize-gluten meal	42.0	0.60	0.80	1.00	1.10	0.20	2.0	4.0	-	0.16	0.40	2400
Meat-cum-bone meal	42.0	0.51	2.40	0.65	1.60	0.29	8.5	2.1	0.30	10.50	5.60	2200

Meat meal	60.0	0.62	2.60	0.70	2.00	0.32	12.3	2.80	0.60	7.30	3.40	2800
Rapeseed extractions	38.0	0.90	2.05	0.72	1.58	0.47	1.50	9.50	-	1.10	0.88	2200
Sesame extractions	44.0	0.81	1.30	1.45	1.44	0.54	1.0	6.1	0.20	2.70	1.40	2450
Single cell protein	40.0	11.56								3.07		2200
Soybean extractions	45.0	0.72	3.00	0.69	1.80	0.61	1.0	8.0	0.40	0.90	0.64	2600

2. Protein and amino acid nutrition

a) **Requirements for Amino Acids:** The protein requirement of chickens can be met easily, but not of AAs. Normally 10 AAs are dietary essentials for chickens, arginine and glycine are additionally needed. Unlike the other farm livestock, the protein metabolic end product in poultry is uric acid and not urea. Biosynthesis of uric acid requires glycine, and which may be produced from keratin in the presence of vitamins B_{12}, biotin and folic acid. Arginine yields urea and ornithine, the later with glycine helps detoxify aromatic compounds in the liver, cysteine and tyrosine are semi essential for these can be obtained from methionine and phenyl-alanine, respectively.

b) **Limiting Amino Acid Concept:** Ratio between the amount of an AA in diet and that of its requirement by the bird gives an idea of its being limited or otherwise. Lysine requirement as percent of dietary protein is less for egg production than for growth hence its deficiency in diet for egg production is not usual. Generally, all of the AAs must be present in diet for efficient feed protein utilization. When necessary, synthetic L-Lysine and D-L Methionine may be added in diet to make up their deficiency.

c) **Amino Acid Toxicity and Inter-relationships:** Excess of an AA in diet is harmful, expensive and may lead to imbalances of other dietary nutrients. A high dietary level of methionine depresses growth of chicks. Arginine and lysine are interrelated in that a high requirement of anyone will increase requirement for another. Glycine and threonine eliminate toxic effects of tryptophan. Glycine also alleviates toxic effects of methionine, leucine and isoleucine. Such factors must be duly considered while formulating diets for chickens to optimize levels of EAAs avoiding any excesses or the deficiencies.

3. Nutrition and feeding of chickens

Chickens vary greatly in respect to their feed and nutrient requirements depending on the purpose they have been reared for. Those intended for egg production have smaller body size but prolific layers. The broiler chicks grow rapidly gaining body weight quickly but the hens lay poorly. Nutrient needs of the two kinds of chickens differ accordingly.

Factors affecting Nutrient Requirements: Genetic improvements over the last several decades have transformed chickens as more efficient converter of feed into muscle mass than its predecessors. The modern strains are more capable of utilizing dietary nutrients for growth and production. Several factors influence birds need for nutrients, and which include:

- Genetic constitution of the bird (Breed/Strain).
- Gender of the bird and production status – males have greater maintenance needs than females, egg-laying hens need more nutrients than non-layers.
- Age of the stock-young birds have less maintenance needs than the old stocks.
- Housing – wire cages or litter floor matters.
- Environmental temperature and humidity bring in stress in birds.
- Feeds and feedstuffs quality – nutrient contents and their availability,
- Non-nutrients, antimetabolites and toxicants,
- Nutrient interrelationships and imbalances- arginine:lysine; energy:protein, Ca:P.
- Disease and gut status.

a) **Feeding egg-type chickens:** Suggested levels of various nutrients in diet for egg-type chickens during the grower, layer and breeder stages have been presented in Table 3 and 5. Chick starter diet containing high protein and high energy is served during the first seven weeks of age followed by grower feed (8-18 wk) with lowering of dietary CP and ME by 20 and 10 per cent, respectively. This allows chicks a good early start followed by pullets grow well to the maturity without going fat. The contents of all other nutrients (amino acids, mineral elements, vitamins) in diet are ensured at levels slightly in excess of their actual requirements in view of uncertainties with respect to actual contents and bioavailability of nutrients therein. After attaining 18 wks of age, such pullets come into lay and switched over to the layers diet (Ph-I) with extra amounts of protein, energy, calcium, linoleic acid, and nearly all of the micronutrients. Dietary CP, ME and Ca levels are raised to 18%, 2600 kcal/kg, and 2.5%, respectively. From ~5% at 19 wk of age, the egg production gradually touches 97% by 52 wk, and the average egg weight from ~30 g increases to ~55 g. It is interesting to note that birds will naturally manage such a remarkable biological change through gradual increase in feed intake from ~60 g at ~19 weeks of age to 100 to 110 g at 52 wk, and 110 to 113 g thereafter as the birds reach peak egg production. It is also necessary to have provision for extra calcium during the high lay period for proper eggshell formation, topping up feeders with calcium grit in the after noons is beneficial. Any extra calcium in the body is usually excreted. Every possible effort must be made to enable hens stay for long in the high-lay period (~ 20 to 30 weeks) to maximize productivity.

It is usual for the hens to continue eating food at the same pace even though egg production started declining after 72 weeks of age. Therefore, it is time to economise on expensive nutrients by lowering the protein contents from 18 to 16% and ME from 2600 to 2400 kcal/kg diet (Ph-II). Exercising quantitative control on feed intake by hens post-peak period is also an effective measure to economizing on the operational costs as also saving hens from going fatty due to extra energy intake. The extra provision of calcarious grit may also be dispensed with gradually with the decreasing egg production rate.

The nutritional requirements of broiler chickens vary greatly depending on such factors as mentioned earlier. The minimum requirement levels of various nutrients in diet for broiler chickens during different growing phases have been set out in Table 4 and 6. Values given for any nutrient are adequate to support optimum growth and normal wellbeing of the elite commercial stocks reared and managed in standard conditions of housing and semi-controlled environment.

b) **Feeding broiler chickens:** Commercial broiler chicks are selected for rapid growth, efficient feed utilization, high survival rate and good body confirmation and to reach the market early by 6 week(wk) of age. Accordingly, such elite stocks are offered high nutrient-density diets with due attention given in respect to all EAAs, trace elements, vitamins and energy to enable them perform optimally in the given situations of housing, management and health care. It has been customary to use two types of chick diets (starter and finisher) but, considering the need to give the chicks a good start, provision of three diets : pre-starter (1-7 d), starter (8-21 d) and finisher (22 to market) is now in vogue. Suggested levels of most nutrients in diet of commercial broiler chicks have been set out in Table 4 and 6. With ~40 g body weight at hatch, the broilers by 6 wk of age are able to attain ~1.9 kg i.e. nearly 48 times the birth weight, something highly impressive performance in about 42 d period. All possible care is, therefore, needed in selecting feedstuffs, designing feed formulae, and mixing/manufacturing the feed. Any laxity in the process of housing, management, water supply, sanitation and health care of the stock may cost dearly.

It's a fact that all feedstuffs in their natural state comprised of any or many micronutrients (vitamins, trace elements) in varying amounts and bioavailable forms. But, how much and how much of that is actually bioavailable is a big question? It is also well known that such micronutrients, though needed in small quantities, play vital roles in the bio system towards optimizing productivity. Being uncertain, the amounts of most micronutrients are generally disregarded while formulating diets. Besides, the requirements for many nutrients might increase substantially under the stressful environment, vaccination, diseases, anti-nutrients/anti-metabolites in diet, possible interactions between nutrients, presence of toxicants and the like situations. Under such circumstances it is obligatory to supplement diets liberally with most micronutrients and not to risk the performance of elite broiler flocks or else it may cost the producer/farmer dearly.

Nutritional management of the commercial broiler chickens and their parent stock needs to be precisely dealt with considering huge developments in their genotypes. Whereas, a commercial female broiler chick at 6 wk of age weighs ~1.8 kg, the breeder pullet of the same age is targeted to weigh ~ 600 g only. Overweight and not underweight is, therefore, a problematic issue during the growing period to which both the dietary protein and energy hold the key. Infact, energy is the most expensive nutrient and it is also the one usually found limiting the performance of birds. Limiting the energy intake markedly affects the production parameters, whereas a similar change in protein intake matters hardly.

At the end of the growing period, nearly 80% of the ingested energy is spent towards the maintenance of pullets just the way for broiler breeder hens from 20 to 70 wks of age. The remainder of the energy (~ 20%) goes in towards the formation of eggs and also increase in body size/weight, if any. The hens preferentially partition nutrients for maintenance and for the egg mass, any deficit is reflected in terms of reduced egg production. Besides, the ambient temperature and bird's feather condition also influence dietary needs of the flock quite considerably.

4. Concept of calorie: protein ratio

Chickens eat feed primarily to satisfy their energy needs. The concept calorie:protein (C:P) ratio, therefore, has some advantage from the standpoint of broiler nutrition for these birds generally over eat. The expression is defined as the ratio of dietary ME (Kcal/kg) divided by per cent crude protein in the diet. The ratios serve as guidelines for the nutritionists/feed formulators to help balance diet in respect of protein and energy contents (Table 3, 4). The C:P ratios of 130, 140 and 160 in pre-starter, starter and finisher broiler diets, respectively have been found practically satisfactory. It must, however, be understood that with an increase in the dietary ME a corresponding increase in the crude protein content is warranted to safeguard against possible protein deficiency that may otherwise arise due to decreased feed intake. Maintaining a proper C:P ratio in diet will not only ensure optimum intake of the two major nutrients (ME and CP) but also that of all other nutrients to optimizing productivity and the overall performance of chickens.

5. Mineral nutrition of chickens

Chickens require 12 different mineral elements in their diet accounting ~ 4% of their body weight, Ca and P making up more than half of the amount. Skeleton formation takes away almost 99% of the Ca leaving only ~ 1% for all other important biochemical activities in the body. The second most abundant and versatile mineral element is P, ~ 80% of which goes in for skeleton formation and the remainder distributed widely throughout the body involving in almost all of the metabolic activities taking place therein.

Utilization and metabolism of Ca and P is primarily influenced by their relative amounts to each other, and also the presence of vitamin D_3 in diet. Bioavailability may differ from source to source, physiological status and age of the flock. Fast-growing chicks utilize dietary Ca and P more efficiently than the grown-ups. Likewise, chickens in good lay utilize more Ca than the non-laying or poorly laying flock. Vitamin D_3 under the influence of a specific protein calbindin promotes Ca uptake from the small intestine, whereas a passive ionic diffusion only suffices when Ca demand is low. The P absorption takes place in the duodenum, greater is the need more efficient is the absorption. Following absorption, the P gets circulated throughout the body quickly, and also withdrawn from the blood whenever needed for bone development or any other bodily functions.

a) **Sources of mineral elements:** Naturally available sources (bone meal, limestone, oyster shell) are good enough to furnish Ca and P in poultry feeding although pure elemental salts (Table 7) may be made use of to make up for any deficiency. Additionally, the calcarious limestone and oyster shell grits help coarsely ground feed into fine slury in the gizzard promoting digestion and quick absorption of dietary nutrients across the gut wall. A ratio of 2:1 Ca and P in diets for growing poultry has for long been found satisfactory. Laying hens need extra Ca for eggshell formation hence provision of up to 3.0-3.5% Ca may be needed as per the situation warrants.

   Though all mineral elements in pure forms are available commercially for use in poultry feeding (Table 7), these are also naturally present in variable amounts in many feedstuffs (Table 9). However, some of these (Ca, P, Mg, Mn, Zn) are formed associated with phytic acid and hence remain largely indigestible and biologically unavailable. About 70% of the P found in plant feedstuffs is in the form of phytates, and only about 30% is in the biologically available form. Due to the absence of natural phytase, poultry are unable to utilize a good amount of dietary P, hence supplementation of commercially available phytase is beneficial.

b) **Significance of common salt:** Sodium chloride (NaCl or common salt), is an inexpensive of all elements, yet an essentially important ingredient contributing to Na and Cl supplies in all poultry diets to support normal growth, wellbeing, production and reproduction. Feeding diets without added salt result in growth retardation, dullness in the growing birds, and ceasation of egg production in the laying stock. Correcting deficiency may restore performance, but not the damage done already, an inexpensive mistake often leading to expensive losses to the poultry industry. Broiler chicks on low or no sodium diets develop ascites, a condition characterized by accumulation of fluid in the lungs and the body cavity eventually leading to death. Adult birds on low-sodium diets resort to packing each other, and also begin to shed feathers – a process known by moulting.

c) **Electrolyte balance:** An electrolyte is a chemical substance that on dissolution in suitable solvent such as water, ionizes quickly and allows electric current to pass through itself. The primary role of electrolyte lies in the maintenance of body ionic-and water-balances which gets altered due to the loss of body water during summer. Panting is the physiological response by birds to get relief from excessive body heat. Most soluble salts (acids or bases) serve natural electrolytes and of these Na, K and Cl are available to the birds naturally through diet and water. Sodium bicarbonate and potassium chloride have been recognized as the best choice in salt selection for use in the diet of broiler chickens during hot humid weather when high cation and low anion levels are recommended. Sodium helps control body fluid amount and enables efficient working of the nerve and muscle tissues. Provision of electrolytes through diet or water encourages birds to consume more water thereby helping them regulate normal body temperature. An electrolyte balance between 170-200 mEq/kg with minimum K level of 0.6% in diet of broiler breeders is beneficial to achieving satisfactory performance.

Strategic nutritional management

Economic turmoil coupled with food and feed scarcity in any part of the Globe isn't a rare phenomenon, India experienced drought many a times. Its aftermath in the form of mismatch in demand and supply of food is invariably accompanied by cost as calations, substandard feed ingredients and feed adulterations beyond imagination. Poultry producers are left with no choice but to compromise with adversity taking all precautions and considering alternatives. Under such circumstances, the knowledge of alternate feed resources with respect to their merits and demerits of usage in poultry feeding, and the presence or absence in them of a number of deleterious substances is obligatory.

a) **Nutrition for healthy gut:** Gut health problems arise due to faulty nutrition, insanitation at places of early chick rearing, dysbiosis and the like. Birds in their intestine harbor bacterial population of both types, beneficial *lactobacillus sp*., and the pathogenic *Escherichia coli*. At times of stress the gut microbial balance may shift in favour of harmful population deploying negative impact on bird's ability to absorb dietary nutrients. The intestinal integrity in terms of epithelial structure and functionality is continually being challenged by numerous entities (feed toxicants, chemicals, endoparasites, microbes, non-starch polysaccharides) and which must be preserved in its natural state for efficient functioning. The immune system must develop well and fast such that Bursa and spleen are responsive enough to the environmental stresses. Use of antibiotics and other growth-promoting compounds, pre- and pro-biotics may extend some protection against pathogens, minor ailments and/or diseases. The damages so caused must be set right quickly through appropriate medication including extra provision of microminerals, electrolytes and vitamins so as to ensure a good start to chicks early in their life.

b) **Nutrition and feathering:** Thickset shine plumage is an attractive feature of chickens of all ages and also an indicator of their sound health, good production and performance. However, despite of proper feeding and management, certain issues relating to poor featherings do crop up in any flock. An understanding of the root causes behind the problem, identifying the real culprit and initiating appropriate remedial measures need to be initiated timely.

   Feathers are largely composed of proteins, especially keratin which is rich in the two sulphur containing amino acids (Cystein and methionine). In general, factors that promote rapid growth of chickens are also the ones induce good feathering. Diets low in protein with an improper amino acid profile are likely responsible for poor feathering, brittleness, discolouration and dullness of the plumage.

   Dietary deficiencies of mineral elements (Ca, Mg, Se, and Zn) are usually found associated with improper feathering (Table 10). Besides, vitamins of the B-group (biotin, folacin, pantothenic acid, B_{12}) significantly influence feather structure, thinning of the web, brittleness and natural sheen of plumage. Due care must, therefore, be observed while formulating diets for any class of poultry from the standpoint of their plumage, which is of great aesthetic value.

c) **Nutrition to boost immunity:** Immunity deals with a complex biosystem endowed with ability to recognize what belongs to the self and what not. Chickens are faced with many external challenges including the disease-causing agents, and interact accordingly to safeguarding health, promote growth and boost up production. Any biological or synthetic product capable of stimulating or suppressing the innate or adaptive qualities of the immune system is referred by immunomodulator and advantageous to those of the commonly used microbials. Escalating concern against chemotherapeutic agents usage in poultry has drawn attention of the farmers, consumers and the industry to this relevant subject necessitating redressal.

Two types of interactions have been noted in poultry: the first being a nutrition-based immunocompetance enabling birds resist microbial infections and overcome the disease and the other being immune-responses that enhance growth and productivity, stimulate metabolic processes and redress nutritional requirements for optimum production efficiency. Accordingly, certain dietary nutrients may be needed in amounts higher to those of the suggested levels, and so termed *"safety margins"*. Potentially useful nutrients to improve immunocompetance in chickens include vitamins C and E; amino acids-arginine and methionine, the latter helps maximize both the cell-mediated and humoral immunity. From the practical point of view several other nutrients (energy, iron, linoleic acid, selenium, vitamins B-group, A and zinc) markedly modulate immune responses in birds, thereby invigorate to resist infections. Due care must, therefore, be observed from this point of view also while designing and formulating practical diets for poultry.

d) **Nutrition and egg size:** The size of an egg has considerable impact on its marketing. Several factors (genetics, age of the bird, sexual maturity, dietary nutrients, and certain drugs/chemicals) may hold the key to egg size. Eggs from pullets freshly coming into lay are usually small, and which tend to increase in size and weight with the laying period. Nutritional management of chickens during the rearing and laying periods also has significant bearing on egg size/weight laid subsequently. Proper feeding enables birds attain a standard body weight so they could normally lay good size eggs. Dietary energy, Amino acids-methionine and cystine, and the EFA linoleic acid can all directly influence the egg size. Reducing the level of anyone of such nutrients in diet will reduce egg size also.

e) **Dietary Form:** When formulating poultry diets, the acceptance and choice of any ingredient rests primarily on four considerations:

- The ease of availability of the raw materials.
- Nutritive quality and feeding value of feedstuffs under consideration.
- Presence or absence of non-nutrients, anti-nutrients or toxicants, in feed ingredients.

- Their relative costs to other similar ingredients or possible alternate feed resources.

Poultry are usually fed diets as mash though crumbs and pellets are gaining in popularity owing to certain benefits these offer over the mash diets. Making poultry mash is a simple process involving a few steps:

- Developing a feed formulation worksheet to prepare a fixed amount.
- Weighing out ingredients one by one as per the worksheet.
- Premixing micro-minerals and vitamins separately.
- Mixing all items together to give a uniform blend.

Manufacturing crumbs and pellets requires specialized machinery and technical expertise to carry out the job efficiently. The process involves huge expenditure and which must be realized in terms of benefits of feeding crumbs or pellets to the flock intended for, so as to be cost-effective exercise. Some of the benefits of feeding crumbs and pellets over the mash are:

- The feed components are bound well avoiding segregation of micronutrients.
- Heat generated during the process inactivates heat-labile anti-nutrients.
- The birds are able to utilize feed better and turn out to be have a superior feed conversion efficiency.
- However, all such benefits need be assessed and evaluated vis-à-vis increased cost of production of crumbs and pellets.

e) **Enhancing feed value:** Poultry lacks the ability to digest and make use of many carbohydrates that exist naturally in any feedstuff. Some of these include non-starch polysaccharides (NSPs) such as cellulose, hemicelluloses (arabinoxylans, galactomannans, B-glucans). In absence of specific enzymes, poultry lacks the ability to deal with and, therefore, doesn't benefit of a considerable amount of nutrients/energy entrapped therein. The largest amount of NSPs (~50%) in typical poultry diets is in the form of arabinoxylans followed by cellulose (~20%) and beta glucans (~5%). Targeting arabinoxylans with high quality xylanase (enzyme feed supplement) will help release a good amount of encapsulated nutrients. Poultry also lacks cellulolytic enzyme system to utilize dietary cellulose. The content of other NSPs being small, any enzyme system may not be cost-effective. Xylanase by far is the most effective and also cost-effective enzyme for improving NSP digestibility in typical poultry rations. Supplemental xylanase in poultry diets will bring in multifold benefits through:

- Breaking the cell walls to free nutrients encapsulated therein.
- Exposing NSPs to digestive action by endogenous enzymes.
- Reducing viscosity of the substrate in the intestinal lumen, thus facilitating absorption of nutrients.
- Enhancing feed value to enable the bird perform better.

Conclusions

Of all livestock, poultry is a delicate species requiring nutritional, housing and health care at their best to enable chicken grow well sustaining environmental changes, produce and reproduce optimally utilizing dietary nutrients efficiently and effectively. Poultry nutritionist and feed technologist have put in tremendous efforts evaluating the goodness or otherwise of very many stuffs worth feeding to poultry. Today a large number of grain, grain-by-product, oilseed meals, plant proteins, animal and marine sources form part of a big inventory.

A huge data is now available in the form of published papers, scientific reports, books and bulletins, scientific reviews and the like for easy reference by the teachers, students, farmers, feed manufacturer to take due advantage while designing diets. Besides, publication brought out from time to time by several agencies (ARC, 1975; NRC, 1994 and BIS, 2007) become valuable reference guide for the academicians, research scholars, farmers and all those regulatory authorities in the poultry world. It is expected that the information laid out in this write-up and suggestions made with respect to the requirements of various dietary nutrients for chickens reared for different purposes will help and enable users accomplish their goals easily and fruitfully.

References

National Research Council, 1994. Nutrient Requirements of Poultry, Ninth Revised Edition, 1994. Washington, DC: The National Academies Press. https://doi.org/10.17226/2114.

BIS, 2007. Nutrient Requirements of Poultry. Bureau of Indian Standards, 5th revision, New Delhi, India.

ARC, 1977. Nutrient requirement of farm livestock, No.1 poultry, Agriculture Research council, London.

Indian Council of Agricultural Research, 2013. Nutrient Requirements of Poultry. Eds. Mandal, A.B., Raju, M.V.L.N., Elangovan, A.V., Bhanja, S.K. and Sahoo, S.K., Indian Council of Agricultural Research, New Delhi.

2

Recent Advances in Amino Acid Nutrition in Chicken

P.K. Shukla

Dean,College of Veterinary Sciences and Animal Husbandry, DUVASU, Mathura, Uttar Pradesh,
Former Joint Commissioner (Poultry), Govt. of India

Introduction

Development of feeding strategies that are more efficient and more eco-friendly by reducing waste is one of the key priorities in poultry production today. Thus, there is a focus on reduction of the crude protein content in a diet fortified with adequate amounts of currently available free amino acids (e.g. L-Lys, DL-Met, L-Thr, L-Val and L-Trp) in order to optimize protein utilization efficiency while maintaining production performance and reducing nitrogen excretion in chicken. Baker *et al* (1978) reported that animals do not need dietary protein to provide amino acids. Since, then numerous studies have been conducted to study amino acid requirement of poultry. They are components of tissue proteins and provision at insufficient levels leads to reduced protein synthesis. Provision of the different essential amino acids is therefore a prerequisite for maintaining optimal rates of protein synthesis. However, optimizing amino acid nutrition requires consideration of the different functions of amino acids, which are recognized to have several significant influences. Amino acids are precursors of important molecules.

Methionine and Lysine are the first two limiting amino acids in a corn soya diet in chicken. Methionine is the source of methyl groups required for all biological methylation reactions, including methylation of DNA and histones involved in epigenetic regulation (Tesseraud *et al*., 2009; Waterland, 2006; Waterland and Michels, 2007). Besides, Met and Cys are required for feather synthesis in birds. There are certain amino acids, which are considered as 'nutritionally essential' in birds. Thr is sometimes supplied in inadequate amounts in low crude protein diets, especially in challenging environmental conditions. Arg cannot be synthesized via the urea cycle. Unlike mammals, Pro cannot be synthesized from Arg, Glu or Gln at sufficient levels in birds. Gly, a precursor for the synthesis of uric acid (nitrogen excretion in uric acid form instead of urea) is not synthesized quickly enough to meet metabolic needs of chicken. It alone or in combination with Ser (because of conversion between these amino acids) must also be present in sufficient quantities in the diet of chicken. Cysteine is required for the synthesis of glutathione and taurine, which are essential compounds for host defense against oxidative stress (Metayer *et al.*, 2010). Studies conducted during the last decade indicate that amino acids act as regulators of various metabolic pathways (Tesseraud *et al.*, 2011; Wu, 2009 and Wu, 2013). Therefore, it is essential to understand the mechanisms by which amino acids regulate protein metabolism to improve control of the use of nutrients and optimize provision of dietary amino acids. In this chapter, we shall discuss about the factors affecting amino acid requirements in chicken, advances in amino acid requirements in broilers and layers and the future studies needed in this field.

Factors affecting amino acid nutrition in broilers and layers

The amino acid requirements of broilers and layers are dependent on various factors *viz*. germplasm, age, diet, condition of the bird and environment. Amino acid requirements differ among strains and lines in same diet and environment. Though there are very less differences in amino acid requirements of laying hens, there are differences in protein requirements of genetically lean and fat chicken (Leclercq and Guy, 1991). Further, male chicken requires a higher level of dietary Lys than females for maximum performance (Han and Baker, 1993). It has been observed that amino acid requirements of broilers decrease with advancing age (Ueno, 1998). Since, deficiency of amino acids in the diet results in an increased feed intake and the efficiency of digestive tract increases with advancing age, the amino acid requirements change with increasing age of the bird. However, in case of layers, amino acid requirement decreases with decrease in egg production. Old layers with high egg production require high amount of amino acids like young layers. Digestibility of crude protein does not vary between young and old layers (Ikeda *et al.*, 1997). Dietary factors include palatability, metabolizable energy, crude protein and availability of amino acids in the diet; deficiency, excess, imbalance and antagonism among amino acids. Amino acid requirement is also influenced by physiological condition of the bird such as age, molting, disease and stress. Further, environment plays a pivotal role in determining amino acid requirements as environmental temperature directly affects feed intake. Till date, different in vivo and in vitro methods have been developed to evaluate the nutritional values of dietary protein and amino acids *viz*. nitrogen balance, protein efficiency ratio, gross protein ratio, net protein ratio, biological value, net protein utilization, plasma amino acid index, chemical score, essential amino acid index etc. In recent years, these methods have been followed by determination of amino acids by advanced techniques like amino acid analyzer and HPLC.

Advances in broiler amino acid nutrition

Using low crude protein diets in broilers often results in inadequate provision of certain amino acids. Another challenge in amino acid nutrition of broilers is formulating balanced diets with increasing number of production criteria (e.g. considering meat quality along with growth performance), and one which improves animal health (importance of 'functional' amino acids is highlighted). Sometimes, Threonine is deficient in low crude protein diets, despite its crucial importance for maintaining intestinal integrity and immune function (Wu, 2009). Digestible Thr:Lys requirement of broilers is estimated to be around 67% and is even higher in critical environmental conditions (Lambert *et al.*, 2015a). Provision of diets deficient in amino acid (i.e. essential amino acids other than Lys) combined with a reduced Lys content favours production of meat with high pH (> 6.0), while more acid meat is produced with higher levels of amino acids (essential amino acids other than Lys) combined with a low Lys content. Recent advances in amino acid nutrition have been mainly in combined approaches of nutritional and metabolic studies. Integrating the data obtained at various levels from the cell to the animal and complete understanding of amino acid metabolism for rational use in nutrition holds a key challenge in near future. This has been well depicted in a review of the role of sulfur amino acids in controlling nutrient metabolism and cell functions (Tesseraud *et al.*, 2009). Till date, numerous studies have been conducted to understand the roles of sulfur amino acids, but future studies are necessary to obtain direct evidence regarding some of their effects on cell functions, nutrient metabolism and physiological responses in birds on early nutrition or stress and disease conditions. It is important to analyze the effects of sulfur amino acids under circumstances affecting oxidative status and gene expression. It has also become necessary to revisit the recommendations for Met and Cys intake in the light of their roles and the intricacies of sulfur amino acid metabolism. In addition, it is also needed that studies should be conducted to understand the integration of the various roles of sulfur amino acids at the whole-body level. These findings are particularly important in birds due to the high Met and Cys requirements for feather synthesis. The content of Cys has to be taken into account when adjusting the provision of Met, while also taking into account their potential interactions with Gly-Ser. Glycine (or Gly+Ser because of equimolar and reversible conversion between them) must also be present in the diet in sufficient quantities, since Gly is not synthesized quickly enough to meet the glycine requirement for synthesis of uric acid. Gly supplementation in low protein diets results in a positive effect in chicken performance of (Dean *et al*., 2006). However, there are still conflicting reports in the literature and it is still difficult to establish Gly+Ser requirements for broilers due to the low number of dose responses available and probably limiting factors or bias in these dose responses (Lambert *et al*., 2015b).Further, it is necessary that the interaction between Gly and Thr is investigated. Right now it appears that quantitative importance of Gly synthesis from Thr is probably dependent on dietary Thr availability (Wang *et al*., 2013; Lambert *et al*., 2015c).

Dietary amino acids are also major determinants of the carcass components of broilers, as abdominal fat content and breast meat yield are influenced by their levels (Moran and Bilgili, 1990; Leclercq, 1995). Lysine is known to have specific effects on carcass composition. Lysine deficiency greatly reduces breast muscle proportion (Tesseraud *et al*., 1996a, b). In fact, neither threonine nor valine exhibits as pronounced an effect as that of lysine on body composition, as demonstrated in experiments in which these three amino acids were studied together in similar conditions (Leclercq, 1998). Interestingly, increasing the level of lysine in the diet of broilers (beyond the requirement for growth) reduced drip loss of breast muscle during storage by increasing its ultimate pH (Berri *et al*., 2008). This result was consistent with the general hypothesis that breast muscle hypertrophy in broilers is accompanied by a decrease in glycogen storage (Berri *et al*., 2007). It has been observed that breast meat traits and the pH is affected by subjecting the broilers to diets varying in amino acid content over a very short period of 3 days before slaughter (Guardia *et al*., 2014). Provision of various amino acids (and the resulting amino acid balance or imbalance) may indeed affect the proportion of nutrients used for glycogen storage and hence the pH. Variations in dietary amino acid profiles significantly affected breast meat lightness that itself is strongly correlated with the water holding capacity of meat and processing yield (Qiao *et al*., 2002; Petracci *et al*., 2004; Zhuang and Savage, 2010). Amino acid provision has been shown to have an impact on the chemical composition of tissues, with a potential effect on meat quality. In fact, Met and/or Cys deficiency not only affects lipid and protein content, also affects amino acid composition of tissue proteins in chickens (Conde-Aguilera *et al*., 2013). It has been noted that provision of sulfur containing amino acid modifies meat susceptibility to oxidation. For example, oxidative stress and lipid per oxidation is more or less significant according to the Met source provided in the diet (DL-Met or hydroxy analog of methionine, DL-HMTBA) (Martinvenegas *et al*., 2006; Swennen *et al*., 2011; Willemsen *et al*., 2011). It has been observed that fully or partially replacing DL-Met by its hydroxyl-analog HMTBA reduces breast meat susceptibility to oxidation (leg and breast meat) and also increases its pH, with positive consequences on storage and processing ability (Mercier *et al*., 2009).

Advances in layer amino acid nutrition

Reducing dietary nitrogen closely meeting the birds' amino acid requirements and decreasing excessive amino acid excretion, pose challenges to nutritionists in the layer industry. In addition, there are challenges from diet cost, to bird health, to the environment. Thus, in amino acid nutrition of the hens, it is important that diets contribute to precision nutrition based on strain of the hen, changes in housing and management. However, laying hen research is limited at universities and research institutions because of facilities and time for proper experimentation to support the shell egg industry. Thus, studies on amino acid nutrition in layers are limited. A 2% reduction in CP, validated in comparison to control layer (18 to 16% CP), was feasible pending an Ile-to-Lys ratio of 82 to 88% (Parenteau *et al.*, 2020). It has also been observed that feeding hens for egg weight demands increased amino acid density (Van Krimpen *et al.*, 2015). Further, dietary amino acids offer some unique benefits for egg operations to manage change. It has been reported that increase in dietary Lys decreases the severity of *Ascaridia galli* infection in layers (Das *et al.*, 2010) and increase in Thr in layer diet improves intestinal function in layers (Dong *et al.*, 2017). Further, it has been noted that increased dietary L-Glu improves bone density in layers (Pereira *et al.*, 2019). Bregendahl *et al.* (2008) conducted a series of experiments to assess ideal protein ratios for Met, Cys, Thr, Val, Ile, Trp, and Arg in Hy-Line W36 hens from 26 to 34 wk of age. Ratios to Lys were established from calculating amount of amino acid needed per hen per day to maximize egg mass, and all amino acid treatments resulted in improved responses, except Arg. As a result, the ratio of Arg to Lys was concluded to be no higher than 107%. Established ratios of all other amino acids tested were Met, 47%; Met 1 Cys, 94%; Thr, 77%; Val, 93%; Ile, 79%; and Trp, 22% and are in agreement with Rostagno *et al.* (2017)., Spangler *et al.* (2019) fed laying Lohmann LSL-Lite hens with Lys from 22 to 47 wk using a blended diet-CP titration formulation design to address digestible Lys requirements of modern strains. It was observed that hens required higher digestible Lys to optimize egg mass and FCR vs. that of egg production. Management practices that favor floor rearing over cages may result in higher Thr-to-Lys requirements to support maintenance requirements, with specific reference to those in support of intestinal health. Dong *et al.* (2017) fed Lohmann Brown hens a low-CP diet supplemented with L-Thr and found intestinal mucin 2, IgA, and IgA expression as measured by mRNA was increased with dietary Thr, indicating potential intestinal health–related benefits by supplementation of dietary Thr. Thus, studies should be undertaken in future to compare Thr requirements in laying hens reared in cages and deep litter system. Broilers reared in used vs. clean litter have increased Thr requirements (Kidd *et al.*, 2003; Corzo *et al.*, 2007).

Another important issue in amino acid nutrition in layers is that there is a concern that in addition to branched-chain amino acid interactions between themselves (i.e., Val, Ile, and Leu), they interact with large neutral amino acids (i.e. Trp) because they share the same brain transporters (Fernstrom, 2005). Peganova *et al.* (2003) fed Lohmann Brown layers diets varying in Val, Ile, Leu, and Trp from 25 to 28 wk of age. Dietary Trp did not interact with the branched-chain amino acids, and it was concluded that 175 mg Trp/hen/day supports the egg mass. However, as dietary Ile was increased from 0.57 to 1.15% of diet, the egg production and egg mass were significantly suppressed but restored in the presence of diets increased in both Val and Leu. The interaction was mediated by excess Ile depressing feed intake, and although Trp increased feed intake, no Trp by Ile interaction occurred (Peganova and Eder, 2003).

It has also been noted that large neutral amino acids impact Trp. Trp requirements for egg production (145 mg/hen/d) and egg mass (155 mg/hen/d) are low when hens are fed high with large neutral amino acids. However, when hens are fed with low large neutral amino acid levels, Trp levels have to be enhanced for egg production (184 mg/hen/d) and egg mass (198 mg/hen/d) (Peganova *et al.*, 2003).

An important aspect in layer amino nutrition is to understand the role of amino acids in maintaining intestinal mucosa integrity. In fact, a significant amount of the hen's amino acid requirement is to maintain intestinal mucosa integrity, and more specifically, to create mucins (Moran, 2017). Mucin chemical arrangement primarily consists of Cys, Thr, Gly, Ser, Pro, and Gln, but Ile and Val are central to the chemical structure of the glycocalyx (Moran, 2017). It is unlikely that intestinal mucosa formation would be impaired from one of the former amino acids being limiting in diet. Hence, one can understand that it is imperative that the nutrient requirements of the intestinal cells (e.g., enterocytes and goblet cells) take priority over other parts of the body for amino acid requirements (Moran, 2016). However, in situations when hens are fed diets low in CP with corn as the primary cereal and marginal in amino acids, as the former tends to result in elevated Leu, which can exacerbate an Ile or Val imbalance; amino acid limitation in the diet may result in whole body cellular pools of amino acids being either low or imbalanced (i.e., Ile and Val) (D'Mello and Lewis, 1970).

Another interesting thing to note is increasing the Arg-to-Lys ratio in broilers during a coccidiosis challenge from 90 to 130% improved FCR and increasing the Arg-to Lys ratio from 110 to 130 decreased mortality (Kidd, 2004). Since, de novo synthesis of Arg in laying hens is incomplete, rendering Arg as an essential amino acid, future studies should focus on assessing requirements for Arg in the diet in diverse managemental and challenging conditions in layers.

Conclusion

Improving the nutrient utilization and optimizing dietary amino acid requirements for production in chicken has always been a sought after topic for studies for nutritionists globally. Reducing the crude protein content of diets for chicken appears to have major benefits for the sustainability of poultry production, but it is practically difficult to achieve in chickens despite the knowledge available on amino acids. This is due to the complex mechanisms involved in the control of metabolism and interactions among amino acids whose importance and implications for nutrition need to be examined and even prioritized. Studies often focus on a few particular areas and it's difficult to integrate and analyze all the data available to propose recommendations.

Ideal protein ratios for dietary amino acids for chicken have resulted in diets balanced in amino acids that support growth, egg production and flock health. However, assessment of ideal protein in chicken warrants research by varying strains and management practices whereby test diets are first limiting in Lysine and second limiting is the amino acid nutrient level in question (Thr, Val, Ile, Trp, Arg etc). A major challenge for future studies in amino acid nutrition in chicken is to improve the integration of data without oversimplification, while taking into account the findings/concepts which are generalizable or dependent on a particular condition such as the experimental design, physiological situations, including early life etc.

References

Baker, D.H., Robbins, K.R. and Buck, J.S. 1978. Modification of the level of histidine and sodium bicarbonate in the Illinois crystalline amino acid diet. Poultry Science, 58: 1122-1131.

Berri, C., Besnard, J. and Relandeau, C. 2008. Increasing dietary lysine increases final pH and decreases drip loss of broiler breast meat. Poultry Science, 87: 480-484.

Berri, C., LE Bihan-Duval, E., Debut, M., Sante-Lhoutelier, V., Baeza, E., Gigaud, V., Jego, Y. and Duclos, M.J. 2007. Consequence of muscle hypertrophy on characteristics of pectoralis major muscle and breast meat quality of broiler chickens. Journal of Animal Science, 85: 2005-2011.

Bregendahl, K., Roberts, S. A., Kerr B. and Hoehler, D.. 2008. Ideal ratios of isoleucine, methionine, methionine plus cystine, threonine, tryptophan, and valine relative to lysine for white Leghorn-Type laying hens of twenty-eight to thirty-four weeks of age. Poultry Science, 87: 744–758.

Conde-Aguilera, J.A., Cobo-Ortega, C., Tesseraud, S., Lessire, M., Mercier, Y. and Van Milgen, J. 2013. Changes in body composition in broilers by a sulfur amino acid deficiency during growth. Poultry Science, 92: 1266-1275.

Corzo, A., Kidd, M. T., Dozier III, W.A., Pharr, G. T. and Koutsos, E. A. 2007. Dietary threonine needs for growth and immunity of broilers raised under different litter conditions. Journal of Applied Poultry Research, 16: 574–582.

D'Mello, J. P. F. and Lewis, D. 1970. Amino acid interactions in chick nutrition: Interrelationships between leucine, isoleucine, and valine. British Poultry Science, 11: 313–323.

Das, G., Kaufmann, F., Abel, H., and Gauly, M. 2010. Effect of extra dietary lysine in Ascaridia galli-infected grower layers. Veterinary Parasitology, 170: 238–243.

Dean, D.W., Bidner, T.D. and Southern, L.L. 2006. Glycine supplementation to low protein, amino acid-supplemented diets supports optimal performance of broiler chicks. Poultry Science, 85: 288-296.

Dong, X. Y., Azzam, M. M. M. and Zou, X. T. 2017. Effects of dietary threonine supplementation on intestinal barrier function and gut microbiota of laying hens. Poultry Science, 96: 3654-3663.

Fernstrom, J. D. 2005. Branched-chain amino acids and brain function. Journal of Nutrition, 135 (6 Suppl): 1539S–1546S.

Guardia, S., Lessire, M., Corniaux, A., Métayer-Coustard, S., Mercerand, F., Tesseraud, S., Bouvarel, I. and Berri, C. 2014. Short-term nutritional strategies before slaughter are effective in modulating the final pH and color of broiler breast meat. Poultry Science, 93: 1764-1773.

Han, Y. and Baker, D.H. 1993. Effects of sex, heat stress, body weight and genetic strain on the dietary lysine requirement of broiler chicks. Poultry Science, 72: 701-708.

Ikeda, T., Yamamoto, A., Fujimura, S., Kadowaki, M. and Ishibashi, T. 1997. Causes of the depression of the protein efficiency with aging on laying hens-especially with dietary protein levels and amino acids absorption. Hokuriku Journal of Zootechnological Science, 56: 827-834.

Kidd, M. T. 2004. Nutritional modulation of immune function in broilers. Poultry Science, 83: 650–657.

Kidd, M. T., Barber, S. J., Virden, W. S., Dozier III, W.A., Chamblee, D. W. and Wiernusz, C. 2003. Threonine responses of Cobb male finishing broilers in differing environmental conditions. Journal of Applied Poultry Research, 12: 115–123.

Lambert, W., Rovers, M., Ensink, J., Tesseraud, S., Corrent, E., De Lange, L., Star, L. 2015c. Interaction between threonine and glycine at low dietary crude protein and the effect on production performance, meat quality and plasma metabolites in broilers. In: 20th European Symposium on Poultry Nutrition, Prague (CZE) 2015/08/2

Lambert, W., Simongiovanni, A., Tesseraud, S. and Corrent, E. 2015a. Threonine requirement of broiler chickens: integrated prediction by meta-analysis. In: 20th European Symposium on Poultry Nutrition, Prague (CZE) 2015/08/25-27, Abstract

Lambert, W., Simongiovanni, A., Tesseraud, S. and Corrent, E. 2015b. Is meta-analysis an effective tool to estimate the glycine plus serine requirement of broiler chickens? In: 20th European Symposium on Poultry Nutrition, Prague (CZE) 2015/08/25-27, Abstract.

Leclercq, B. 1995. Broiler quality: considering the trio of genotype, quality and dietary amino acids. OECD-Workshop "Growth and quality in broiler production" from 7th-9th June 1994 in Celle. Archiv für Geflügelkunde, 59: 37-40.

Leclercq, B. and Guy, G. 1991. Further investigations of protein requirement of genetically lean and fat chickens. British Poultry Science, 32: 789-798.

Leclercq, B., 1998. Specific effects of lysine on broiler production: comparison with threonine and valine. Poultry Science, 77: 118-123.

Martin-Venegas, R., Geraert, P.A. and Ferrer, R. 2006. Conversion of the Methionine Hydroxy Analogue, DL-2-Hydroxy- (4-Methylthio) butanoic Acid, to Sulfur-Containing Amino Acids in the Chicken Small Intestine. Poultry Science, 85: 1932-1938.

Mercier, Y., Berri, C., Baéza, E., Bordeau, T., Chartrin, P., Ercerand, F. and Geraert, P.A., 2009. Improvement of muscle oxidative stability and processing yield in relation with dietary methionine sources. In: Poultry Science Association 98th Annual meeting. Raleigh, North Carolina (USA) 2009/07/20-23. Abstract 117.

Métayer-Coustard, S., Mameri, H., Seiliez, I., Crochet, S., Crépieux, P., Mercier, Y., Geraert, P.A. and Tesseraud, S. 2010. Methionine deprivation regulates the S6K1 pathway and protein synthesis in avian QM7 myoblasts without activating the GCN2/eIF2α cascade. Journal of Nutrition, 140: 1539-1545.

Moran, E. T. 2016. Gastric digestion of protein through pancreozyme action optimizes intestinal forms for absorption, mucin formation and villus integrity. Animal Feed Science and Technology, 221: 284–303.

Moran, E. T. 2017. Nutrients central to maintaining intestinal absorptive efficiency and barrier integrity in fowl. Poultry Science, 96: 1348–1363.

Moran, E.T. and Bilgili, S.F. 1990. Processing losses, carcass quality, and meat yields of broiler chickens receiving diets marginally deficient to adequate in lysine prior to marketing. Poultry Science, 69: 702-710.

Parenteau, I. A., Stevenson, M. and Kiarie, E. G. 2020. Egg production and quality responses to increasing isoleucine supplementation in Shaver white hens fed a low crude protein corn-soybean meal diet fortified with synthetic amino acids between 20 and 46 weeks of age. Poultry Science, 99: 1444–1453.

Peganova, S. and Eder, K. 2003. Interactions of various supplies of isoleucine, valine, leucine and tryptophan on the performance of laying hens. Poultry Science, 82: 100-105.

Peganova, S., Hirche, F. and Eder, K. 2003. Requirement of tryptophan in relation to the supply of large neutral amino acids in laying hens. Poultry Science, 82: 815–822.

Pereira, A. P. A. E., Murakami, C., Stefanello, Iwaki, L. C. V. and Santos T. C. 2019. Productive performance, bone characteristics, and intestinal morphology of laying hens fed diets formulated with L-glutamic acid. Poultry Science, 98: 2500–2508.

Petracci, M., Betti, M., Bianchi, M. and Cavani, C. 2004. Color variation and characterization of broiler breast meat during processing in Italy. Poultry Science, 83: 2086-2092.

Qiao, M., Fletcher, D.L., Smith, D.P. and Northcutt, J.K. 2002. Effects of raw broiler breast meat color variation on marination and cooked meat quality. Poultry Science, 81: 276-280.

Rostagno, H. S., Albino, L. F. T., Hannas, M. I., Donzele, J. L., Sakomura, N. K., Perazzo, F. G., Saraiva, A., Teixeira de Abreu, M. L., Rodrigues, P. B., Oliveira, R. F., Barreto, S. L. T. and Brito, C. O. 2017. Page 311 in Brazilian Tables for Poultry and Swine-Composition of Feedstuffs and Nutritional Requirements. 4th ed. Department of Animal Science, Federal University of Viçosa, MG, Brazil.

Spangler, H., Utterback, P., Parsons, C. M. and Tillman, P. 2019. Determining the digestible lysine requirement of 22- to 47-week-old Lohmann laying hens using an increasing protein titration methodology. Poultry Science, 98: 1706–1715.

Swennen, Q., Geraert, P.A., Mercier, Y., Everaert, N., Stinckens, A., Willemsen, H., Li, Y., Decuypere, E. and Buyse, J. 2011. Effects of dietary protein content and 2-hydroxy-4-methylthiobutanoic acid or dl-methionine supplementation on performance and oxidative status of broiler chickens. British Journal of Nutrition, 21:1.

Tesseraud, S., Everaert, N., Boussaid-Om Ezzine, S., Collin, A., Métayer-Coustard, S. and Berri, C. 2011. Manipulating tissue metabolism by amino acids. World's Poultry Science Journal, 67: 243-252.

Tesseraud, S., Maaa, N., Peresson, R. and Chagneau, A.M. 1996a. Relative responses of protein turnover in three different skeletal muscles to dietary lysine deficiency in chicks. British Poultry Science, 37:641-650.

Tesseraud, S., Métayer Coustard, S., Collin, A. and Seiliez, I. 2009. Role of sulfur amino acids in controlling nutrient metabolism and cell functions: implications for nutrition. British Journal of Nutrition, 101: 1132-1139.

Tesseraud, S., Peresson, R., Lopes, J. and Chagneau A.M. 1996b. Dietary Lys deficiency greatly affects muscle and liver protein turnover in growing chickens. British Journal of Nutrition, 75: 853-865.

Ueno, K. 1998. Research of Arginine and Lysine requirement for Broilers. PhD. dissertation, Niigata University.

Van Krimpen, M. M., Veldkamp, T., Van Riel, J. W., Khaksar, V., Hashemipour, H., Blok M. C. and Spek, W. 2015. Estimating Requirements for Apparent Faecal and Standardised Ileal Digestible Amino Acids in Laying Hens by a Meta-Analysis Approach. Wageningen UR Livestock Research Report 848, Wageningen, The Netherlands.

Wang, W., Wu, Z., Dai, Z., Yang, Y., Wang, J. and Wu, G. 2013. Glycine metabolism in animals and humans: implications for nutrition and health. Amino Acids, 45: 463-477.

Waterland, R.A. 2006. Assessing the effects of high methionine intake on DNA methylation. Journal of Nutrition, 136: 1706S-1710S.

Waterland, R.A. and Michels, K.B. 2007. Epigenetic epidemiology of the developmental origins hypothesis. Annual Revision of Nutrition, 27: 363-388.

Willemsen, H., Swennen, Q., Everaert, N., Geraert, P.A., Mercier, Y., Stinckens, A., Decuypere, E. and Buyse, J. 2011. Effects of dietary supplementation of methionine and its hydroxy analog DL-2-hydroxy-4-methylthiobutanoic acid on growth performance, plasma hormone levels, and the redox status of broiler chickens exposed to high temperatures. Poultry Science, 90: 2311-2320.

Wu, G., 2009. Amino acids: metabolism, functions, and nutrition. Amino Acids, 37: 1-17.

Wu, G., 2013. Functional amino acids in nutrition and health. Amino Acids, 45: 407-411.

Zhuang, H. and Savage, E.M. 2010. Comparisons of sensory descriptive flavor and texture profiles of cooked broiler breast fillets categorized by raw meat color lightness values. Poultry Science, 89: 1049-1055.

3

Recent Advances in Organic Minerals in Poultry Nutrition

Chandra Deo and Divya Sharma

Principal Scientist, Central Avian Research Institute, Izatnagar, Bareilly Uttar Pradesh

Introduction

Minerals are essentially required for growth maintenance, egg and meat production, health, nutrient metabolism, physiological function, reproduction, skeletal growth and development and maintenance of normal immune function. There are 25 essential minerals, seven are major minerals, as they are present in relatively higher amount in the body than the trace minerals and need to be supplemented in higher quantities in the feed. These major minerals are calcium, phosphorus, magnesium, sodium, chloride, potassium, and sulphur. The micro minerals are present in small quantities in the body and their requirements in the diet are below 100 mg/kg. The 18 trace minerals are iron, copper, zinc, manganese, iodine, selenium, cobalt, molybdenum, chromium, tin, vanadium, fluorine, silicon, nickel, arsenic, aluminium, lead and rubidium. Among these, the first nine micro minerals have been identified to play a significant role in birds. Total minerals in diet include feed sources and supplementary sources. Drinking water also supplies certain minerals to some extent. However, some of the essential minerals, except under certain specific conditions, are meet out through dietary sources like magnesium, potassium, molybdenum, tin, vanadium, fluorine, silicon, nickel, arsenic, aluminium, lead and rubidium. Thus those minerals are not generally considered for dietary supply. Other minerals (calcium, phosphorus, sodium, chloride, iron, copper, zinc, manganese, iodine and selenium) are apt to be deficient in diet. Cobalt as such has no role in poultry but as component of vitamin B_{12} (cyanocobalamin), it plays an important role. Chromium plays important role in reducing stress. Sulphur usually is not deficient unless sulphur containing amino acids are deficient in diet.

The supplemental sources of minerals can be classified in two broad categories viz. inorganic and organic. Inorganic sources of the minerals are the carbonate, sulphate, oxide or chloride salts. The bioavailability of minerals also differs due to salt. Inorganic salts usually have low bioavailability mainly due to the antagonism between themselves or other minerals, feed ingredients and nutrients, which results in reduced absorption. The solution commonly used is to increase the concentration or the quantity of the inorganic trace minerals in poultry diet, which further results in reduced mineral bioavailability and high residues in litter, causing danger to environment and no benefit to the animal. The other category is organic sources, often referred to as chelated minerals. However, the term chelated minerals may not be always appropriate.

The chelates minerals have been classified into three groups. Group I includes those chelates that serve to transport and to store metal ions. In this type of chelates, the mineral binds with a ligand, which has physical and chemical properties for facilitating chelates for absorption, transportation in the blood, and passing across cell membranes where those are deposited to meet the requirement, e.g. amino acids, ethylene diamine tetra acetate (EDTA), etc. Group II chelates include those which are essential for metabolism like haemoglobin, myoglobin, cytochrome enzymes, vitamin B12, etc. The third group (group III) includes those chelates that interfere with the availability of essential minerals, like phytate, oxalates, etc. The ideal chelating compounds are those which will facilitate the release of minerals in the ionic form in the intestinal wall (site for absorption) or absorption as an intact chelate. Such chelates prevent conversion of minerals into insoluble form in the intestine, or prevent adsorption on an insoluble colloid. On chelation with amino acids or hydrolysed proteins they become more stable and less reactive in the digestive tract. The inorganic minerals may interact with fibre, phytate, tannin, oxalate, silicates or other minerals in the gastro-intestinal tract, which may interfere with their absorption. Such interaction can be prevented by using organic minerals. Common organically bound trace minerals used in poultry nutrition are iron, copper, zinc, manganese, chromium and selenium. Supplementation of organic mineral complexes is reported to improve the bio-availability of minerals in majority of the studies but the results on improvement in growth performance of birds are not always consistent. Improved bio-availability of minerals also reduces their poultry excreta minerals content and thus environment friendly. There are different categories of organic trace minerals such as metal specific amino acid complexes, metal amino acid complexes, metal amino acid chelates, metal proteinates, metal poly saccharide complexes, metal propionates and yeast derivative complexes. Research has indicated that these organic sources of minerals are more bio-available than their inorganic counterparts due to the following reasons: these complexes are absorbed more efficiently in the gut, less interaction between competing minerals for absorption sites and the ring structure protects the mineral from unwanted chemical reactions in the gut. The most commonly used organically complexed minerals include zinc, copper, manganese, iron, selenium and chromium.

Categories of organic trace minerals: The Association of American Feed Control Officials (AAFCO, 1998) has categorized organic trace minerals as below:

i. **Metal (specific amino acid) complexes:** Supplements produced by complexing a soluble metal salt with a specific amino acid e.g. zinc methionine, which is produced by combining zinc sulphate with methionine. Similarly copper-lysine and manganese-methionine are such complexes. These complexes are most effective and efficiently absorbed in gut among all the organic minerals.

ii. **Metal amino acid complexes**: Single metal atom (zinc for instance) complexed with several single amino acids in a single blend (viz. zinc methionine, zinc lysine, zinc leucine, zinc cystine etc). Each individual complex molecule is having one metal ion and one amino acid but has a variety of amino acids in the blend.

iii. **Metal amino acid chelates:** These are formed from the reaction of a metal ion from a soluble metal salt with amino acids having a mole ratio of one mole of metal to one to three (preferably two) moles of amino acids to form coordinate-covalent bonds. The molecular size of such chelates should not exceed 800 Dalton. Nowadays trace mineral glycinate using glycine as a ligand is getting popular as glycine is readily absorbed in gut and gets transported right into the cells.

iv. **Metal proteinates:** Chelation of a soluble mineral salt with amino acids and/or hydrolyzed protein. The final product may contain single amino acids, dipeptides, tripeptides or other protein derivatives. The molecular size of metal proteinates is sometime higher than the desired size resulting in decreased bioavailability of minerals. Moreover, the products do not very high stability constant because of its ligand size as such molecules are easily broken apart especially with change in pH, resulting in the loss of heterocyclic chelate ring structure. These proteinates are generally less expensive but are not much beneficial over single amino acid chelates.

v. **Metal polysaccharide complexes:** These are prepared by coating the metal with polysaccharide molecules. These are larger molecules based on chains of simple sugars which are highly soluble in the digestive tract.

vi. **Metal propionates:** These mineral products are result of combining soluble metals with soluble organic acids like propionic acid. The resultant products are highly soluble and are generally disassociate in solution. Metal propionate minerals are highly soluble, and dissociate at a rate that is approximately equal to the need or availability of the respective metal transport sites throughout the GI tract.

vii. **Yeast Derivative Complexes:** Other sources of organic trace elements that show promise are mineral enriched yeast. Presently the most common is selenium yeast with selenium complexed with a methionine molecule (selenomethionine). Chromium enriched yeast also has gained popularity for improving animal production.

Absorption of organic minerals

After intake of the organic minerals from the feed, mineral absorption process can occur in any region of the intestine, but metals are usually absorbed in the duodenum region of the digestive tract. After gastric hydrolysis these inert complexes of minerals reaches the intestinal lumen where ligand bounded to the minerals act as their transporter and protect them from interacting with the different antagonists and vitamins present in the diet. Most antagonists present in the feed include sulphates, oxides, fibre, high sulphur containing dried distillers grains, cotton seed hulls and other fermented feeds and the minerals in hard water, notably sulphur and calcium. These ligand-mineral complexes get absorbed through the enterocytes while the inorganic minerals only get absorbed when there is any inorganic metal transporter otherwise they will be excreted in the faeces. Commercial organic trace minerals are prepared in such a way that provide natural protection and are more likely to be absorbed and used. They do not interact with antagonists or vitamins. Inorganic trace minerals, however, can readily interact with antagonism between themselves or other minerals, feed ingredients and nutrients and these interactions leave inorganic trace minerals bound and unavailable to the birds.

Bioavailability of organic trace minerals

Formulation of poultry diets with inclusion of inorganic sources such as carbonate, sulphate, oxide or chloride salts can result in poor bioavailability of the minerals due to numerous chemical antagonisms and interactions with other components in the diet. For the past 20 years, trace mineral research has focused on bioavailability enhanced with the development of new sources, mainly of organically bound origins (chelates).Studies have been carried out with the development of microbial phytase enzyme, which partly counteract the negative interaction with phytate, which binds minerals affecting their bioavailability and excretion rates. Poultry nutritionists can achieve higher bioavailability of trace minerals by using organic sources in which the minerals are chemically bound to an amino acid, organic acid, protein and carbohydrate. The quantity of minerals present in feed is not necessary that available to the birds, but it is necessary to how much minerals are bioavailable to the birds that determines the effectiveness of trace minerals for growth and production traits in poultry. Therefore, knowledge of the bioavailability of trace minerals from different sources is essential for economic feed formulation to improve performance of birds. Bioavailability can be defined as the degree to which an ingested nutrient in a particular source is absorbed in form that can be utilized in metabolism by the normal livestock and poultry. Birds absorb, digest and use mineral chelates better than inorganic form of minerals. This means that lower concentrations of organic trace minerals can be used in poultry feeds. In addition, birds fed chelated sources of essential trace minerals excrete lower amounts of minerals in their poultry excreta and so there is less environmental contamination. Mineral chelates also offer health and welfare benefits in poultry nutrition. Various work reported on bioavailability of different minerals from organic and inorganic sources are given in Table 1.

Table 1: Bioavailability of different minerals from organic and inorganic sources

S.No.	Organic minerals	Bioavailability	References
1.	Proteinates and amino acid chelates	Higher bioavailability and lower excretion of mineral in organic forms of mineral as compared to inorganic source.	Wedekind and Baker (1990). J of Anim. Sci. 68:684-689.
2.	Copper and Zinc Complex with lysine	Bioavailability of organic minerals is higher (120% and 106%) than inorganic source sulphate form (100%).	Aoyagi and Baker (1993). Poult. Sci.72:165-171.
3.	Organic Zinc	Higher bioavailability indicates more zinc was deposited in bone tissue from organic sources as compared to inorganic sources.	Cao *et al.* (2000). J of Anim. Sci. 78: 2039-2054.
4.	Zn Propionate	Higher relative bioavailability of Zn on the basis of tibia bone Zn content as compared to inorganic source Zn oxide and Zn sulphate.	Yogesh Kumar (2007) M.V.Sc. Thesis IVRI, Deemed unversity
5.	Cu Propionate	Higher relative bioavailability of Cu on the basis of tibia bone Cu content as compared to inorganic source Cu sulphate.	ShariqIqbal (2010). M.V.Sc. Thesis IVRI, Deemed unversity
6.	Zn Propionate	Higher Zn retention and lower Zn excretion in organic source Zn propionate as compared to inorganic source Zn sulphate.	ShariqIqbal (2010). M.V.Sc. Thesis IVRI, Deemed unversity

7.	Mnproteinate	Higher relative bioavailability of Mnproteinate (139%) as compared to inorganic source Mn sulphate (100%) in bone.	Brook *et al.* (2012). J of Appl. Poult. Res. 21:126-130
8.	Zn proteinate	Higher relative bioavailability of Zn on the basis of tibia bone Zn content.	Brook *et al.* (2013). J of Appl. Poult. Res. 22:153-159.
9.	Chelated Zinc	Higher expression of the metallothionine (indicator of zinc status) in intestinal tissue than the inorganic salt.	Varun *et al.* (2017). J of Curr. Microbiol. App. Sci. 6(7); 845-849.

Factors influencing utilization of organic minerals

There are several factors that may affect the utilization of trace minerals from organic complexes.

i. **Age of bird:** The efficiency of utilization of organic zinc decreases as the birds ages increases, suggesting that there may be less benefit in using organic zinc sources in feed for adult birds. This is probably due to increased diet uptake and the subsequent intake of trace minerals as birds mature.

ii. **Dietary protein contents:** A high protein diet significantly increased the apparent absorption of zinc and deposition in bone, but zinc requirement by birds fed a high protein diet did not decline due to this improved zinc bioavailability. In contrast, birds fed a low protein diet had a reduced zinc requirement.

iii. **Dietary calcium, phosphorus and environmental temperature:**Calcium retention increased with the addition of zinc to swine diets, but zinc had no influence on phosphorus retention, nor was retention of absorbed zinc affected by increased dietary calcium concentration. Most of studies on the biological availability of trace minerals have been conducted in temperature control environments suitable for bird growth. However, high environmental temperatures have been shown to increase mineral excretion and reduce minerals retention.

iv. **Trace mineral interactions:** A number of negative interactions can occur such as excess of one trace mineral will interfere with another trace mineral's availability. The most common antagonism occurs between zinc and copper. High levels of dietary zinc will inhibit copper absorption, hepatic accumulation and deposition in the egg. Ratios greater than 4:1 of zinc:copper can be considered antagonistic. High levels of copper and iron can interfere with zinc availability and potentially could induce anemia. Excess dietary phosphorus will interfere with manganese availability in poultry. Other factors such as water, equipment and or soil conditions for crops may also contribute excessive trace minerals to the birds.

Mineral toxicity

There are various parameters to investigate the bird response to the supplementation of inorganic trace minerals, the minimum levels associated with deficiencies, optimum levels are to meet the requirements and excess levels, which would result in toxicity. There are wide ranges between optimum and toxic levels of Calcium (Ca), Phosphorus (P), Copper (Cu),Iron (Fe), Manganese (Mn), Zinc(Zn) and selenium(Se) in broilers and layers diet, but relatively narrow ranges between minimum and optimum levels. There is evidence to suggest that organic trace minerals are less toxic than inorganic minerals.

Organic trace minerals in chicken production

Birds more efficiently absorb, digest and use organic minerals complexes than inorganic form of minerals. It means that lower concentrations of organic trace minerals can be used in poultry feeds. In addition, birds fed organic sources of essential trace minerals excrete lower amount in their faeces, so there is less environmental contamination. Organic minerals also offer health and welfare benefits in poultry nutrition such as decreased mortality and stress. The most commonly used organically-complexed mineral includes zinc, manganese, copper, iron, selenium and chromium.

i. **Zinc (Zn):** Zinc is an essential trace mineral required for growth, bone development, feather development, enzyme structure and function, immunomodulation, reproduction and appetite for all avian species. Deficiency of zinc in young chicks leads to retarded growth, shortening and thickening of leg bone and enlargement of hock joint, scaling of skin especially on the feet, poor feathering, reduce immunomodulation, reduced feed utilization and loss of appetite and in severe cases mortality and in adult birds deficiency of Zn causes reduced hatchability, embryonic abnormalities, reduced feed intake and utilization, reduced egg production, poor feathering and delayed in sexual maturity. Zinc sources have been the most studied of these compounds and a number of researchers have reported improvements in broiler growth rate and/or feed conversion with organic zinc sources. Studied conducted at CARI, Izatnagar (Iqbal *et al*., 2011) reported that a dietary combination of 40mg Zn and 16 mg Cu per kg either organic or inorganic forms of mineral was found sufficient for optimum growth performance and carcass quality traits of broiler chicks from 0-6wks of age. However, better immune response was found at a dietary combination of 80mg Zn and 16 mg Cu/kg diet with organic sources. Similarly in another experiment (Kumar *et al*., 2013), indicated that the optimum supplemental level of Zn should be 60-80mg/kg diet for broiler chickens to get better immune response. However, the Zn sources did not significantly influence Zn utilization. Most of the growth and carcass yield factors were found to be non –significant due to different Zn sources either organic or inorganic. Stanley *et al*. (2012) indicated that organic Zn (Bio-Plex) significantly increased egg production and decreased mortality of laying hens, but significantly reduced egg weight, albumen weight and shell weights in post molt hens. In contrast, Swiatkiewicz and Koreleski (2008) reported no effect of organic Zn amino acid complexes on egg production. However, in older layers, organic Zn positively affected eggshell breaking strength.

ii. **Manganese (Mn):** Manganese is an integral component of enzymes which are involved in the anti-oxidative defense system, metabolism of amino acid, protein, lipid and carbohydrate, maintenance of normal immune system, development of bone organic matrix, essential for insulin synthesis, necessary for mucopolysaccharides formation that are activated for the glycosyl transferase, involved in normal function of central nervous system and maintenance of normal reproduction. Deficiency of Mn in young birds leads to poor growth, reduced bone development, skeletal abnormalities and state of perosis, in this condition both legs may be affected. Perosis condition is characterized by thickened and enlarge hock joint, twisting and bending of tibia and tarso-metatarsus bone, thickening and shortening of long bones and slipping of achilles tendon from its condyle. Deficiency of Mn in adult birds causes lower egg production, reduced hatchability, poor egg shell qualityand nutritional chondrodystrophy in embryonic chicks characterized by poor growth, protruded abdomen, round head, parrot beak and edema. In surviving chick's incoordination of movement and pulling of the head towards the back similar to star gazing conditioned may be seen. Excess dietary levels of calcium, phosphorus and iron decrease the utilization of manganese in poultry. The phytic acid along with fibre has also been correlated to a decrease the manganese absorption in poultry. Abdallah *et al.* (2009) reported that significantly higher body weight and better feed conversion efficiency was observed in 100% organic mineral source than those observed in inorganic source of minerals. Yildiz *et al.* (2011) observed that organic source of manganese as manganese proteinate exhibited better weight gain, egg weight, percentage un-damage eggs and tibia bone quality parameters than that recorded in inorganic source manganese sulphate.

iii. **Copper (Cu):** Copper is an essential trace mineral for poultry, present in many enzyme systems in the body such as superoxide dismutase, cytochrome oxidase, and lysyl oxidase, or ceruloplasmin where it serves as a co-factor. Copper is also a component of blood proteins, one being erythrocuprein, found in erythrocytes where it is important in oxygen metabolism. Copper also occurs in certain pigments, especially turacin a pigment of feathers. It is present in most body cells, particularly in the liver which in the main body storage site. There are reports indicating that the Cu is involved in fat metabolism. Supplementary Cu reduced the incidence of oily bird syndrome. Copper deficiency in young chicks could cause severe health problems including growth depression, disability of bones, poor feathering and anemia. Birds being unable to absorb iron mobilize it from tissues and utilize it in hemoglobin synthesis may be due to copper deficiency. Copper deficiency results in a wide range of sign in different animal species, and indeed in the same species different situations are noted. However, anemia is a common sign noted for all animals, as is growth depression, bone disorders (fragile long bones and lameness), depigmentation of hair, wool, fur and feathers etc. Copper deficiency in laying hens causes shell-less and misshapen eggs and in breeder stock reduced egg production and hatchability, embryonic mortality is increased during second and third day of incubation. Das *et al.* (2010) reported that the substitution of inorganic Cu sulphate with organic Cu proteinate in broiler chickens diet positively affected body weight gain, feed conversion ratio and nutrient utilisation. Jageda *et al.* (2012) reported that supplementation of copper sulphat in growing pullet diet @ 50, 100 and 150 ppm, The organic copper source copper proteinate exhibited decreased plasma cholesterol, low-density lipoprotein (LDL) and triglyceride in comparison to supplementation of inorganic source Cu sulphate. Deo *et al.* (2018) reported that supplementation of copper sources (copper sulphate, CuS; copper chloride, CuCl and copper propionate, CuP) and their levels (8, 100, 150 and 200 mg/kg) in broiler diet to study the growth, carcass yield and serum cholesterol contents. Results suggested that a dietary copper concentration of 200 mg/kg through supplementation of organic copper (copper propionate) in broiler diet is more effective in promoting growth, feed conversion efficiency, carcass yield and reducing serum cholesterol concentration in comparison to inorganic source copper sulphate and copper chloride. Pekel and Alp (2011) comparing the efficacy of inorganic (Cu sulphate) and organic (Cu lysine or Cu proteinate) sources of Cu used ata high dietary level (250 ppm), did not find any beneficial effects of organic Cu in terms of egg production, egg mass, feed conversion ratio, egg quality, egg yolk cholesterol, plasma total cholesterol, high-density lipoprotein cholesterol, triglycerides and glutathione-peroxidase activity.

iv. **Iron (Fe):** Iron is an essential component of haemoglobin and myoglobin. It also plays a key role in several enzymes (oxidases, oxygenase, peroxidase, and catalase) and electron transport (cytochrome).Iron plays a role for pigmentation of feathers along with lysine and folic acid in coloured feather chickens. Deficiency symptoms of iron causes macrocytic and hypochromic anaemia, depressed body weight, loss or gain of appetite and poor feathering. The requirement of iron in feed increases during blood loss (parasite infection), feed contain tannins, gossypal and phytin and excess dietary concentration of phosphorus, manganese and copper. There has been a considerable research indicating reduction of recommended levels of organically complexed minerals in broiler chicken diets without any negative effects on growth performance (Bao *et al*., 2007). Pierce *et al*. (2005) reported that Supplementing organically complexed minerals at 25% of NRC requirement of Cu, Zn & Fe had no negative effect on body weight gain and feed intake. Park *et al.* (2004) reported that Fe content of egg can be increased by supplementing organic iron supplements. Fe-Methionine was most effective source I enriching Fe in egg followed by Availa-Fe and lowest in inorganic source $FeSo_4$. Inkee Paik *et al*. (2009) conducted an experiment to determine the efficacy of dietary iron-soy proteinate and iron methionine chelate on the performance of laying hens and iron content in egg yolk. Results suggested that iron content in egg yolk could be effectively increased by supplementing 100ppm iron as iron soy-proteinate for 5weeks. No significant difference was found in Fe content of egg yolk between iron soy-proteinate and iron methionine.

v. **Selenium (Se):** Selenium is an essential trace element protecting the cellular and sub-cellular membrane from oxidation. Enzyme glutathione peroxidase plays an important role as an antioxidant. It acts in the cytoplasm and helps to remove free radicals. Selenium also plays a role in reproductive function, development of immune system and ageing. Selenium is closely associated with vitamin E and one can spare the other. Deficiency of selenium causes exudative diathesis, characterised by subcutaneous accumulation of green-blue fluid on breast and abdomen and tissue haemorrhage, white muscle disease or muscular dystrophy caused by deficiency of selenium, vitamin E and sulphur containing amino acids characterised by dystrophy (development of white striations) of skeletal muscles especially breast muscle. Selenium deficiency is associated with impaired immune competence, reduced egg production, decreased hatchability and increased embryonic mortality. Feed ingredients contain variable concentrations of Selenium, but most of them are deficient in selenium contents. Physiological requirement of selenium is very low, but if not met, antioxidant system is compromised with detrimental consequences for animal health. Surai (2006) reported that selenium has a positive effect on egg shell quality including shell breaking strength via the modulation of organic matrix formation. Payne *et al.* (2005) also reported higher Se content in eggs of layers fed Se-methionine. Advantage of organic selenium in broiler diet increased selenium transfer to the muscles and the build-up of selenium reserve in the body which improve chickens resistance to various stresses and a positive effect on immunity, gut health and meat quality (Fisinin *et al.,* 2008; Surai and Fisinin, 2014). Ozkan *et al.* (2007) reported that dietary supplementation with inorganic or organic selenium@ 0.15mg/kg diet did not affect the body weight of broiler reared at optimum temperature.

vi. **Chromium (Cr):** Last two decades chromium has been considered as an important micro-mineral in poultry production. It required for protein, lipid, carbohydrate and nucleic acid metabolism. It also activates certain enzyme system and stabilizes protein. Chromium is known to increase the insulin sensitivity and reduce the plasma glucose concentration in broilers. Insulin controls the metabolism of carbohydrate, protein, lipid and stimulates the uptake of amino acids, protein synthesis and glucose utilization. Chromium supplementation in broiler diet reduced plasma glucose and non-steroid fatty acid concentration. Chromium acts as a co-factor of insulin activity and the presence of this mineral is required for proper glucose metabolism and growth in poultry. Dietary chromium increased serum insulin, decreased corticosterone level and glucose concentration in laying hens. Dietary supplementation of chromium improved the utilization of dietary energy through stimulation of insulin action and thus could help to maintain the productivity of birds even if the dietary energy level is low. Organic source of chromium is more bioavailable than inorganic source. Feeding of Cr-methonine @ 200 ppb increased body weight by 11.5% while at 400 ppb level the increase in body weight gain was 2.5% (Ohh and Lee; 2005). Body weight gain was also higher in broiler birds fed diets supplemented with 0.5 ppm Cr from organic than inorganic source (Mohammed *et al.,* 2014). Feeding of Cr-aminoniacinate @ 47 ppm in layer diet, increased egg production by 1.6% (Piva *et al.,* 2003). Kroliczewska *et al.* (2005) evaluated the effect of Cr-enriched yeast supplementation on performance of broilers and suggested that supplementation of Cr either at 300 or 500µg/kg of diet did not affect feed conversion ratio up to 21 days but supplementation of 500µg Cr/kg significantly improved feed conversion ratio at 22-42 days of age. Further, feed conversion ratio of the entire trial (1-42 days of age) was reported higher in 500µg Cr/kg diet supplemented group in comparison to 300µg Cr/kg diet supplemented group and control diet.

Conclusion

Minerals form an important component of balanced diet and use of organic-based minerals (50% or 100%) in poultry diet improves number of total eggs and hatching eggs, fertility rate, total hatchability, hatchability of fertile eggs, progeny livability, body mass and carcass yield of offsprings. Birds more efficiently absorb, digest and utilize organic mineral complexes than inorganic form of minerals. Hence, lower concentrations of organic trace minerals can be used in poultry feeds. In addition, birds fed organic sources of essential trace minerals excrete lower amount in their faeces, so there is less environmental contamination.

References

AAFCO, 1998. Official publication of the Association of American Feed Control Officials incorporated (Ed. Paul. M. Bachman). pp. 237-238.

Abdallah, G., El-Hussein, O.M. and Abdel-Latif, K.O. 2009. Influence of Some Dietary Organic Mineral Supplementations on Broiler Performance. International Journal of Poultry Science, 8: 291-298.

Aoyagi, S. and Baker, D. 1993. Nutritional evaluation of copper-lysine and zinc-Iysinecomplexes for chicks. Poultry Science.72:165-171.

Bao, Y.M., Choct, M., Iji, P.A. and Bruerton, K. 2007. Effect of organically complexed copper, iron, manganese and zinc on broiler performance, mineral excretion and accumulation in tissues. Journal of Applied Poultry Research, 16: 448-455.

Brooks, M. A., Grimes, J. L., Lloyd, K. E., Valdez,F. and Spears, J. W. 2012. Relative bioavailabilityin chicks of manganese from manganese proteinate. Journal of Applied Poultry Research 21:126-130.

Brooks, M.A., Grimes, J. L., Lloyd, K. E., Verissimo, S. and Spears, J. W. 2013. Bioavailability in chicks of zinc from zinc proteinate.Journal of Applied Poultry Research 22:153-159.

Cao, J., Henry, P. R.,Guo, R., Holwerda, R.A., Toth J. P.,Littell R.C., Miles R. D. andAmmerman C. B. 2000. Chemical characteristics and relative bioavailability of supplemental organic zinc sources for poultry and ruminants. Journal of Animal Science, 78:2039–54.

Das, T.K., Mondal, M.K., Biswas, P., Bairagi, B. and Samanta, C.C. 2010. Influence of level of dietary inorganic and organic copper and energy level on the performance and nutrient utilization of broiler chickens. Asian-Australian Journal of Animal Science 23: 82-89.

Deo Chandra, Mandal, A.B. and Tyagi, Praveen K. 2018. Response of supplementary sources and levels of copper on the performance of broiler chickens. Animal Nutrition and Feed Technology. 18:89-96.

Fisinin, V. I., Papazyan, T. T. and Surai, P. F. 2008. Selenium in poultry nutrition. In: Vol. 1. pp. 221-261. Wageningen Academic Publishers, Wageningen, Netherlands. Current Advances in Se Research and Applications (Surai, P.F. and Taylor-Pickard, J. eds.). Vol. 1. pp. 221-261. Wageningen Academic Publishers, Wageningen, Netherlands.

Iqbal S., Deo, C., Mandal, A.B., Tyagi, P.K. and Awachat, V.B. 2011. Response of feeding different sources and concentrations of zinc and copper on performance of broiler chickens. Indian Journal of Poultry Science, 46(3):330-336.

Iqbal, S. 2010. Effect of supplementary sources and concentrations of zinc and copper on performance of broiler chickens.M.V.Sc. (Poultry Science) Thesis, IVRI Deemed University, Izatnagar, 243122 (UP).

Jegeda, A.V., Oduguwa, O.O., Oso, A.O., Fafiolu, A.O., Idowu, O.M.O. and Nollet, L. 2012. Growth performance, blood characteristics and plasma lipids of growing pullet fed dietary concentrations of organic and inorganic copper sources. Livestock Science, 145: 298-302.

Kroliczewska, B., Zawadzki, W., Skiba, T. and Mista, T. 2005. Effect of chromium supplementation on chickens broiler growth and carcass characteristics. Acta Vet Brno, 2005: 74:543–549.

Kumar, Y. 2007. Response of broiler chickens to dietary supplemental zinc levels and sources. M.V.Sc. (Poultry Science) thesis, IVRI Deemed University, Izatnagar, 243122 (UP).

Kumar, Y., Deo, C., Shrivastava, H.P., Mandal, A.B., Wadhwa, A. and Singh, I. 2013. Growth performance, carcass yield and immune competence of broiler chickens as influenced by dietary supplemental zinc sources and levels. Agriculture Research, 2(3):270-274.

Mohammed, H.H., El-Sayed, B.M., Abd El-Razik, W.M., Ali, M.A. and Abd El-Aziz, R.M. 2014. The Influence of Chromium Sources on Growth Performance, Economic Efficiency, Some Maintenance Behaviour, Blood Metabolites and Carcass Traits in Broiler Chickens. Global Veterinaria, 12 (5): 599-605.

Ohh, S.J. and Lee, J.Y. 2005. Dietary Chromium-methionine chelate supplementation and animal performance.Asian-Australasian Journal of Animal Sciences. 18(6): 898-907.

Ozkan, S., Basmacyoolu-Malayoolu, H., Yalcyn, S., Kardab, F., Kocturk, S., Cabuk, M., Oktay, O., Ozdemir, S., Ozdemir, E. and Ergul, M. 2007. Deitary vitamin E (α-tocopherol acetate) and selenium supplementation from different source; performance, ascites related parameters and antioxidant status in broiler reared at low and optimum temperatures. British Poultry Science.48:580-593.

Paik, I., Hankyu, L. and Park, S. 2009. Effect of organic iron supplementation on the performance and iron content in the egg yolk of laying hens. Journal of Poultry Science.46:198-202.

Park, S.W., Namkung, H., Ahn, H. J, and Paik, I. K. 2004. Production of iron enriched eggs of laying hens. Asian- Australasian journal of Animal Science.17:1725-1728.

Payne, R. L. and Southern, L. L. 2005. Changes in glutathione peroxidase and tissue selenium concentrations of broilers after consuming a diet adequate in selenium. Poultry Science, 84: 1268-1276.

Pekel, A.Y. and Alp, M. 2011. Effects of different dietary copper sources on laying hen performance and egg yolk cholesterol. The Journal of Applied Poultry Research 20: 506-513.

Pierce, J. L., Shafer, B. L., Power, R. and Dawson K. A. 2005. Nutritional means to lower trace mineral excretion from poultry without compromising performance. Poultry Science, 84 (Suppl. 1): 11.

Piva, A., Meola, E., Gatta, P.P., Biagi, G.C., Mordenti, A.L., Luchansky, J. B., Silva, S. andMordenti, A. 2003.The effect of dietary supplementation with trivalent chromium on production performance of laying hens and the chromium content in the yolk. Animal Feed Science and Technology, 106: 149-163.

Stanley, V. G., Shanklyn, P., Deley, M., Gray, C., Vaughan, V., Hinton, A. Jr and Hume, M. 2012. Effects of organic selenium and zinc on the aging process of laying hens. Agrotechnology 1: 103, doi:10.4172/2168-9881.1000103.

Surai, P. F. 2006. Selenium in Nutrition and Health. Nottingham University Press, Nottingham.

Surai, P. F. and Fisinin, V. I. 2014. Selenium in poultry breeder nutrition: An update. Animal Feed Science and Technology, 191: 1-15.

Swiatkiewicz, S. and Koreleski, J. 2008. Effect of zinc and manganese source in the diet for laying hens on eggshell and bones quality.VeterinarniMedicina 53: 555-563.

Varun, A., Karthikeyan, N., Muthusamy, P., Raja, A., Wilfred Ruban, S. 2017. Real time PCR based expression of Metallothionein and evaluation of Zn bioavailability in chickens fed zinc oxide and zinc methionine. International Journal of Current Microbiology Applied Science, 6(7): 845- 849.

Wedekind, K. J. and Baker, D. H. 1990. Zinc bioavailability in feedgrade sources of zinc.Journal of Animal Science, 68: 684–89.

Yildiz, A.O., Cufadar, Y. and Olgun, O. 2011. Effects of dietary organic and inorganic manganese supplementation on performance, egg quality and bone mineralisation in laying hens. Revue de MedecineVeterinaire, 162: 482-488.

4

Application of Biotechnology in Poultry Nutrition

Jaydip R. and Monika M.

ICAR - Central Avian Research Institute, Bareilly, Uttar Pradesh

Introduction

Conventional practises of raising livestock had been practised for several years on a worldwide basis to satisfy the protein needs. Increasing human population, income growth and increase of urbanization, pressurizes serious demand on the quantity and attribute of livestock products. The feed stuffs such as maize, soya, groundnut, etc. used in livestock especially for poultry possesses a great competition for human food. This limited feed resources compelled to intensify the expense of poultry feeds and also the production cost (Ravindran & Blair, 1991). In order to equalize both the poultry business growth accompanied with shortage of raw ingredients scientists and researchers are forced to explore an alternative. Application of unconventional feed stuffs also not much practically possible as most of them contain anti-nutritional factors, which impose a great disadvantage in their complete utilization. Under these circumstances, a substitute should be sought in poultry nutrition and feed improvement to combat the present and future hindrances in the sector. To substantiate the longer production with the existing demand of raw materials, a new intensive technology including biotechnology can be implemented as an alternative. Presently, biotechnology has ability to dispense with wide-scope for improved productivity for livestock which facilitates the path to alleviate poverty, provides nutritious food with security and also plays a great contribution in the sustainable use of natural resources (Bimrew *et al.,* 2014). Furtherance, in feed technology using biotechnological appliances leads to produce protected forms of proteins, amino acids and fats, so that respective nutrients can be targeted perfectly. Various enzymes, prebiotics and probiotics can be attuned to strengthen the plane of nutrition by proper utilization of nutrients from the feed to inhibit the enteric pathogenic bacteria. Using biotechnology, hybrid varieties of plants and fodders were developed with less or no anti-nutritional factors, ensuring food safety also. Further, biotechnology also improves nutrition aspects of feed, livestock health and also reduces the environmental waste. Improving productivity can be predominantly due to enhanced digestibility or nutrient amenability from feeds or selective breeding for feed efficiency. Biotechnology is a generally defined term that encompasses a wide range of different techniques which turn raw material into something nutritious or sustainable (Bayer *et al.,* 2005). With this background the emphasis of this chapter is to emphasize on the applicability of biotechnological concepts in poultry to derive a potential output in production.

Biotechnology: General Aspects

With the intention of strengthening the efficiency of production to feed an expanding human population the new science of biotechnology has been explored by many people. The phrase biotechnology is acquired from two Greek text: "Bios"- meaning "*life*", living being or organic nature and "Technologia"-meaning "*systematic approach*". In accordance with Convention on Biological Diversity, biotechnology means: *"any technological application that uses biological systems,* dwelling *organisms or derivatives, to construct or alter products or processes for certain purposes."* Scope of biotechnology application in poultry production are often considered as biological, chemical and physical techniques that influences poultry's health, nutrition, breeding and reproduction (Ben Salem *et al.,* 2017). The enforcement of biotechnological methods for poultry will help to achieve socio-economic goals rapidly especially doubling the farmer's income. This could be pursued by utilising vast scope of opportunities to boost the poultry production through increased growth factor, carcass quality and reproduction, improved nutrition and feed utilization. Biotechnology can strengthen the soundness of poultry feed, health promotion and welfare of birds, and reduced waste through more efficient utilization of resources. In this book chapter, we will now discuss implementation of biotechnology in different aspect of poultry nutrition.

1. **Postbiotics:** Due to awareness of consumers antibiotics arbitrary use raised the concern of antibiotic vestiges in the poultry derivatives such as meat and eggs (Shareef *et al.*, 2009). Also, it leads to emergence of antibiotic-resistant among bacterial populations (Shazali *et al.,* 2014), causing detrimental effect on the well-being of poultry and humans (Ajuwon, 2015). By reviewing the above demerits, approaches on natural alternatives are gaining focus with the safe and pathogen-free food products. One such option is probiotics. Probiotics are a desirable bacterium that proliferate actively and competes with pathogenic microorganisms for nutrients in the host digestive system (Cheng *et al.,* 2019). These probiotics act as an antagonist to pathogens by increasing challenge for nutrients or by secretion of antimicrobial substances against pathogens (Mousavi Khaneghah *et al.,*

2020). Despite their proven benefits, still worries about their biosafety aspects; ease of microbial production, handling and storage; route of probiotic administration; stability; and survival of the probiotic in the host and tolerance for bile are there. Moreover, these probiotic microorganisms may alter the physicochemical, microbiological, and tactile characteristics of the inoculated food. *The antimicrobial substances produced by probiotic bacteria are called as postbiotics*. Postbiotics are extremely safer and it also decreases the pathogen's growth in the food with the augmentation of improving health status of consumers. Postbiotics are the substances or metabolites of probiotic organisms, produced when they die which tends to have great impact on host health.

The word 'postbiotics' is now acquainted to bioactive compounds, and the view of postbiotics can be broadened to (a) soluble bioactive factors (metabolic products) developed during the growth and fermentation of food grade microorganisms in complex microbiological cultures (cell-free supernatants [CFS]), foods or intestines that have certain positive effect to the food or host (b) cell compounds, and (c) substances produced by the sequel of microorganism on food ingredients (e.g., bioactive peptides), whereas the term para-probiotics (ghost probiotics) is characterised as intact or ruptured nonviable and inactivated cells from beneficial microorganisms (Aguilar Toala *et al.,* 2018; Barros *et al.,* 2020). Postbiotics extracted from probiotics contain several bioactive metabolites such as organic compounds, short-chain fatty acids, sugars, antimicrobial peptides, enzymes, vitamins, cofactors, immune-signalling compounds, and complex agents (Rajakovich & Balskus, 2019). Solution called CFS containing biological substances developed by target microorganisms and used as postbiotics in almost every food safety-related research. Several strains of probiotics can be considered and their postbiotic substances recurrently show similar or corresponding beneficial impacts to the consumers (Aguilar-Toala *et al.,* 2018). Postbiotics reduce risks closely linked with the handling of live microorganisms without compromising probiotic effects on living cells. In comparison to probiotics, in the context of handling and storage, metabolites are relatively more robust and are outrageous will never transfer antimicrobial resistance traits to other bacteria. Postbiotics also have advantage by virtue of being clear in chemical structure, safety dose parameters and longer storage life which can influence the physiological function of host (Shenderov, 2013). Postbiotic metabolites of probiotics will be collected as per the standard biotechnology method portrayed by Kareem *et al*. (2016). Then in vitro characterization of postbiotics such as pH, mineral profile, free radical scavenging activity, antimicrobial activity, anti-inflammatory potential & biochemical activity of the postbiotics is done. A study has been conducted at Central Avian Research Institute by Beulah *et al.,* 2021, isolated postbiotics from *Lactobacillus planatarum*, found better production performance to the birds fed with postbiotics than pro and antibiotics supplemented groups.

2. **Nucleotides in Poultry Nutrition:** The term "alternative chicken" is gaining attention now a day's implies that the chicken has been raised with the diet free from antibiotic growth promotors, anti-coccidials and other feed stuff inclusions. But, these birds have to compromise on their performance, nutrient uptake and are easily susceptible to enteric disease-causing pathogens. With an eye to counterbalance these losses, alternatives have to be considered. Nucleotide supplementation serves as an excellent alternative (Swiatkiewicz *et al.,* 2013). Nucleotides are the core units of nucleic acid (DNA & RNA). This structure comprised of combination of sugar, ribose or deoxyribose, a nitrogenous base such as purine or a pyrimidine and with one or more phosphate group. These nucleotides are synthesised in the cell by pathways such as de novo pathway (from amino acid precursors such as glutamine, formate, glycine and aspartic acid). They are further recycled via salvage pathway (breakdown of nucleic acids, nucleosides are reutilized for biosynthesis of nucleotides). Nucleotides play as a pioneer of nucleic acids, source of energy for cells, acts as a component for various coenzymes, mediate hormonal action and also connected with the amalgamation of DNA and RNA (Dina kruger et al., 2018). Nucleotides exert its great action on intestinal cell development, maintains cell integrity, increase intestinal villi length, promoting better nutrition absorption, reinforce the immune condition of the broilers thereby improving the overall broiler quality performance. Nucleotides are also very important for growth, reproduction, nutrition of the broiler birds. It aids faster recovery of birds from injuries, improve disease challenges, also acts on the enterocytes where it exerts in action on the intestinal development, maturation and repair from damage caused due to stress (high stocking density with dirty litter) and pathogens. Beneficial impact of nucleotide supplementation can be visualized in the challenging conditions such as infectious condition, stress or challenge due to environmental change. Various findings (Jung & Batal, 2012; Wu *et al.,* 2108) supported the positive effect of nucleotides on the broiler diet by increasing body weight with better FCR, increasing villus height in duodenum.

   Frankic *et al.,* 2006, suggested that nucleotides can repair the DNA damage that occurred in the immune cells when fed with the mycotoxin challenge.

Nucleotide supplementation in poultry is expected to strengthen the immune system (Boza & Martinez Augustin, 2002). In poultry, nucleotide inclusion in the basal diet has also been shown to shoot-up the immune response of broilers by boosting leukocyte and macrophage activity (Dil & Qureshi, 2002). Studies also proved that bird's mortality was decreased by approximately 30 per cent under stressful conditions upon nucleotides feeding (Rutz *et al.,* 2008). Frankic *et al.,*2006, have revealed that mycotoxin-challenged chickens are healed by feeding nucleotides. This could be by virtue of nucleotides that help to repair DNA damage caused by mycotoxin in immune cells.

3. **Nanotechnology in poultry:** Nutrition is a significant portion (around 60–65 per cent) of poultry inputs. Nanotechnology could be an exciting emerging technology with a great capacity to revolutionize India's agriculture and livestock market, and throughout the globe. Nanotech is a novel technology which creates materials and changes structure, enhances quality and texture of foodstuffs at the molecular level and includes a major effect on production, processing, transportation, storage, safety and security of food along with to meet up the necessitate ever-increasing demand for feed to some extent due successful interventions in feed technology. Nano-feed additives can help boost feed performance, reduce feed costs and raise the yield and quality of poultry-based products. Nano form of supplementation magnifies the effective surface which intensifies the absorption and therefore the use of minerals which prevails to a diminution in the considerable quantity of supplements addition and eventually to a reduction in feed costs and increase the yield and attribute of products made from poultry (Rokade *et al.,* 2020). Nano-feed additives and novel detoxifying nano-materials are expected to bring value in feeding strategies owing to their positive influence on efficiency in intensive poultry production.

   Nano is a Latin word meaning little old man or dwarf and in 1952, Nobel laureate of physics Richard Feynman gave the idea of nanotechnology a first in southern California. In 1980 Eric Drexler made nanotechnology popular in the true sense of the term. Particles measuring between 1 and 100 nano meters in diameter are known as nano particles. The term "nano" relates to a milliards of a meter (10^{-9} m), or one millionth of a millimetre. This not only reinforces poultry immunity, resistance to oxidation, and growth, together with reduced antimicrobial substance use and manure odour, which is conducive to improving environment. Nanotechnology could also be accustomed to protect the environment through the use of replacement (evincible) energy supplies and filters or accelerant to reduce pollution and to clean up existing pollutants that have indirect bearings for human food or feed supplies. "It is also possible to use nanotechnology to widen the nutritional value of a food by increasing biological accessibility of certain nutrients." In addition to high bioavailability and biodegradability properties it offers a scientific advantage with its rapid and specific moves. Nano trace metals can enter the poultry body by direct penetration; its consumption rate is therefore of much excellency than that of common inorganic trace metals. Many researches display that the utilization coefficient of the inorganic trace element was around 30 percent, while the utilization coefficient of the nano trace element was nearly 100 percent (Rokade *et al.,* 2020). All of these benefits have significant effects on farm poultry production and also economic losses, as well as healthier food and feed production. The facility to produce and manipulate nanoscale matter has created opportunities for new directions and with unprecedented accuracy to interact with biology. Recently trace minerals are used successfully in the diets of poultry in the mould of nanoparticles to meet the mineral requirements. From a different perspective, feeding such antibiotics at low levels in poultry for a sustained period of time is normal practice in the poultry industry to increase feed efficiency for birds. Yet, recently, attributable to the potential growth of antibiotic-resistant bacteria and their residues in poultry processing, an in-feed antibiotic has been banned. Nano type of supplementation improves the surface area which could potentially increase the uptake and thus the use of minerals leading to a drop in the lots of nutrients and eventually a decrease in feed costs. The growing concern about the possible contribution of phosphorus in poultry excreta to surface water eutrophication has led to increased pressure to limit the abundance of excess phosphorus in poultry ration, thereby reducing the phosphorous faecal production. Mineral nanoparticles, especially in large-scale poultry farming, will be profitable in curtailing the voiding of unused minerals which reduce the environment. Mineral nanoparticles can significantly minimize the excretion of leftover minerals, particularly for large commercial poultry, to mitigate environmental damage. Because, of their incredibly small size and unique physical properties the nanoparticles are considerably different from their standard forms. The physiological routes of nutrient delivery and transport between tissue and cell membranes can be bypassed by nanoparticles. Nanotechnology is increasingly being applied in the domain of veterinary medicine and poultry production, and various compounds are being used as supplementary sources of trace minerals (Na_2O, MgO, Al_2O_3, SiO_2, K_2O, CaO, TiO_2, and Fe_2O_3) in diets. Furthermore, applicability of nanotech in poultry has shown improvement in immunity, resistance to oxidation and growth, and reduced use of antibiotics and manure odour, ultimately improving the environment (Rokade *et al.,* 2019). Due to the enforcing of agents with several ways of antibacterial action, bacteria's resistance to traditional antibiotics can be reduced by using nanotechnologies.

4. **Nutrigenomics in poultry:** Nutrigenomics helps to analyze the genomic influence of nutrition on animals/birds. It can be executed by measuring the alterations in gene activity that occurs due to modifications in diet. Nutrigenomics guides in profound understanding of importance of nutrition on bird's health, performance and production (Swiatkiewicz *et al*., 2014). It indirectly explains us all the biological changes that prevail in the cell, in response to modification made in the diet. The nutrients which are added in the diet produces a dietary signal in the cell which can be detected by cellular sensors. These dietary signals greatly influence gene and protein expressions via metabolite productions. The key components and other biologically active food constituents in the body has a central role in gene expression profile patterns (Swiatkiewicz *et al.,* 2014). The quantam of gene expression, protein expression and metabolite productions occur because of dietary nutrients can be examined in the body cells, tissues and organisms as dietary signatures. Dietary signatures impart brief idea about the dietary nutrients changes and its impact in the body homeostasis (Benitez and Ovilo, 2017). Sometimes gene chips, can also be used to ascertain the effects of certain dietary supplements and its role in transforming the gene interaction in the body. By knowing the target genes, we can manipulate the gene action which results in promotion of favourable genes and simultaneously suppression of bad ones.

Nutrigenomics, how would it function? Nutrigenomics is nothing but the amalgamation of various sciences with the intention of perceiving the impact of nutrients on the body's physiological reactions. In nutrigenomics, nutrients are stimuli to particular cells in the body, the cell responds by transmitting biochemical information from DNA or genes (the science of genomics) to RNA (the science of transcriptomics) while interpreting the information of such a nutrient, which is then converted into specific proteins (the science of proteomics) and eventually decides metabolic pathways (the science of meta-transcriptomics) (Moody, 2001). The flow of information in this series depends upon all biological processes. While these processes are governed by the basic genetic make-up, these pathways may be influenced by external determinants such as disease threats, environmental contaminants or particular nutrients. Nutrigenomics is the basis of the better perception of the genome of human beings and animals. Although facilities have been available for several years to appraise the expression of individual genes, only the invention of gene chips (DNA microarrays) has allowed researchers to measure the expression of stacks of genes simultaneously. Gene chips are merely a series of thousands of particular DNA sequence microscopic spots. Researchers may extract relevant messenger RNA (mRNA) derived from tissue at any point, rather than assessing the significantly impact of a particular nutrient on animal's output or the physiological response at the end of the analysis. The quantity of mRNA present pertains to the relative quantity of identified gene copies, calculated using gene chips. Using contrasting colour labels, determination of gene regulations such as up-regulated, down-regulated or unaffected as a consequence of a particular dietary modification, it can be made possible (Jung & Batal, 2012).

Nutrigenomics forms the basis of contour of all the genes and its action. It helps in careful selection of nutrients for fine tune genes and DNA present in every cell and every tissue of the animal. This molecular technology allows for the rapid evaluation and precision of nutritional strategies in poultry industry. It guides us how using nutrition in order to get the best outcome from our animals/birds, what nutrients can be used or what combination will be best? Or how long duration the nutrients can be given? to get better efficacy, production performance with better health. It pays a great way for researchers to concentrate on the nutritional aspects of both humans and poultry.

a) *Nutrigenomics in early life*: Studies showed that nutrigenomics study is greatly important in the neonatal and early life period. Nutrigenomics could perhaps help us to better interpret how nutrition programs work by exposing changes in gene expression linked to early-life nutrition. For example, for the first 96 hr post-hatch, feeding 100% of the NRC (normal) suggested for trace elements shown beneficial effects on gene expression, including after birds have changed into low mineral diets (20% of NRC recommendations) (Brennan *et al.,* 2013a). In this study, elevated concentrations of minerals fed during the post-hatch period have been shown to significantly boost cycline D1 (gene expression), a biological function vital for the cell cycle regulation, development and repair of the intestinal lumen. In adult birds receiving a normal diet after hatching, there were upregulation of nutrients both actively and passively in the intestines, leaded by expression of family of transporters i,e., solute carrier proteins. But, there was no influence on performance results in the analysis (Brennan *et al.,* 2013). However, considering the importance of proper intestinal function and health, these changes are considered beneficial. Overall, this research has shown that post-hatch feeding can shift long-term patterns of gene expression that can have long-life effects on bird health.

b) *Nutrigenomics in Gut health:* Gut health care is very important in poultry for proper feed digestion and assimilation of nutrients from the feed. Promoting proper GI function aids, optimal health and growth of the birds. At GI tract there are various commensal organisms or microbes, Nutrigenomics assist us to comprehend how nutrients influences intestinal health through interaction with gut cells and microbiota in the intestine. Microgenomics – molecular technology in which advanced DNA sequencing of intestinal gut can be done to study the GIT microbial community. A study conducted by Gopi *et al.,* 2020, in CARI indicated that nucleotide supplemented community birds showed greater improvement in efficiency, due to the increase in villi height by the effect of nucleotides in yeast extract. This improves nutrient digestibility capacity as the absorptive surface area is increased.

c) *Nutrigenomics in Broilers:* Due to rapidly increasing live weight of present broilers, optimization of proper diet/feed is very important. Nutrigenomics can be included in broilers diet which can aid to improve poultry production like correlating nutrition, genetics in breeding programs, helps to improve bird performance, better FCR, better health and meat quality. Recently, Jiang *et al.* (2014) stated in his study that nicotinic acid plays a major role in lipid metabolism in two broiler strains of female chicken. The results of the experiments discloses that presence of nicotinic acid in feed at varying extents regulates the expression of hepatic genes A-I (ApoA-I) and Apolipoprotein B (Apo B) accordingly. In addition to bioactive ingredients, a series of micronutrients and vitamins are also recognised as health factors. Vitamin E is also a transcriptional regulator of the lipid oxidation genes in broiler chicken and antioxidant genes which lower stress and improve the quality of meat. Analysis of data from Nutrigenomics also expressed that when chicken fed with diet containing algae can mitigate the anxiety in chicken through nutrigenomics. Similarly, the transporter genes of broiler chicken can also be activated by the availability of various mineral's especially zinc, and the phenomenon of gene expression are directly linked to the portion of zinc present in feed. While selenium acts as a key gender-specific control regulator for poultry. Nutrigenomic results combined with performance data in whole-animal studies (e.g., weight gain, egg production) assist us to conclude the effect of nutrients on animals and on their production. Nutrigenomics offers the opportunity to accurately identify the nutrients or nutrient combinations that are suitable and to achieve optimum value. With the assistance of Nutrigenomics, we envisaged enhanced poultry economics derived from optimized feeding approaches that lead to better feeding efficiency and bird's health.

5. **Metagenomics application in poultry:** The systematic profiling of microbial community in chicken gut is very important. Microbiota in GI tract performs a paramount role in the digestibility of feed and uptake of nutrients, indirectly plays a major function in promoting health and defence mechanism of chicken. Clear apprehensive idea regarding microbiota is necessary with regards to type, number of micro-organisms in the gut, as gut composition differs from one bird to the other. The conventional techniques (e.g. Culture based techniques) will be more biased and fails to describe the complete characterization and properties of microbes. So, a holistic approach such as Metagenomics or Microbial ecogenomics can be carried out to study the ecological/biogeochemical role of microbes in unique habitats. Meta-genomics is a Greek word, "meta" means transcendent (combo of separate analysis); "genomics refers to the study of genome. The word metagenomics first introduced by Jo Handelsman, Jon clarly, Robert M Goodman in 1998. Metagenomics is the study of genetic makeup retrieved from environmentally related sample directly without the requirement of cultivating invitro. It can be put forward as the envisioning genetic materials from host associated microbiota to identify the microbial diversity and function (Banik and Brady, 2008). Metagenomics facilitates the evaluation and utilization of the taxonomic and metabolic diversity of microbial communities at ecosystem-level. Poultry gut contains millions of diverse microorganisms. Most of these microbes are underexplored and constitute an immense pool of genetic and metabolic diversity that has not been addressed. Metagenomic study is basically of two types: Sequence based approach involving the filtering of clones from direct isolation of DNA from a particular environment using the 16s rRNA gene which is the highly conserved bacterial gene acts as phylogenetic anchor for sequencing the entire microbiota (Hoff *et al.*, 2008). This type of study offers us to identify and establish the abundance and diversity of microbial species in a specific sample. On contrary the Functional based approach screens for a specific trait or phenotype like enzyme activity, heat or stress tolerance followed by the identification of phylogenetic origin (Dinsdale *et al.,* 2008). Recent advancements in the gene sequencing using technologies and Next Generation Sequencing resulted in the genesis of large data sets of varied microenvironments even including the gastrointestinal tract of many species. The GIT of bird is like a metabolism system for nutrients.

6. **Role of microbiota in nutrient metabolism in chicken**

a) *Polysaccharide metabolism:* The major portion of polysaccharide metabolism carried out at paired caeca of poultry (Stanley *et al.*, 2014), but chicken do not have a complete metabolic pattern to process and produce readily available forms of polysaccharides. Study conducted by Sergeant *et al.*, 2014 reported that 20% of the genes in the chicken GIT microflora metagenome were lacking the key enzymes such as carbohydrate esterase, polysaccharide lyase, and glycoside hydrolase. In addition to that, proteins associated with carbohydrate metabolism were most frequently identified in the chicken GIT microbiota metaproteomic study (Tang *et al.*, 2014). The significant association was observed between metagenomic and metaproteomic analysis done by Tang *et al.*, 2014 at chicken microbiome composition and protein expression.

b) *Nitrogen Metabolism:* Results obtained via subsystems-based annotations (SEED) database, conducted by Qu *et al.*, 2008 explained that genes in intestinal microbiota of poultry explores nine percent of protein & amino acid metabolism and one percent nitrogen as nutrient derivations. When, chicken GIT microbiota undergoes metabolising nitrogen sources, results in the degradation and biosynthesis of peptides. The amino acids which ever synthesised by the microbes will be absorbed by the birds as effective protein utilization. Nearly half of the nitrogen sources were processed into ammonia, which was eventually released into the atmosphere and this excretion has significant impact on the chicken's health. This adverse protein fermentation also produces biogenic amines, nitrogenous toxins which can trigger inflammation, increase stress and ultimately affects the welfare of the birds.

c) *Fatty acids and lipid metabolism:* The metabolism of NSPs (commonly present in grains) by microbes such as Firmicutes, Bacteroides, and Proteobacteria were usually detectable in the chicken ceca, produces SCFA. Clostridiales is the major contributor of SCFA metabolism. These SCFA play a vital role in reducing pH so that growth of acid-sensitive pathogens will be inhibited. It also promotes growth of epithelial cells and mineral absorption in the host (Sergeant e*t al.*, 2014). In the whole intestine metagenomic study, conducted by Qu *et al.*, 2008, there exists only 1% to 2% gene associated with fatty acid and lipid metabolism. The experiment performed by Yeoman *et al.*, 2012, explained that when polyunsaturated linoleic acid undergoes metabolism process results in the release of a by-product such as Conjugated linoleic acid (CLA), which affects the yolk quality leading to embryonic death.

Through culture-independent metagenomic research, increased awareness of the chicken GIT microbiome has focused on understanding the complexity of microbial populations and their importance in chicken metabolism and health. In order to ascertain better quantity and quality of productivity, more

GIT microbiota studies will analyze and identify the role of the microbe in modulating poultry production under different environmental conditions, such as nutrients, stress and welfare. Identification and monitorization of key genes concerned with metabolism and health of the birds using metagenomic data of chicken GIT microbiota finds a new pathway to tackle the deficiencies and improve the performance. It also gives an idea of introducing beneficial or low pathogenic organisms which possess genes for better nutrient digestibility. Furthermore, the metagenomic techniques combined with bioinformatic tools has to be done for the sound analysis of gut microbiota of chicken.

7. **Genetically modified (GM) crops:** The main aim of production of genetically modified crops is to enhance the nutritional properties of the crops, minimise the presence of anti-nutritional factors, adjustment of desirable substances in the crops are positive concern. eg In GM crops fortification of essential elements such as amino acid groups, dietary fatty acids with decreased number of harmful compounds such as phytate in seeds. Due to this advantage, the utility of GM crops as feed materials to poultry adds great positive impact on production. Mutagenic plants have been designed to reduce the phytate concentration. Mutant cross-breed corn type such as high available phosphorus maize variety, developed using LPA1 gene shown reduced phytic acid in the seeds. The advantage of this variety leads to decreased requirement of dicalcium phosphate supplementation in comparison to conventional maize, with no compromise on laying performance (Ceylan *et al.,* 2003). It also displayed higher clutch period, egg weight, feed consumption and also feed efficiency. Study performed by Snow *et al*., 2003 showed that bird's fed with HAP (High Availability Phosphorus) diet excreted very less total phosphorus content compared to control birds in both broilers and layers. Similarly, mutation made in the legume crop such as soybean (high level of phytase) leads to the development of low-phytate soybean meal (LPSBM) enclosed 0.13-0.16% phytate P, as contrary to the 0.34-0.37% in traditional soybean meal (Powers *et al*., 2006). Broilers supplied with LPSBM displayed greater phosphorus bioavailability than the conventional Soya bean Meal. Likewise, when diet having LPSBM fed to duck, digestibility of both energy and amino acids were greater than the conventional SBM. Nyannor and Adeola, 2008 found that when genetically modified maize with the assertion of Escherichia coli-derived phytase gene fed to broiler birds, birds exhibited superior weight gain, feed conversion ratio also increases the dry matter, P, Ca and N retention. When birds with solely grains, in such as the requirement of amino acid may be failed to achieve especially amino acid such as lysine, methionine should be considered.

Using genetic engineering fortification of in-dispensable amino acids to the crops can be done so that additional supply of those amino acids is not mandatory. By inserting the cordapA gene from *Corynobacterium glutamicum*, a popular soil bacterium, into the maize genome, genetically modified high lysine maize (LY038) variety was created (Lucas *et al.*, 2007). The transgenic enzyme reflection in LY038 maize can be substantiated by the intensified performance and accumulation of free available lysine in the germ. A protein rich soybean containing significantly more crude protein and essential amino acids compared to traditional soybeans was developed through genetic engineering methods. Edwards et al. (2000) in an experiment, investigated the nutritive benefits of meals extracted from GM high protein soybeans performed on caecectomized cockerels. The results showed that the meal derived from GM soybeans, which included more digestible Lys, Met, Thre and Val, as shown in the balance trial, had a higher metabolizable energy level than traditional soybean meal.

In oilseed plants, comprehensive research of modifying the constituents of oilseed plants to accomplish an increased concentration of nutritionally high-value, long-chain polyunsaturated fatty acids n-3 (LC PUFA n-3) and, more laterly, genes encoding microbial desaturases and elongase enzymes have been investigated systematically (Truksa *et al.,* 2009; Venegas-Caleron et al., 2010). Enhancing the amount of stearidonic acids (SDA, C18:4, n-3), eicosapentaenoic acids (EPA, C20:5 n-3) and docosahexaenoic acids was the primary purpose of this transgenesis (DHA, C22:5 n-3). In a myriad of health aspects, the LC PUFA n-3 plays a vital role while still being inadequate in the human nutrition. A high content of β-glucan and low concentration of metabolizable energy mean that barley is less likely to be employed in poultry diet feed component. The results of a study conducted on chickens showed that when added to a barley-based diet, the malt of GM barley exhibiting a thermo-tolerant Bacillus β-glucanase appreciably minimized the quantity of sticky excreta and obtained an average daily gain analogous to that of maize-based diets. By embedding transgenes expressing human lactoferrin (LF) and lysozyme (LZ) into the grain, rice was genetically modified. These are active compounds whose properties are antimicrobial and immune-stimulating. In chickens, two experiments were performed to valuate the effectiveness of GM LF or LZ rice as a replacement for antibiotics in poultry diets (Humphrey *et al.,* 2002). The birds fed a diet with 5 percent LF + 10 percent LZ rice had a much better FCR and thinner lamina propria in the small intestine in the first experiment than those fed with 20 percent traditional rice. Chicks fed a diet with 10 percent LZ + or 5 percent LF + 10 percent LZ rice in the second study had a considerably lower food consumption and a significantly better feed efficiency than those fed with 15 percent regular rice. It was shown that the influence of GM rice was similar to that of the antibiotics operated in the study, namely bacitracin + roxarsone, because both the diet containing GM rice and the diet incorporating antibiotics enhanced the villus height in the duodenum compared to the controls, decreased the widths of the GI tract lamina propria and dropped significantly the number of leukocytes (Humphrey *et al.,* 2002). These results highlighted the prospects of GM LF and LZ rice in broiler diets as a replacement for antibiotics (Humphrey *et al.,* 2002)

Conclusion

Conventional nutritional practices needs to be changed because of increasing human population, urbanization, shrinking land with ever increasing demand of poultry products. Also, there are challenges of environment friendly sustainable farm practices. Therefore, to substantiate the longer production a new intensive biotechnology application should be explored. All the above technologies mentioned in this chapter will very well address the issues of poultry nutrition and also it will help in enhancing overall welfare and production of poultry.

References

Aguilar-Toalá, J. E., Garcia-Varela, R., Garcia, H. S., Mata-Haro, V., González-Córdova, A. F., Vallejo-Cordoba, B., & Hernández-Mendoza, A. 2018. Postbiotics: An evolving term within the functional foods field. Trends in Food Science andTechnology, **75**: 105–114.

Ajuwon, K.M. 2015. Toward a better understanding of mechanisms of probiotics and prebiotics action in poultry species. Journal of Applied Poultry Research. 25(2): 277-283.

Banik, J.J. and Brady, S.F. 2010. Recent application of metagenomic approaches toward the discovery of antimicrobials and other bioactive small molecules. Current Opinion in Microbiology, 13(5): 603-609.

Barros, C. P., Guimarães, J. T., Esmerino, E. A., Duarte, M. C. K. H., Silva, M. C., Silva, R., Cruz, A. G. 2020. Paraprobiotics and postbiotics: Concepts and potential applications in dairy products. Current Opinion in Food Science, 32: 1–8.

Bayer, T. S. and Smolke, C. D. 2005. Programmable ligand-controlled ribo regulators of eukaryotic gene expression. Nature biotechnology, 23(3): 337-343.

Rakia Ben Salem Mohamed, Abbassi, Vanesa García, Raquel García-Fierro, Javier Fernández, Hajer KilaniIlmen, Jaouani Monia, Khayeche, Lilia Messadi, María R. Rodici. 2017. Antimicrobial drug resistance and genetic properties of Salmonella enterica serotype Enteritidis circulating in chicken farms in Tunisia. Journal of Infection and Public Health, 10: 855-860.

Benítez, R., Núñez, Y. and Óvilo, C. 2017. Nutrigenomics in farm animals. J Invest Genomics, 4, p.1.

Bimrew, A. and Yeshambel, M. 2014. Exogenous enzymes in nutrient digestion and health of non-ruminant: Carbohydrases enzyme.

Boza, J.J. and Martinez-Augustin, O. 2002. Role and function of nucleotides in infant nutrition. In Nestle Nutrition Workshop Series (Vol. 47, pp. 165-184).

Brennan, K. M., R. S. Samuel, D. E. Graugnard, T. Ao, R. Xiao,A. H. Cantor, and A. J. Pescatore. 2013. Organic Trace minerallevels in the first 96-h post-hatch impact growth performance andintestinal gene expression in broiler chicks. Biol Trace Elem Res.156: 166–174.

Cheng, D., Song, J., Xie, M. and Song, D. 2019. The bidirectional relationship between host physiology and microbiota and health benefits of probiotics: A review. Trends in Food Science and Technology, 91: 426-435.

Dil, N. and Qureshi, M.A. 2002. Different expression of inducible nitric oxide synthethase is associated with differential toll-like receptor-4 expression in chicken macrophages from difference genetic backgrounds. Veterinary Immunology and Immunopathology, 84: 191-207

Dinsdale, E.A., Edwards, R.A., Hall, D., Angly, F., Breitbart, M., Brulc, J.M., Furlan, M., Desnues, C., Haynes, M., Li, L. and McDaniel, L. 2008. Functional metagenomic profiling of nine biomes. Nature, 452(7187): 629-632.

Frankiè, T., Pajk, T., Rezar, V., Levart, A. and Salobir, J. 2006. The role of dietary nucleotides in reduction of DNA damage induced by T-2 toxin and deoxynivalenol in chicken leukocytes. Food and chemical toxicology, 44(11): 1838-1844.

Hoff, K.J., Tech, M., Lingner, T., Daniel, R., Morgenstern, B. and Meinicke, P. 2008. Gene prediction in metagenomic fragments: a large scale machine learning approach. BMC Bioinformatics, 9(1): 1-14.

Humphrey, B.D., Huang, N. and Klasing, K.C. 2002. Rice expressing lactoferrin and lysozyme has antibiotic-like properties when fed to chicks. Journal of Nutrition, 132(6): 1214-1218.

Jiang, RR, Zhao GP, Zhao JP, Chen JL, Zheng MQ, Liu RR and Wen J. 2014. Influence of dietary nicotinic acid supplementation on lipid metabolism and related gene expression in two distinct broiler breeds of female chickens. Journal of Animal Physiology and Animal Nutrition, 98: 822-829.

Jung, B. and Batal, A.B. 2012. Effect of dietary nucleotide supplementation on performance and development of the gastrointestinal tract of broilers. British Poultry Science, 53(1): 98-105.

Jung, B. and Batal, A.B. 2012. Effect of dietary nucleotide supplementation on performance and development of the gastrointestinal tract of broilers. British Poultry Science, 53(1): 98-105.

Kareem, K.Y., Loh, T.C., Foo, H.L., Asmara, S.A. and Akit, H. 2017. Influence of postbiotic RG14 and inulin combination on cecal microbiota, organic acid concentration, and cytokine expression in broiler chickens. Poultry Science, 96(4): 966-975.

Kruger, D. and Werf, M.V.D. 2018. Benefits of nucleotide supplementation in poultry. Ohly Application Note, pp.1-3.

Lucas, D.M., Taylor, M.L., Hartnell, G.F., Nemeth, M.A., Glenn, K.C. and Davis, S.W., 2007. Broiler performance and carcass characteristics when fed diets containing lysine maize (LY038 or LY038× MON 810), control, or conventional reference maize. Poultry Science, 86(10): 2152-2161.

Moody, J.D., Freeman, J.P., Doerge, D.R. and Ceriglia, C.E. 2001. Degradation of phenanthrene and anthracene by cell suspensions of Mycobacterium sp. strain PYR-1. Applied Environmental Microbiology, 67(4): 1476–1483.

Khaneghah, A.M., Abhari, K., E°, I., Soares, M.B., Oliveira, R.B., Hosseini, H., Rezaei, M., Balthazar, C.F., Silva, R., Cruz, A.G. and Ranadheera, C.S. 2020. Interactions between probiotics and pathogenic microorganisms in hosts and foods: A review. Trends in Food Science and Technology, 95: 205-218.

Perry, J.N. 2003. Genetically-modified crops. Science and Christian belief, 15(2): 141-164.

Powers, W.J., Fritz, E.R., Fehr, W. and Angel, R. 2006. Total and water-soluble phosphorus excretion from swine fed low-phytate soybeans. Journal of Animal Science, 84(7): 1907-1915.

Qu, A., Brulc, J.M., Wilson, M.K., Law, B.F., Theoret, J.R., Joens, L.A., Konkel, M.E., Angly, F., Dinsdale, E.A., Edwards, R.A., Nelson, K.E. and White, B.A. 2008. Comparative metagenomics reveals host-specific metavirulomes and horizontal gene transfer elements in the chicken cecum microbiome. PLoS One 3: e2945.

Rajakovich, L. J., & Balskus, E. P. 2019. Metabolic functions of the human gut microbiota: The role of metalloenzymes. National Product Reports, 36(4): 593– 625.

Ravindran, V. and Blair, R. 1991. Feed resources for poultry production in Asia and the Pacific region. I. Energy sources. World's Poultry Science Journal, 47(3): 213-231.

Rokade J.J., Gopi M., Monika M., Hable A.A. And Madhupriya. 2020. Application of nanoparticles and nanotechnologies in poultry production. International Journal of Agriculture Sciences, 12(3): 9497-9500.

Rutz, F., Xavier, E.G., Anciuti, M.A., Roll, V.F.B. and Rossi, P. 2008. The role of nucleotides in improving broiler pre-starter diets. Gut efficiency; the key ingredient in pig and poultry production, p.155.

Sergeant, M.J., Constantinidou, C., Cogan, T.A., Bedford, M.R., Penn, C.W. and Pallen, M.J. 2014. Extensive microbial and functional diversity within the chicken cecal microbiome. PloS one, 9(3): e91941.

Shareef, A.M., Jamel, Z.T. and Yonis, K.M. 2009. Detection of antibiotic residues in stored poultry products. Iraq Journal of Veterinary Science, 23(1): 45–48.

Shazali, N., Foo, H.L., Loh, T.C., Choe, D.W. and Rahim, R.A. 2014. Prevalence of antibioticresistance in lactic acid bacteria isolated from the faeces of broiler chicken in Malaysia. Gut Pathogy, 6, 1.

Shenderov, B.A. 2013. Metabiotics: novel idea or natural development of probiotic conception. Microbial ecology in Health and Disease, 24(1): 20399.

Swiatkiewicz, S., Arczewska-Wlosek, A., and Jozefiak, D. 2014. Immuno-modulatory efficacy of yeast cell products in poultry: a current view. World's Poultry Science Journal, 70.

Tang, Y., Underwood, A., Gielbert, A., Woodward, M.J. and Petrovska, L., 2014. Metaproteomics analysis reveals the adaptation process for the chicken gut microbiota. Applied and environmental microbiology, 80(2): 478-485.

Truksa, M., Vrinten, P. and Qiu, X. 2009. Metabolic engineering of plants for polyunsaturated fatty acid production. Molecular Breeding, 23(1): 1-11.

Venegas-Calerón, M., Sayanova, O. and Napier, J.A. 2010. An alternative to fish oils: metabolic engineering of oil-seed crops to produce omega-3 long chain polyunsaturated fatty acids. Progress in lipid research, 49(2): 108-119.

Wu, C., Yang, Z., Song, C., Liang, C., Li, H., Chen, W., Lin, W. and Xie, Q. 2018. Effects of dietary yeast nucleotides supplementation on intestinal barrier function, intestinal microbiota, and humoral immunity in specific pathogen-free chickens. Poultry Science, 97(11): 3837-3846.

5

Nano-biotechnology in Poultry Nutrition: The Hindsight

S.K. Bhanja and S.V.S. Verma

ICAR - Central Avian Research Institute, Izatnagar-243 122, Bareilly (UP), India

Introduction

The Indian poultry industry has emerged as one of the fastest growing segments in the Agriculture Sector, contributing significantly to the national GDP. The 20th Livestock Census in 2019 estimated the total poultry population in the country at 851.81 million with an increment of about 16.8 % over the last one in 2012. The Indian poultry industry is annually growing at around 6.0% for the past four decades and is expected to touch 1066.2 million by 2030. The Per capita availability of meat and eggs is expected to increase accordingly so as to meet requirement projections made by the National Institute of Nutrition (NIN), by the year 2031. To be able to realize such goals, the Indian Poultry may require approximately 57.84 million tons of feed for the egg and broiler stocks (Mandal and Bhanja, 2017). As much of the expenses on poultry production accounts to the feed and feeding, any substantial savings in this regard would help farmers raise their farm profits. Scientific investigations have been continuing in various laboratories to search and research new resources worth feeding to poultry and their real nutritional worth. Simultaneously, efforts are also being made to enhance effective utilisation of various nutrients in the unconventional feeds through feed processing, supplementation with digestive enzymes, making up deficiencies of essential nutrients so as to enhance the biological value of the feed. Besides, application of nanotechnology has also emerged as a scientific tool to improve the feeding value of the diet and exhibited tremendous potential in the agriculture, feed and food sector. In the bio system, many activities are performed on nano-scale thereby reducing cost of operations, saving nutrients and enhancing production efficiency. The nanomaterials can be synthesized purposefully to perform a specific function. The nanoparticles in the medical field assist drug transportation to the target site, thus helping both an effective and economical usage of expensive chemicals. In the animal production systems, supplementation of nutrients, probiotics, drugs, diagnostic compounds, hormonal immuno-sensors and the like form part of efficient management tools to animal reproduction. Similarly, nanotechnology has wide applicability in animal feeding by improving nutrient absorption, nutrient transport, obviating antagonism amongst bivalent cations thereby helping efficient uptake and better utilization of nutrients.

What Nanoparticles are?

A nanoparticle (NP) is a minute part of any substance that may range between 1 to 100 nanometre in size. Nanoparticles can exhibit significantly different physical and chemical properties than those of their bigger counterparts. Most nanoparticles are made up of only a few hundred atoms, their material properties change with time on the atomic scale. This is due to an increase in the surface area:volume ratio, resulting in the material's surface atoms dominating the material performance. Because of this feature nanoparticles possess unexpected optical, physical and chemical properties owing to being small enough to confine to their electrons and produce quantum effects.

Classification of Nanoparticles:

The origin, shape, structure and the purpose for administration do influence the classification of nanoparticles (Table 1).

Table 1: Various types of nanoparticles based on their structure and usage

S.No.	Nanoparticle type	Description
1.	Polymeric nanoparticles	The fabricated polymers, e.g. polyethylene glycol (PEG) and the other type trademark polymers whose structure rely upon polysaccharides, fall under this category, and include inulin and chitosan.
2.	Liposomes	They are spherical biodegradable non-destructive polyethylene glycolated particles, having a two-fold layer of phospholipid shell encasing the non-water dissolvable contents. The outside surface is coated by an external poly ethylene glycol layer which protects the particles from body immune defense. Liposomes are very useful for the delivery of both water soluble and water insoluble components.
3.	Fullerenes and Bucky tubes	Fullerenes are carbon nanoparticles resemble the shape of little ball that able to communicate effectively with pathogens or cells. The buckytubes are round and hollow structures which can be utilized as bio-sensor for different elements identification like immunoglobulins. Because of their needle-like structure nanotubes can enter the cells for the purpose of disease treatment.

4.	Nanoshells	They are round shaped connected with outer gold layer and used for analysis of malignant tumors by irradiation with Infrared laser, and can also be utilized as an adjuvant for radiotherapy.
5.	Quantum dots	They are exceptionally little gems (2 to 10 nm), possessing the semi conduction when exposed to light and this feature enables them to be used for opto-electronic purposes. Cadmium, zinc and selenium are used in semiconductor parts. Generally quantum dots can be used for diagnostics and immunodiagnostics purposes.
6.	Solid-lipid nanoparticles	They comprise of a lipophilic center which helps them into cancer treatment. Different hydrophilic medications or antibodies can we'll be conjugated to their outer hydrophilic shell. They are capable to cross the blood brain barrier thus, effectively delivering the medications inside the central nervous system.
7.	Dendrimer	They are polymers with hyper-branched nanomaterials and can exceptionally dissolve in aqueous solution. They are utilized fundamentally in cancer treatment. Many studies confirmed that dendrimer-loaded nanocomposites are very effective antimicrobial agents against *Pseudomonas aeruginosa, E-coli* and *Staphylococcus aureus*.
8.	Nano emulsion:	Nano-emulsions offer promising usage and bactericidal and virucidal medications. In addition, nano-emulsion can serve as vehicles for the antigens delivery.
9.	Metallic/ mineral nanoparticles:	There are different types of metals used in the nano system. These nanoparticles possess a metallic centre that is coated by a protected layer. In addition, various antibodies and chelated radionuclide are loaded on metallic nanoparticles. Particles are attached to polyethylene glycol which protects them and also maintains a strategic distance from non-specific binding. Some metallic nanoparticles especially bimetallic nanoparticles were utilized for disease treatment including silver/gold nanoparticles, silver–selenium, or gold-platinum etc. Various mineral NP, such as calcium, zinc, copper, selenium, and chromium, have been studied in different farm animals including poultry.

Classification of Nanoparticles according to their origin

Nanoparticles can be categorized into different types based on their ability to carry different ingredients and react to different environmental conditions. They can be divided into three broad categories, inorganic, organic, and hybrid type based on the chemical characteristics of the nanoparticles

1. *Inorganic nanoparticles:* Generally, they are safe, biocompatible and less cytotoxic. They have novel electrical and optical characteristics which can be adjusted during assembling. This group includes different inorganic materials, for example, gold, silver, iron oxide and calcium phosphate
2. *Organic nanoparticles:* Organic nanoparticles are used to enhance the nutritive value of feed systems. Nanoparticles have been designed to

deliver vitamins or other nutrients in feed without affecting the taste or appearance. These nanoparticles encapsulate the nutrients and carry them via the gastrointestinal tract (GIT) into the bloodstream, increasing their bioavailability. Organic nanomaterials include proteins, fat and sugar molecules. Nutraceuticals consisting of feed additives derived from plants are also organic nanomaterials used in feed.

3. *Hybrid nanoparticles:* They are composed of more than one type of nanoparticle, e.g. mixture of polymeric NP and liposomes that results in a polymer-lipid hybrid system. They have a core of biodegradable hydrophobic polymers loaded with hydrophilic drugs for simultaneous release of the drugs.

Nanomaterial synthesis and characterization

Over the last decade, novel synthesis approaches/methods for nanomaterials such as metal nanoparticles, quantum dots, carbon nanotubes, graphene, and their composites have been an interesting area in nanoscience and technology. To obtain nanomaterials of desired sizes, shape & functionalities, two different fundamental principles of synthesis (i.e., top down and bottom up methods) have been applied (Fig.1). In the former, nanomaterials/nanoparticles are prepared through a diverse range of synthesis approaches like lithographic techniques, ball milling, etching, and sputtering. The bottom up approach in which nanoparticles are grown from simpler molecules includes many methods like chemical vapor deposition, sol–gel processes, spray pyrolysis, laser pyrolysis, and atomic or molecular condensation. The morphological parameters of nanoparticles (e.g., size and shape) can be modulated by varying the concentrations of chemicals and reaction conditions (e.g., temperature and pH).

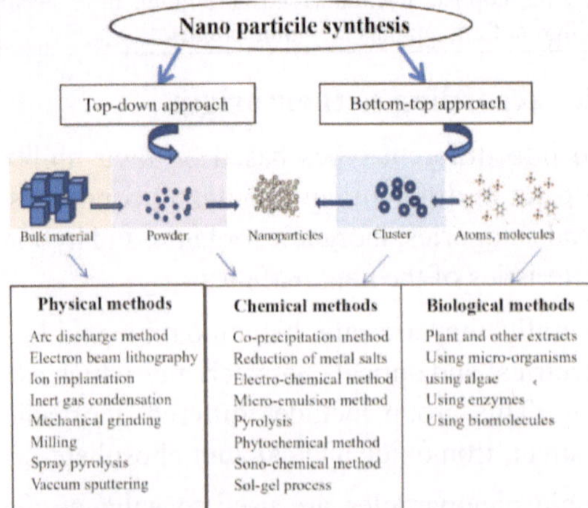

Fig. 1: Different approaches for synthesis of nano particles

The nanomaterials synthesized through the above mentioned methods, however, do have certain issues with respect to stability, accumulation, toxicity, recycling, regeneration features and the like. To counter such limitations, 'Green synthesis' approaches/methods have been developed. Basically, in Green synthesis the materials/nanomaterials are produced through regulation, control, clean up, and remediation procedures (Sintubin *et al*., 2009). Green synthesis of metallic nanoparticles has been adopted to accommodate various biological materials (e.g., bacteria, fungi, algae, and plant extracts). Among the available green methods of synthesis for metal/metal oxide nanoparticles, utilization of plant extracts (especially in leaves such as ketones, aldehydes, flavones, amides, terpenoids, carboxylic acids, phenols, and ascorbic acid) is a rather simple and easy process to produce nanoparticles at large scale relative to bacteria and/or fungi mediated synthesis. These products are known collectively as biogenic nanoparticles.

Different characterization techniques have also been employed in the analysis of various physicochemical properties of NPs. These include techniques such as X-ray diffraction (XRD), X-ray photoelectron spectroscopy (XPS), infrared (IR), Scanning Electron Microscopy (SEM) and Transmission electron Microscopy (TEM), Particle size analysis and the like, details of which presented and discussed by Khan *et al*. (2019).

Absorption and bioavailability of nano minerals

Owing to their small size, NPs are easily absorbed through to the gastro-intestinal epithelium. The uptake of NP through mucosal layer is, however, dependent on the surface charge and pH of the adjacent environment. The cationic NP can be trapped within the glycosylated areas of mucin, whereas anionic nanoparticles diffuse through the epithelial surface. The NPs either absorbed through epithelial villi into the circulation which subsequently transported to the liver and spleen or pass into the hepatic circulation crossing through M-cells in the Peyer's patches enterocytes. Due to the smaller pore size (0.6 to 5 nm) of tight junctions, paracellular transport (passage of substances across the epithelium through the intercellular spaces) of NP is usually limited under normal physiological conditions. Nano-minerals have the potential to enter the blood, brain, lung, heart, kidney, spleen, liver, intestine and stomach after crossing the small intestine. But their uptake rate in the intestinal epithelia and other body tissues differs substantially. The particle sizes less than 300 nm can reach the blood circulation, whereas particles smaller than 100 nm can penetrate various tissues and organs and takes part in transcellular transport (passage of substances through the cells). Paracellular transport does not include any transporter or energy expenditure for transporter, the absorption being concentration-dependant is not very efficient. Tight junctions act as gate keeper for paracellular transport, limiting the entry of macromolecules. Transcellular absorption involves either diffusion across concentration gradient or active carrier-mediated transportation utilizing energy or through endocytosis (Hassan *et al*., 2020; Patra and Lalhriatpuii, 2020).

Nano-minerals and bird performance

Broiler chickens: Amongst the nano-minerals, nano-Zn has been employed extensively. Feeding nano-Zn (60 or 90 mg/kg diet in the form of Zn.O, Zn.SO4 or Zn-methionine) increased their body weight gain, feed intake, feed efficiency, bone dimensions, bone weight, total ash, liver and muscle Zn concentration, antioxidant status of broiler chickens and also reduced their body fat and cholesterol contents (Ahmadi *et al*., 2013; Mohammadi *et al*., 2015; Dukare *et al*., 2020). However, increasing the nano-Zn concentration beyond 120 mg/kg in diet tended to lower performance. Zinc oxide nano-particles supplementation at 30-120 ppm /Kg broiler feed significantly decreased serum enzyme activity (ALT, AST, and LDH), LDL, cholesterol and triglyceride levels, but increased the HDL, total antioxidant capability, SOD and catalase activity as compared to those of birds fed the supplemented diets (Ahmadi *et al*., 2013). Nano-ZnO also increased mRNA expressions of insulin-like growth factor-1 and growth hormonegenes in broiler chickens compared to those fed inorganic or organic sources of Zn.

Similarly, the CuO in NP form was found more efficient in enhancing growth performance and immunity of broiler chickens as compared to using the conventional sources of Cu (Lianqin *et al*., 2007; Sharif *et al*., 2020). Supplemental nano-Se up to 0.30 mg /Kg diet improved body weight gain and feed conversion ratio of broilers as compared to those fed Se in inorganic form but beyond that level no beneficial effect was recorded (Zhou and Wang, 2011; Mohapatra *et al*., 2014). Nano-Se supplementation also reduced the drip loss percentage without altering performance, immune organ index (thymus, bursa, and spleen) or meat color in broilers (Cai *et al*., 2012).

The dietary Fe sulfate In NP form improved weight gain and feed conversion (Sizova *et al*., 2016), increased jejunal villi width and it's surface area in broiler chickens evaluated at 21 and 42 days of age (Laledashti *et al*., 2020). The nano Fe when employd in compound feed, and also with additional amino acids, significantly increased the performance of broilers. Adding nano Fe in poultry diet (4 mg/kg) resulted in an increase in the blood erythrocytes, NO-metabolites content in the liver by 3.1-3.5% and body iron concentration in birds by 5.3% (Miroshnikov *et al*., 2017). Besides, intramuscular injection of Fe-NP (2 mg/kg body weight) improved body weight gains, hematological picture, and increased retention of Fe in the body tissues in broiler chickens (Yausheva *et al*., 2016).

NP-Mn_2O_3 or MnO supplementation helped to reduce the Mn requirement of the birds from 100 to 50 or 10 mg/kg without affecting their growth performance or the oxidation process in liver and the breast muscles with improved ileal digestibility of Mn while decreased Cu accumulation in the liver and breast muscles (Jankowski *et al.*, 2019). Dietary supplementation of MnSO4 in NP form resulted in improved tibial bone characteristics (length, volume, breaking strength, diameter and weight) studied by Patra and Lalhriatpuii (2020). Nano-Ca phosphate at 50% of the recommended level, resulted in improved body weight gain without altering feed conversion ratio, carcass characteristics and biochemical parameters similar to those at 100% DCP supplemented level (Samanta *et al.*, 2019). A study conducted by Omara *et al.* (2020) revealed no significant difference in body weight, feed intake, tibial ash weight and percentage in the di-calcium phosphate and the Nano P fed group of birds, thereby indicating almost similar phosphorus bioavailability from such sources.

Though, there being no recommendations on the feeding of metals like silver, gold or chromium from either the NRC, 1994 or ICAR, 2013, a study on feeding supplemental Ag NPs (4 mg/kg) suggests improved body weight gain and better feed conversion ratio in broiler chickens (Elkloub *et al.*, 2015). Silver, with antimicrobial effect on harmful gut microbiota may have led to better nutrient absorption as manifested in form of improved weight gain, feed intake and feed conversion ratio of such broiler chickens (Andy *et al.*, 2011). *In-ovo* administration of 50 ppm hydrocolloids of Ag NPs and alloys with Cu and Pd did not increase oxidative damage to liver DNA, blood biochemicals and the liver enzymes (Sawosz *et al.*, 2009). Other studies also reported no effects of AgNPs on serum SGOT, SGPT, ASP, ALT, AP, glucose, triglycerides, and cholesterol levels (Sawosz *et al.*, 2009; Andi *et al.*, 2011; Saki and Salary, 2015; Rath, 2018), but HDL cholesterol reduced in birds fed supplemental Ag NP at 8 and 12 ppm/kg diet (Ahmadi and Kurdestany, 2010). Dietary Ag NPs induced oxidative stress and adversely affected the structure and peroxidation value of lipids accumulated therein and leading to rupturing of the cell membranes (Fig. 2).

Feeding chromium NPs at 0.5 mg/kg diet improved breast and thigh muscle protein content, average daily gain and feed efficiency ,and lowered the cholesterol and fat content in the thigh muscles of broiler chickens (Zha *et al.*, 2009). Increasing the amount to 0.8 mg/kg diet was found to improve meat quality of quail broilers, as was evident from reduced malondialdehyde concentration in the thigh muscle and also the unaltered hematological parameters (Yarmohammadi *et al.*, 2020).

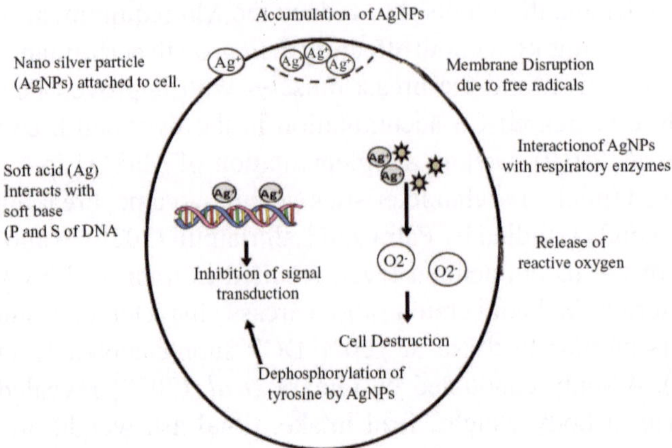

Fig. 2: Action of silver nano particles (AgNPs) inside the animal cell

It is evident from such studies that feeding nano-minerals to poultry at low concentrations has the potential to improve growth performance as also the quality of meat as compared to using the conventional mineral sources. Data in Table 2 shows a comparison of mineral requirement figures given by the NRC, 1994 and ICAR, 2013, vis-a-vis those of mineral nanoparticles.

Table 2: Comparison of inorganic and nano-minerals requirements for the meat and egg type chickens

Nutrient Amount	NRC, 1994		ICAR, 2013		Nano minerals*	
	Broilers	**Layers**	**Broilers**	**Layers**	**Broilers**	**Layers**
Ca (%)	0.90-1.00	3.25-3.40	1.0	3.40-3.80	0.50	
Av. P (%)	0.35-0.45	0.25	0.45	0.28-0.36	0.24	
Mn (mg/Kg)	60.0	20.0	100.0-120.0	40.0-50.0	10.0	
Zn (mg/Kg)	40.0	35.0	100.0-120.0	40.0-50.0	60.0-90.0	40.0-80.0
Fe (mg/Kg)	80.0	45.0	80.0	45.0-55.0	4.0-7.0	
Cu (mg/Kg)	8.0	?	20.0	5.0-8.0	0.5-1.5	
I (mg/Kg)	0.35	0.035	2.0-3.0	0.03-0.04	-	
Se (mg/Kg)	0.15	-	0.3	0.05-0.08	0.30	0.50
Ag (mg/Kg)	-	-	-	-	4.0	
Cr (mg/Kg)	-	-	-	-	0.3-0.8	

(-) Indicate no recommended value

(*) Values derived from research reports

Layer chickens and egg quality: In recent times, the production of designer or enriched eggs has caught up the attention of nutritionists, wherein the response of egg laying chickens to certain nano-minerals in diet has been evaluated. Changes, if any, on the composition of eggs laid by such birds have also been evaluated. Supplemental Zn in nano form at 40 and 80 mg /kg diet increased the egg yolk Zn contents (Alagawany *et al*., 2018) and improved egg production, Haugh unit, eggshell thickness and strength, tibial ash content and strength (Tsai *et al*., 2016; Olgun and Yildiz, 2017; Abedini *et al*., 2018). Supplementation of diet with nano-Zn proved advantageous in producing the designer eggs and enhanced keeping quality. The malondialdehyde content in eggs also reduced on feeding birds 80 mg Zn/kg diet added through ZnO in nano form (Abedini *et al*., 2017).

Dietary Se has a well recognised role in egg production and immunity in poultry, and reports suggest even more favorable responses of employing it in the nano form. Nano-Se (0.3-0.5 mg/kg diet), raised the egg Se content, improved bird performance in terms of egg production and feed conversion without altering egg weight, feed intake (Radwan *et al*., 2015; Qu *et al*., 2017; Meng *et al*., 2019) and also improved the glutathione peroxidase (GPx) activity and the total antioxidant status (Qu *et al*., 2017). Injecting 40μg nano-Se and nano-ZnO in birds lessened negative effects of heat stress by increasing the GPx activity, superoxide dismutase (SOD), and antioxidants and reduced the corticosterone, cortisol, T3 and T4 in such eggs (Shokraneh *et al*., 2020). Dietary nano-selenium also improved the fatty acid profile in eggs by reducing the ratio of saturated to unsaturated acids, decreased total lipids and cholesterol, increased its HDL fraction in egg yolk and plasma of laying hens (Shokraneh *et al*., 2020).

Nanominerals and Immunity

Bird immunity is an important problem in raising flocks successfully and with optimal bird productivity, more so in stressful challenging situations. Dietary provision of mineral elements in nano forms has shown better immune responses in poultry. ZnO in the form of NPs enhanced cellular immunity as was evident from increased serum IgY concentration, total lymphocyte count, macrophages, phagocytic activity and the ndex (Hafez *et al*., 2020). Nano-Zn supplementation at 0.06 mg/kg in the basal diet improved immune status of broiler chickens to the level of those fed 15 mg organic Zn /kg diet (Sahoo *et al*., 2014). Supplementation of ZnO-NP in broiler ration increased relative weight of lymphoid organs (Mohammadi *et al*., 2015; Esfahani *et al*., 2015), inhibited fungal growth (*Aspergillus flavus, A. ochraceus and A. niger*) and also mycotoxin production (Hasan *et al*., 2013). Certain possible mechanisms of bactericidal actions by metal oxide NP was creation of reactive oxygen species inside the bacterial cells (e.g., hydroxyl, hydroperoxide, and superoxide radicals) and that may damage lipid cell membranes, the organelles of bacteria or alter permeability of bacteria on entering the plasma membrane resulting in cell death. Addition of Cu-NP to drinking water @ 10 mg/l improved bird immunity as compared to those of birds fed the conventional CuSO4 in diet (El-kazaz and Hafez, 2020). El-Kassas *et al*. (2018) reported that birds fed CIO in NPs form exhibited significantly higher immune response as evidenced by increased phagocytic activity (PA), lysozyme serum activity, and upregulation of immune-modulator genes including NF-κβ, PGES, IL-1β, TGF-1β, IFN-γ, BAX and CASP8 as compared to CuO.

A provision of nano-Ag @ 50 micro gm /egg on 18th day of incubation was found effective in modulating the post-hatch immune response and expression profile of immune cytokines without affecting hatchability and subsequent performance of broiler chicks (Bhanja *et al*., 2015; Goel *et al*., 2017). Rath (2018) and Goel *et al.* (2017) reported that *in- ovo* injection of AgNPs enhanced the in vivo immune response to PHA-P (Cell-mediated immunity) and SRBC (Humoral immunity) in comparison to the control group. Saki and Salary (2015) have also reported about the enhanced cell-mediated immunity in terms of mean skin thickness sensitive to phytohaemagglutinin in chicks treated with AgNPs, and which also can increase cell immunity by stimulating heat shock protein (HSP) synthesis, without pro-inflammatory pathway activation as evidenced from lack of influence of AgNPs on the expression of NF-kB, a transcriptional factor involved in defense of the organism (Sawosz *et al*., 2010).

Nanoparticles and Gut health

Nano-Ag supplementation at 4 mg/kg in the diet of broiler chickens reduced caecal *Escherichia coli* with no significant effect on *Lactobacillus* count (Elkloub *et al*., 2015). AgNP is an effective killing agent against broad spectrum gram-positive and gram-negative bacteria including antimicrobial resistant strains (Burrel *et al*., 1999). Dietary colloidal AgNPs @ 0,5,15,25 mg/Kg diet had no effect on the intestinal microflora and duodenal morphology in quails (Sawosz *et al*. 2007), but improved intestinal microflora through increased *Lactobacillus*, and decreased *E. coli* count (Hassanabadi *et al*., 2012). In another study, Rath *et al*. (2018) also reported *in-ovo* injection with AgNPs reduced the coliform counts in the ileum, and lactic acid bacteria in the caecum of chicks. A provision of AgNPs via the drinking water effectively reduced lactose negative *enterobacteria* on 22 day and coliform bacteria on 36 day in the small intestinal contents of broiler chicks. Nano-Ag in water @25 mg/L increased the lactic acid bacteria population without any adverse effect on enterocytes in the duodenal villi (Sawosz *et al*., 2007). Nano-Ag treatment of the litter material lowered the number of *Escherichia coli*, *Streptococcus*, *Salmonella*, and total mesophilic bacteria. ZnO-NP was found to be effective against both gram positive and gram-negative bacteria (Patra, 2019) as well as spores that are resistant to high temperature and pressure.

Antimicrobial activity of Nanoparticles

The usage of antibiotics in poultry feeding has primarily been prophylactic or growth promoters in poultry. This has been a great concern due to possible emergence of drug resistance in microbes as well as in poultry products. There is a possibility of using nano-minerals as antibiotic alternatives due to their antimicrobial properties, particularly the silver nanoparticles (Bhanja *et al*., 2019; Patra, 2019). The mode of action of silver is presumed Ag+ions dependent, strongly inhibiting bacterial growth through suppression of respiratory enzymes and electron transport components and also interference with DNA functions (Li *et al*., 2006). AgNPs have also exhibited virucidal activity against broad-spectrum viruses and, in most cases, a direct interaction between the nanoparticle and the virus surface proteins could be seen. Besides the direct interaction with viral surface glycoproteins, metal nanoparticles may also gain access into the cell and exert their antiviral activity through interactions with the viral genome, DNA or RNA (Fig. 3).

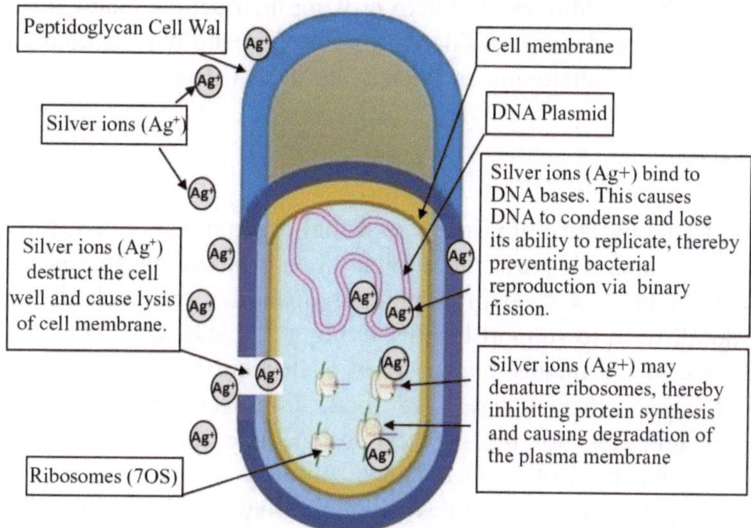

Fig. 3: Action of silver nano particles (AgNPs) inside the bacterial cell

The silver NP and the oxide NP inactivate proteins that are responsible for transport of nutrients into microbial cells, thus decreasing the membrane permeability and eventually causing cellular death. Another explanation about antimicrobial action of metal oxide NP is that the microorganisms carrying a negative charge are electromagnetically attracted towards metal oxides carrying a positive charge, subsequently leading to oxidation and death of microbes. The antibacterial activity depends on the size of NP, better results being obtained with smaller size (Shrivastava *et al*., 2007). The nanoparticles act by attacking the respiratory chain and cell division, finally leading to cell death. In addition, the STEM (Scanning Transmission Electron Microscopy) confirms the presence of silver in the cell membrane and inside bacteria. The antiviral property of AgNPs was evident in the detailed challenge study conducted by Rath (2018), where AgNPs along with amino acids or trace elements successfully countered the ND virus challenges. However, additional research is needed to determine the exact mode of antiviral mechanism and the highest safe dose in broilers, to augment the resistance to lethal avian viruses without creating new risk to humans or the environment.

Other applications of Nanoparticles

Nano materials are also used in microencapsulation of feed components to protect them from oxidation and break down by light and oxidation. Further, it keeps them away from the lysis by enzymes in the digestive system such as proteases, promote stability at various pH values, effective dispersion and mixing of the lipophilic additives, and help prolong their action. Nano silica and nano magnesium oxide are considered a powerful nano anti mycotoxin that bind successfully to aflatoxins and inactivate them (Moghaddam *et al.*, 2010).

Conclusions

Feeds, food and feeding are the primary essential requirements universally for all living beings and, it's provision, a highly complex complicated issue. Providing the right kind of food in sumptuous quantities and biologically useful forms do all want to support healthy living at the least cost. Drawing a positive balance in the quality and costs of such requisites is, therefore, essential to effective efficient usage of food. Improvement of reliable and eco-friendly processes for the synthesis of metallic nanoparticles is a significant step in the field of applied nanotechnology. Trace minerals are normally used in very minute quantities in animal nutrition but issues like lower bioavailability, antagonism, and higher excretion rates from the body come in the way of their real efficiency. Nano-technology offers opportunities to mediate such issues and helps improve bioavailability of trace minerals. Although, limited literature reports are available on potential usage and effects of nano-particles in poultry nutrition, some convincing evidences suggest that feeding of trace minerals (zinc, copper, silver, selenium, iron, chromium, and manganese) in diets for broiler chickens, laying hens, turkeys, and quails. Excellent antimicrobial activities exhibited by the nano-particles of Ag, Cu, and Zn, against major poultry pathogens like *Salmonella* and *Campylobacter*, indicate their potential role in effective efficient poultry production. Recent studies have also demonstrated modulation of gut health by nano-particles through increasing abundance of beneficial microbes (*Lactobacillus and Faecalibacterium*) and production of short-chain fatty acids, which open new vistas of future research.

References

Abedini, M., Shariatmadari, F., Torshizi, M. K., Ahmadi H. 2018. Effects of zinc oxide nanoparticles on performance, egg quality, tissue zinc content, bone parameters, and antioxidative status in laying hens. Biological Trace Element Research, 184: 259-267.

Abedini, M., Shariatmadari, F., Torshizi, M. K., Ahmadi, H. 2017. Effects of a dietary supplementation with zinc oxide nanoparticles, compared to zinc oxide and zinc methionine, on performance, egg quality, and zinc status of laying hens. Livestock Science, 203: 30-36.

Ahmadi, F. and Kurdestani, A.H. 2010. The impact of silver nanoparticles on growth performance, lymphoid organs and oxidative stress indicators in broiler chicks. Global Veterinaria, 5: 366-370.

Ahmadi, F., Ebrahimnezhad, Y., Sis, N. M., Ghiasi, J. 2013. The effects of zinc oxide nanoparticles on performance, digestive organs and serum lipid concentrations in broiler chickens during the starter period. International Journal of Biosciences, 3: 23-29.

Alagawany, M., Farag, M. R., Dhama, K., Patra, A. 2018. Nutritional significance and health benefits of designer eggs. World's Poultry Science Journal, 74: 317-330.

Andi, M. A., Hashemi, M., Ahmadi, F. 2011. Effects of feed type with/without nanosil on cumulative performance,relative organ weight and some blood parameters of broilers. GlobalVeterinaria, 7: 605-609.

Bhanja, S. K., Hotowy, A., Mehra, M., Sawosz, E., Pineda, L., Vadalasetty, K.P., Kurantowicz, N., Chwalibog, A. 2015. In ovo administration of silver nanoparticles and/or amino acids influence metabolism and immune gene expression in chicken embryos. International journal of Molecular Sciences, 16: 9484-9503.

Bhanja, S.K., Mehra, M. and Goel, A. 2019. Application of silver nanoparticles in poultry production. Indian Journal of Poultry Science, 54(3), pp.185-192.

Burrell, R. E., Heggers, J. P., Davis, G. J., Wright, J. B. 1999. Efficacy of silver- coated dressings as bacterial barriers in a rodent burn sepsis model. Wounds, 11: 64-71.

Cai, S. J., Wu, C. X., Gong, L. M., Song, T., Wu, H., Zhang, L.Y. 2012. Effects of nano selenium on performance, meat quality, immune function, oxidation resistance, and tissue selenium content in broilers. Poultry Science, 91: 2532-2539.

Dukare, S., Mir, N. A., Mandal, A. B., Dev, K., Begum, J., Rokade, J. J., Biswas, A., Tyagi, P. K., Tyagi, P. K, Bhanja, S. K. 2020. A Comparative study on the antioxidant status, meat quality, and mineral deposition in broiler chicken fed dietary nano zinc viz-a-viz inorganic zinc.Journal of Food Science and Technology, 2020.

El-Kassas, Seham., Abdo, Safaa, E., El-Naggar, Karima., Abdo, Walied., Kirrella, Abeer, A. K., Nashar, Toufic, O. 2018. Ameliorative effect of dietary supplementation of copper oxide nanoparticles on inflammatory and immune responses in commercial broilers under normal and heat-stress housing conditions. Journal of Thermal Biology, 78: 235-246.

El-kazaz, S. E., Hafez, M. H. 2020. Evaluation of copper nanoparticles and copper sulfate effect on immune status, behavior, and productive performance of broilers. Journal of Advanced Veterinary and Animal Research, 7: 16-25.

Elkloub, K., Moustafa, M. E., Ghazalah, A. A., Rehan, A. A. A. 2015. Effect of dietary nanosilver on broiler performance. International Journal of Poultry Science, 14: 177-182.

Esfahani, M., Farhad, A., Mohammad, A. A. 2015. The effects of different levels of Curcuma longa and zinc oxide nanoparticles on the quality traits of thigh and breast meat in broiler chickens. International Journal of Biosciences, 6: 296-302.

Goel, A., Bhanja, S.K., Mehra, M., Majumdar, S., Mandal, A.B. 2017. In ovo silver nanoparticle supplementation for improving the post-hatch immunity status of broiler chickens. Archives of Animal Nutrition, 71(5): 384-394.

Hafez, A., Nassef, E., Fahmy, M., Elsabagh, M., Bakr, A., Hegazi, E. 2020. Impact of dietary nano-zinc oxide on immune response and antioxidant defense of broiler chickens. Environmental Science and Pollution Research, 27: 19108-19114.

Hassan, A. A., Howayda, M. E., Mahmoud, H. H. 2013. Effect of zinc oxide nanoparticles on the growth of mycotoxigenic moulds. Studies in Chemical Process Technology, 1: 66-74.

Hassan, S., Hassan, F. U., Rehman, M. S. 2020. Nano-particles of Trace Minerals in Poultry Nutrition: Potential Applications and Future Prospects. Biological Trace Element Research, 195(2): 591-612.

Hassanabadi, A., Hajati, H. and Bahreini, L. 2012. The effects of nano-silver on performance, carcass characteristics, immune system and intestinal microflora of broiler chickens.In Proceedings of 3rd International Veterinary Poultry Congress, Tehran, Iran. pp. 55-65.

Indian Council of Agricultural Research. 2013. Nutrient requirements of poultry. Directorate of Knowledge Management in Agriculture, ICAR, New Delhi, pp 58.

Jankowski, J., Ognik, K., Stêpniowska, A., Zduñczyk, Z. and Koz³owski, K. 2019. The effect of the source and dose of manganese on the performance, digestibility and distribution of selected minerals, redox, and immune status of turkeys. Poultry Science, 98: 1379-1389.

Khan, I., Saeed, K. and Khan, I. 2019. Nanoparticles: Properties, applications and toxicities. Arabian Journal of Chemistry, 12(7): 908-931.

Laledashti, M. A., Saki, A. A., Rafati, A. A., Abdolmaleki, M. 2020. Effect of in-ovo feeding of iron nanoparticles and methionine hydroxy analogue on broilers chickens small intestinal characteristic. ActaScientiarum Animal Sciences, 42: e46903.

Li, M., Mizuuchi, M., Burke, T. R., Craigie, R. 2006. Retroviral DNA integration: reaction pathway and critical intermediates. The EMBO Journal, 25: 1295-1304.

Lianqin, Z., Xiangdi, T., Fenghua, Z., Jinquan, S., Zhipeng, L. 2007. Effect of dietary nano-CuO dosage on immune function in broiler. China Poultry, 29: 20-23.

Mandal, A.B. and Bhanja, S.K. 2017. Nitrogen Use Efficiency in Poultry Husbandry—Indian Perspective. In book “The Indian Nitrogen Assessment” edited by Abrol, Y. P., Adhya, T K., Aneja, V. P., Raghuram, N., Pathak, H. Kulshrestha, U., Sharma, C. and Singh, B., Elsevier publication, UK, pp 249-266.

Meng, T., Liu, Y., Xie, C., Zhang, B., Huang, Y., Zhang, Y., Yao, Y., Huang, R., Wu, X. 2019. Effects of different selenium sources on laying performance, egg selenium concentration, and antioxidant capacity in laying hens. Biological Trace Element Research, 189: 548-555.

Miroshnikov, S.A., Yausheva, E.V., Sizova, E.A., Kosyan, D.B. and Donnik I.M. 2017. Research of opportunities for using iron Nanoparticles and amino acids in poultry nutrition. International Journal of Geomate, 13 (40): 124-131.

Moghaddam, S. H., Jebali, A., Daliri, K. 2010.The use ofMgO-Sio2 nano-composite for adsorption of aflatoxinin wheat flour samples.Nanocon, 10: 12–14.

Mohammadi, F., Ahmadi, F., Amiri, A. M. 2015. Effect of zinc oxide nanoparticles on carcass parameters, relative weight of digestive and lymphoid organs of broiler fed wet diet during the starter period. International Journal of Biosciences, 6: 389-394.

Mohammadi, V., Ghazanfari, S., Mohammadi-Sangcheshmeh, A., Nazaran, M. H. 2015. Comparative effects of zinc-nano complexes, zinc-sulphate and zinc-methionine on performance in broiler chickens. British Poultry Science, 56:486-493.

Mohapatra, P., Swain, R. K., Mishra, S. K., Behera, T., Swain, P., Behura, N.C., Sahoo, G., Sethy, K., Bhol, B. P., Dhama, K. 2014. Effects of dietary nano-selenium supplementation on the performance of layer grower birds.Asian Journal of Animal and Veterinary Advances, 9: 641-652.

National Research Council. 1994. Nutrients requirements of poultry, 8th revised ed., Washington, DC, USA, National Academy Press.

Olgun, O., Yildiz, A. O. 2017. Effects of dietary supplementation of inorganic, organic or nano zinc forms on performance, eggshell quality, and bone characteristics in laying hens. Annals of Animal Science, 17: 463-476.

Omara, I. I., Mou, C.T., Persia, M. E. and Wong, E.A. 2020. Effects of available phosphorus source and concentration on performance and expression of sodium phosphate type IIb cotransporter, vitamin D-1á-hydroxylase, and vitamin D-24-hydroxylase mRNA in broiler chicks. Poultry Science, 99: 1822-1831.

Patra, A. K. 2019. Are nanomaterials potential new generation antimicrobial feed additives in livestock? Indian Journal of Animal Health, 58(Special 2): 105-120.

Patra, A., Lalhriatpuii, M. 2020. Progress and Prospect of Essential Mineral Nanoparticles in Poultry Nutrition and Feeding-a Review. Biological Trace Element Research, 197(1): 233-253.

Qu, W., Yang, J., Sun, Z., Zhang, R., Zhou, F., Zhang, K., Xia, Y., Huang, K., Miao, D. 2017. Effect of selenium nanoparticles on antioxidative level, egg production and quality and blood parameter of laying hens exposed to deoxynivalenol. Journal of Animal Research and Nutrition, 21: 1.

Radwan, N. L., Eldin, T. S., El-Zaiat, A. and Mostafa, M. A. 2015. Effect of dietary nano-selenium supplementation on selenium content and oxidative stability in table eggs and productive performance of laying hens. International Journal of Poultry Science, 14 (3): 161–176.

Rath, P. K. 2018. Investigation on in ovo supplementation of nano silver (AgNPs) and critical nutrients for enhancing immunocompetence in broiler chickens. Ph D Thesis submitted to ICAR-Indian Veterinary Research Institute, Deemed University, Izatnagar, UP-243122, India, pp. 1-97.

Rath, P. K., Bhanja, S. K., Mehra, M., Goel, A. and Aswathi, P. B. 2018. Effect of in ovo supplemented silver nanoparticles on the gut morphology and hemato-serological parameters in broiler chickens. Indian Journal of Poultry Science, 53(2): 181-189.

Sahoo, A., Swain, R. K., Mishra, S. K. 2014. Effect of inorganic, organic and nano zinc supplemented diets on bioavailability and immunity status of broilers. International Journal of Advanced Research, 2: 828-837.

Saki, A. A. and Salary, J. 2015. The impact of in ovo injection of silver nanoparticles, thyme and savory extracts in broiler breeder eggs on growth performance, lymphoid-organ weights, and blood and immune parameters of broiler chicks. Poultry Science Journal, 3(2): 165-172.

Samanta, G., Mishra, S. K., Behura, N. C., Sahoo, G., Behera, K., Swain, R. K., Sethy, K., Biswal, S., Sahoo, N. 2019. Studies on utilization of calcium phosphate nano-particles as source of phosphorus in broilers. Animal Nutrition and Feed Technology, 19: 77-88.

Sawosz, E., Chwalibog, A., Szeliga, J., Sawosz, F., Grodzik, M., Rupiewicz, M., Niemiec, T., Kacprzyk, K. 2010. Visualization of gold and platinum nanoparticles interacting with Salmonella enteritidis and Listeria monocytogenes. International Journal of Nanomedicine, 5: 631-637.

Sawosz, E., Binek, M., Grodzik, M., Zielinska, M., Sysa, P., Szmidt, M., Niemiec, T., Chwalibog, A. 2007. Influence of hydrocolloid silver nanoparticles on gastrointestinal microflora and morphology of enterocytes of quails. Archives of Animal Nutrition, 61: 444-451.

Sawosz, E., Grodzik, M., Zielinska, M., Niemiec, T., Olszanska, B., Chwalibog, A. 2009. Nanoparticles of silver do not affect growth, development and DNA oxidative damage in chicken embryos. European Poultry Science, 73: 208–213.

Sharif, M., Rahman, M. A., Ahmed, B., Abbas, R. Z., Hassan, F. U. 2020. Copper Nanoparticles as Growth Promoter, Antioxidant and Anti-Bacterial Agents in Poultry Nutrition: Prospects and Future Implications. Biol Trace Elem Res. 2020 Nov 20. doi: 10.1007/s12011-020-02485-1.

Shokraneh, M., Sadeghi, A. A., Mousavi, S. N., Esmaeil Khani, S., Chamani, M. 2020. Effects of in ovo injection of nano-selenium and nano-zinc oxide and high eggshell temperature during late incubation on antioxidant activity, thyroid and glucocorticoid hormones and some blood metabolites in broiler hatchlings. Acta Scientiarum Animal Sciences, 42: e46029.

Shrivastava, S., Bera, T., Roy, A., Singh, G., Ramachandrarao, P., Dash, D. 2007. Characterization of enhanced antibacterial effects of novel silver nanoparticles. Nanotechnology, 18:225103.

Sintubin, L., De Windt, W., Dick, J., Mast, J., Van Der Ha, D., Verstraete, W., et al. 2009. Lactic acid bacteria as reducing and capping agent for the fast and efficient production of silver nanoparticles. Applied Microbiology and Biotechnology, 84, 741–749. doi: 10.1007/s00253-009-2032-6.

Sizova, E. A., Miroshnikov, S. A., Lebedev, S. V., Êudasheva, A. V., Ryabov, N. I. 2016. To the development of innovative mineral additives based on alloy of Fe and Co antagonists as an example. Agricultural Biology, 51: 553-562.

Tsai, Y. H., Mao, S.Y., Li, M. Z., Huang, J. T., Lien, T. F. 2016. Effects of nano size zinc oxide on zinc retention, eggshell quality, immune response and serum parameters of aged laying hens. Animal Feed Science and Technology, 213: 99-107.

Yarmohammadi, A. B., Sharifi, S. D., Mohammadi-Sangcheshmeh, A. 2020. Efficacy of dietary supplementation of nanoparticles-chromium, chromium methionine and zinc-proteinate, the n performance of Japanese quail under physiological stress. Italian Journal of Animal Science, 19:1123-1134

Yausheva, E.V., Miroshnikov, S.A., Kosyan, D.B. and Sizova, E.A., 2016. Nanoparticles in combination with amino acids change productive and immunological indicators of broiler chicken. Agricultural Biology, 51(6), pp.912-920.

Zha, L. Y., Zeng, J. W., Chu, X. W., Mao, L. M., Luo, H. J. 2009. Efficacy trivalent chromium on growth performance, carcass characteristics a tissue chromi in heat-stress broiler chickscks. Journal of the Science of Food and Agriculture, 89:1782-1786.

Zhou, X., Wang, Y. 2011. Influence of dietary nano elemental selenium on growth performance, tissue selenium distribution, meat quality, and glutathione peroxidase activity in Guangxi Yellow chicken. Poultry Science, 90: 680-686.

6

Gut Health
What's New in Chicken Nutrition?

Deben Sapcota and Dimpi Choudhury

Department of Poultry Science, College of Veterinary Science
Assam Agricultural University, Guwahati, Assam

Introduction

Improvement of growth rate and feed efficiency through formulating effective diets are mostly considered for its effect on gut health. Several factors need to be well thought-out such as genetic makeup of the birds, feed source and quality, environmental condition and disease incidence. Apart from these factors, maintenance a good gut ecosystem or enhancement of it is essential for the welfare, optimum performances and productivity of birds. When the gut function is impaired, digestion and absorption of nutrients is hampered and thus the health and performance of birds will be affected drastically. It will also have a detrimental effect on feed efficiency and greater susceptibility to diseases leading to economic loss. Dysbacteriosis is an imbalance in the gut microbiota as a consequence of an intestinal disruption and has impact on economic and welfare issues (Bailey, 2010).

The demand for poultry and poultry products has increased exponentially in recent decades and it is estimated that production will reach 130 million tons of chicken meat in 2021, when it will become the most commonly consumed meat in the world (FAO, 2017). Hence, a well-functioning and healthy gut is the keystone for the optimum performances of the birds. As a result the intestinal tract is arguably the most important organ. Intestinal mucosa of chicken plays an important role in providing an effective barrier from the intestinal content and other internal organs and helps in digestion and absorption of nutrients. Of these factors the microbiota in the gut ecosystem seem to have essential roles as they aid in the development of gut morphology, transform the immune responses, offer protection from intestinal pathogens as well as support digestion and utilization of the nutrients (Rinttila¨ and Apajalahti, 2013). Yegani and Korver (2008) suggested that gut ecosystem is highly affected by diet, in which the changes in dietary composition may result in the alteration of the microbial ecosystem in the gut. In addition to that, some feed ingredients have showed to alter the gut microbiota and immune system which may be advantageous for the chicken.

Development of the Gastro-intestinal tract and Maturation of the Intestinal Microbiota

The embryonic small intestine size and weight increases at a much greater rate than body weight during incubation period. The small intestine continues to increase in weight more rapidly than the rest of body mass even after hatching along with enzymatic and absorptive activities which plays a major role in inducing early growth (Sklan, 2001). Early access to nutrients initiates growth rapidly about 24 hours after ingestion of exogenous feed for the first time after hatch. The digestive system of a chicken is simple, short, and extremely efficient. The mucosal layers of esophagus and crop are lined with incompletely keratinized stratified squamous epithelial cells which secrets mucus and is an important source of carbon, nitrogen, and energy for commensal as well as pathogenic bacteria inhabiting the gut mucosa (Pan and Yu, 2014).

The initial colonization of the gastrointestinal tract of birds occurs from the point of hatching or even before, by entry of microorganisms through the pores of the eggshell. Once hatched, the gastrointestinal tract of chickens becomes successively colonized by microorganisms like *Enterobacteriaceae* at first days of age and then *Firmicutes* at approximately from 7 days of age (Ballou, *et al.,* 2016). A sequence of growth of microorganisms take place and population density and complexity increases as the birds grow, until microbiota reaches a state of maturation and density stabilizes. In commercial chicken production, development times and density of intestinal microbiota species can vary greatly depending on the genetic conditions of the birds and other farm management factors (Ding, 2017). The environment of the crop, proventriculus and gizzard is slightly acidic and therefore, it forms a protective barrier for passage of pathogenic and zoonotic bacteria, to pass through the gut. Microflora composition of the crop is mainly dominated by Grampositive, facultative anaerobes *Lactobacilli* responsible for crop colonization (Classen *et al*., 2016). Besides that, Sarra *et al*. (1992) revealed that the crop has the ability to colonize *lactobacilli* to produce an amylolitic enzyme with a pH and temperature optimum of 5.2 to 6.3 and 40 to 50◦C, respectively.

Compositions of poultry gut ecosystem and its role

The gastrointestinal tract of poultry is habitat to a multifarious and dynamic microbial community (Zhu *et al.,* 2002). Researchers have found 640 distinct species and 140 bacterial genera in the GIT of poultry, where about 90% of the species are yet to be described (Yadav and Jha, 2019). Composition and density of microbiota depends on the microbial composition of the inoculum introduced at hatch, first diet and host intestinal epithelium. The initial bacteria grow very fast and the sterile environment soon becomes inhabited by 10^8 and 10^{10} bacteria per gram of digesta in ileum and cecum, respectively in 1–3 days (Apajalahti, 2002). Some of the commonly found microbes in the gastrointestinal tract of poultry are *Lactobacillus sp., Bacteroides sp., Eubacterium sp., Clostridium sp., Escherichia coli, Streptococcus sp., Prevotella sp., Fusobacterium sp., Selenomonas sp., Megasphaera sp., and Bifidobacterium sp.*

Some of the major roles are to help in the development of gut structures, boost immune responses, offers protection from pathogens, as well as in digestion and utilization of nutrients. Gut microbiota has also some direct and indirect harmful effects on chickens such as decrease in digestibility of fat, increase in cell turnover rate, production of toxic metabolites from the protein fermentation and may also lead to poor growth performance.

Gut microbiota provides nutritional compounds to the chicken in the form of fermentation end-products and other secreted products such as Short Chain Fatty Acids (SCFAs) such as acetate, propionate, butyrate, and lactate along with certain enzymes, amino acids, B and K vitamins. SCFAs also stimulate the gut epithelial, cell proliferation, differentiation and increase the villus height, thereby increasing the absorptive surface area. Acetate and propionate also act as an energy substrate for tissues (De *et al.*, 2014)

Lactobacillus producing bacteriocin Reuterin was found effective in inhibiting the growth of Salmonella, Shigella, Clostridium, and Listeria. (Naidu *et al.*, 1999). The digestive process is strongly linked to gut microbiota; nutrient absorption, feed digestibility, energy harvest and therefore productivity are influenced by microbiota composition and diversity. (Stanley *et al.,* 2013; Mancabelli *et al.* 2016). In this chapter, we will discuss some important feed costituents/feed additives and their application in the development and maintenance of gut ecosystem.

1. **Dietary protein:** Dietary protein is an important nutritional factor for maintaining gut ecosystem and immune homeostasis in the gastrointestinal tract. It efficiently modifies the microbial composition of the gut and modulates the production of antimicrobial peptides that hinder in the growth and production of pathogenic organisms by obstructing adhesion to the intestinal mucosa.

2. **Fiber and non-starch polysaccharides:** Dietary fibers have been found to influence the gut microbial ecosystem (Jha and Berrocoso, 2015). Dietary fiber polysaccharides and oligosaccharides are composed of relatively small numbers of monosaccharides e.g. glucose, galactose,

arabinose, xylose, fructose, mannose, rhamnose fucose and some of their uronic acid forms. Based on chemistry and accessibility of specific dietary fiber, it presents a huge potential to change gut microbiota. The unique ability of fiber to escape digestion and absorption provides the opportunity to regulate intestinal morphology, interact with nutrients of the digesta, interact with intestinal microflora, and modulate general digestive organ activity, resulting in changes in nutrient utilization and growth performance. However, inclusion of specific insoluble fiber types such as cellulose at 3–5% in the diet has often proven to improve nutrient utilization by modulating gastric secretions from the proventriculus and muscular activity of the gizzard (Sacranie *et al.*, 2012). Factors such as fiber type and particle size are determinant factors that stimulate the muscular activity of the gizzard, resulting in increased size of the same along with proventriculus as well as in improved feed conversion. Dietary fibre can also increase pancreas enzymatic activity and reverse peristalsis that can lead to an increase in nutrient digestibility. The presence of water-soluble non-starch polysaccharides (WS-NSP) leads to a change in gut microbiota population and diversity. Mathlouthi *et al.*, 2002 found an increase in Lactobacillus and coliforms along with other facultative bacteria population when the bird's diet was switched from corn-based to wheat or barley-based. In case of WS-NSP rich diets, the increase in viscosity of digestive content and transit time is noticed along with a higher production of short chain fatty acids which beneficially regulate ileal motility (Cherbut, 2003)

3. **Dietary fat:** Dietary fat type and level can affect digestion and microbiota (Danicke *et al.*, 1999) and coccidiosis can also affect the digestion of many nutrients, but specially fats (Ravidran *et al.*, 2016). However, it is important to maintain a minimum of 1% fat in the diet to stimulate gastric function and slow release of digesta from gizzard to the small intestine (Svihus, 2014).

   Care must be taken to avoid levels of mycotoxins in feedstuffs and rancid fats that exceed recommended limits (Murugesan *et al.,* 2015). Mycotoxins are able to compromise several functions of GIT resulting in decreased nutrient absorption by decreasing available surface area. Consequently, measures must be implemented by feedstuff to minimize grain damage and conditions that could increase mold or insect spoilage. Diets with a peroxide value of 74 or greater should be rejected, because they result in poorer feed conversion (McGill *et al.,* 2011). Proper storage conditions and transportation should be evaluated in order to control rancidity. The addition of antioxidants and mycotoxin binders to feed can reduce the effects of mycotoxins and peroxide (Yegani and Korver, 2008), thus ensuring optimal digestion and to maintain a healthy microbial ecosystem of the birds.

4. **Antibiotics and antimicrobials:** A subtherapeutic dose of antibiotics has been widely used in poultry industry for decades to improve the growth performance of chicken (Huyghebaert *et al.*, 2011). Antibiotics are either synthetic drugs or are obtained from natural sources and are acknowledged before to improve feed conversion and growth, and reduce morbidity and mortality due to clinical and subclinical diseases. Antibiotics may reduce the microbial load in the gut leading to more nutrient availability for the host. However, many controversies have been raised with the rising incidence of antibiotics resistance in chicken due to irregular use and overuse of these antibiotics (Kabir, 2009). Other negative impacts of the use of antibiotics as a growth promoter, have forced poultry farmers to stop or limit their use in feed. Use of antibiotics as prophylactic dose in animal feed has been banned in European Union (EC Regulation, No. 1831/ 2003) while others are considering or have imposed strict regulation on use or gradual ban in poultry farming. This ban has already added pressure to introduce immediate alternatives to antibiotics to maintain the balance of the gut as well as to improve the overall performance of the birds (Huyghebaert *et al.* 2015).

5. **Nutraceutical:** There are a number of feedstuffs that provide beneficial function leading to the development of the concept of nutraceuticals. In general, nutraceuticals can be defined as food or food components that have a role in modifying and maintaining normal physiological functions that support the healthy host (Das *et al.*, 2012). These nutraceuticals also help in protecting the host against infectious diseases (Cencic and Chingwaru, 2010). Nutraceuticals may range from isolated nutrients (vitamin, mineral, amino acids, fatty acids, etc.), herbal products (polyphenols, herbs, spices, etc.), dietary supplements (probiotics, prebiotics, synbiotics, organic acids, antioxidants, enzyme, etc.) to genetically modified foods.

6. **Probiotics:** Probiotics also referred as direct-fed microbial (DFM), are single or mixed cultures of living non-pathogenic microorganisms, which, when administered in adequate amounts present a health benefit on the host. Their mode of action involves multiple mechanisms, including competitive exclusion, promoting gut maturation and integrity, regulating the immune system, preventing inflammation, improving metabolism, improving growth, improve the fatty acid profile and oxidative stability in fresh meat, and neutralizing enterotoxins.

The species currently being supplemented as probiotics are mostly *Lactobacillus bulgaricus, Lactobacillus acidophilus, Lactobacillus casei, Lactobacillus helveticus, Lactobacillus lactis, Lactobacillus salivarius, Lactobacillus plantarum, Streptococcus thermophillus, Enterococcus faecium, Enterococcus faecalis, Bifidobacterium spp* and *E coli.* some of these are illustrated in Table 1.

Table 1: Examples of probiotic effects on the gut microbiota and immune system of chicken

Strain/type application	Biological activities	References
L.reuteri, L.gallinarum, L .brevis, L .salivaris	Lactobacillus and bifido bacter population is increased and E.coli counts are decreased in caeca.	Mookiah *et al*. (2014)
L. acidophilus	Induced T-helper-1 cytokines in caecal tonsil cells	Brisbin *et al*. (2010)
L. salivarius	Induced anti-inflammatory responses (interleukin [IL]-10 and transforming growth factor [TGF]-b) in caecal tonsil cells	Brisbin *et al*. (2010)
L.plantarum, L.bulgaricus, L.acidophilus, L.rhamnosus, B.bifidum, S.thermophilus, E. faecium, A. oryzae and C. pintolopessi	Increased antibody titre against Newcastle disease (ND). Increased the geometric means haemagglutination inhibition (HI) titres of birds	Khan *et al*. (2011)
Saccharomyces boulardii	Increase in intestinal villus height and crypt depth in the jejunum and ileum and goblet cell number.	Kumari and Susmita (2014)
Synbiotic 11 Lactobacillus strains plus IMO	Increased the caecal populations of lactobacilli and bifidobacteria and decreased the caecal E.coli	Mookiah *et al*. (2014)
Commercial synbiotics (BiominImbo)	Increased the LAB population and reduced E. coli and total coliform populations in the intestine	Amerah *et al*. (2012)
Bifidobacterium-based symbiotic product	Reduced C. jejuni concentration in poultry faeces	Baffoni *et al.* (2012)

Some other probiotics are microscopic fungi such as strains of yeast *Saccharomyces cerevisiae* spp. The dose and nature of probiotics administrated differ due to variation in the physiological state of the birds. Different species and/or strains of probiotics have different immunomodulatory activities and the ability of probiotics to induce cytokine production, which leads to modulation of immune responses (Brisbin *et al.,* 2010). Specifically, *Bacillus* sp. increased body weight and *Pediococcus pentosaceus* had higher average SCFAs content.

They also identified that cecal microbiota, Bacteroidetes abundance was directly correlated with the content of propionate, butyrate, and isobutyrate, whereas the abundance of *Firmicutes* positively correlates acetate production in the cecum.

Competitive exclusion (CE) is a concept where newly hatched chickens could be protected by dosing with a suspension of a healthy intestinal microbiota from a healthy adult host. This is also referred as Nurmi concept. This concept was originally developed to control *Salmonella* in chickens but now a days it has been expanded to involve other pathogenic bacteria like *E coli*, *C. perfingens, Listeria, Camylobacter* spp. In contrast to actual CE products which are non-defined mixed cultures, probiotics are defined cultures and CE products are not used to establish a complex intestinal microbiota but only to introduce one or few bacterial strains into the gut. Wide scale interest in the use of CE products has increased in recent years with the rise in negative effects of use of antimicrobials.

7. **Prebiotics:** Prebiotics are non-digestible feed ingredients that beneficially affect the host by selectively altering the composition and metabolism of the gut microbiota. The capacity of prebiotics to increase the number of microbes in the gut is constructive for the host health against the pathogens in the gastrointestinal tract. The most common prebiotics used in poultry are oligosaccharides, including inulin, fructooligosaccharides (FOS), mannanoligosaccharides (MOS), galactooligosaccharides (GOS), soya-oligosaccharides (SOS), xylo-oligosaccharides (XOS), pyrodextrins, isomaltooligosaccharides (IMO) and lactulose. The mechanism of action of prebiotics is determined by the nature and type of prebiotics. Dietary supplementation with FOS also decreases *C. perfringens* and *E. coli* and increases *Lactobacillus* diversity in the chicken gut. MOS have receptor properties for fimbriae of *E. coli* and *Salmonella spp.* which binds to them and excretes them with the digesta flow. Prebiotics tends to enhance defense mechanism thus boosting immunity via increasing the production of short chain fatty acids which leads to an acidic environment in the gut and suppresses pathogens, also recover some lost energy from competition with bacteria (Kim *et al*., 2017). Some examples of prebiotic effecting on the gut microbiota and immune system of chicken are given in Table 2.

Table 2: Examples of prebiotic effects on the gut microbiota and immune system of chicken

Type of prebiotics	Biological activities	References
FOS	Reduced intestinal colonization by Salmonella	Bailey *et al.* (1991)
FOS or MOS	Decreased populations of C. perfringens and E. coli in the gut	Kim *et al.* (2011)
FOS	Provided nutrients for the growth of beneficial bacteria in the gut	Alloui *et al.* (2013)
FOS	Increased the population of Bifidobacterium in the small intestine and colon. Increased the population and diversity of lactobacilli in the ileum	Kim *et al.* (2011)
Inulin	Increased Bifidobacterium counts and decreased *E. coli* counts in caecal contents	Nabizadeh (2012)
GOS	Increased Bifidobacterium spp. and decreased Campylobacter spp. in the faecal samples	Baffoni *et al.* (2012)
IMO	Increased the caecal populations of lactobacilli and bifidobacteria and decreased the caecal E. coli	Mookiah *et al.* (2014)
FOS or MOS	Affected the heterophil:lymphocyte ratio and basophil levels	Kim *et al.* (2011)
FOS and MOS	Increased serum concentration of IgA	Kim *et al.* (2009)
MOS	Increased serum concentration of IgG and IgM	Cetin *et al.* (2005)
Commercial prebiotic (Fibregum and Raftifeed- IPE))	Increased serum concentration of IgA and IgM, and enhanced systemic immune capacity in chickens	Vidanarachchi *et al.* (2013)
FOS	Enhanced the IgM and IgG antibody titres in plasma	Janardhana *et al.* (2009)
Prebiotic-based MOS and b-glucan	Increased the relative weight of spleen, decreased the heterophil-to-lymphocyte ratio and increased antibody titres against S. enteritidis	Sadeghi *et al.* (2013)

8. **Organic acids or Acidifiers:** Organic acids are the common constituents of the plant and animal tissues. Organic acids have been found to possess antimicrobial properties helpful in controlling the population of pathogenic bacteria in the gut of birds (Partanen and Mroz, 1999). The capacity of organic acids to transform from undissociated to dissociated form, higher pKa value and hydrophobicity of acids may determine its effectiveness as antimicrobial agents in the gut microbiota of birds. In the undissociated form, these can freely diffuse through the semi-permeable membrane of the bacteria into the cell cytoplasm (Van Immerseel *et al.*, 2006). The mode of action of organic acids includes reduction of pH, feed buffering capacity, energy provision and antimicrobial action. Organic acids can be classified

into three types- Short chain fatty acids, Medium chain fatty acids and Tricarboxylic acids. The common medium chain fatty acids are lauric acid, capric acids, caprylic acids and caproic acids. Lauric acid has the greatest antimicrobial effect of all medium chain fatty acids and it is active against Gram positive bacteria. Whereas, examples of Short chain fatty acids are acetic acids, propionic acids and butyric acids. Tricarboxylic acids are citric acids, malic acid and fumaric acid. Other organic acids widely used are benzoic, sorbic and lactic acids.

When the pH reaches around 7, the acid will dissociate and suppress bacterial cell enzymes (e.g., decarboxylases and catalases) and nutrient transport systems (Huyghebaert *et al.*, 2011). Use of organic acids or acidifiers improves protein digestion by reducing the buffering capacity of feed. Thereby ultimately enhance healthier gut ecosystem by reducing availability of undigested protein for pathogenic bacteria.

9. **Enzymes:** Poultry diets are mostly comprised of corn and soyabean based meals and these ingredients tend to have various anti nutritive factors which have adverse effects on the health of the chickens. The different anti-nutritive factors such as non-starch polysaccharides (NSP) and protease inhibitors can hinder normal digestion and absorption processes of nutrients in the digestive tract. In this circumstance, the exogenous enzymes are mostly used to correct the lack of specific endogenous enzymes for digesting certain nutrients in various feed ingredients or to hydrolyse anti-nutritional factors present in the feed ingredients. Commonly used exogenous enzymes in poultry diets are β-glucanase, xylanase, amylase, α-galactosidase, protease, lipase, and phytase.

   Adeola and Cowieson (2011) revealed that carbohydrase (such as Xylases, gluconases) supplementation increased the proportion of lactic and organic acids, reduced ammonia production, and increased fatty acids concentration which is indicative of hydrolysis fragmentation of NSP and supporting growth of beneficial bacteria and also allow to obtain energy from the diet. Phytases enhance the release of phosphorus and trace minerals from plant phytate breaks it down before it binds the protein, avoiding the anti-nutritive effect and improving nutrient uptake for a better functioning gut. Ultimately, this results in less availability of undigested protein, reducing protein fermentation and potentially reducing ammonia production. Proteases and lipases act by breaking down protein and fat. Xylanase in the diet reduced the number of *Coliform* and *Salmonella*, and increased the number of *Lactobacillus* in the ileum of chicken (Nian *et al.*, 2011).

To obtain the maximum benefit, the use of multiple enzymes is suggested as the combination of the enzymes as cocktail enzymes or tailored enzymes can be used to target different anti-nutritive compounds in the feedstuffs. It should also be noted that the beneficial effect of enzyme combination may be dependent on the diet composition (Meng *et al.*, 2005) and how the enzymes work together to hydrolyze their respective substrates is crucial to maximize the efficacy of enzyme combinations.

10. **Phytobiotics:** Phytobiotics are plant-derived natural bioactive compounds that can be added to the poultry feed to improve the performance of the birds. The active compounds of phytobiotics are mostly terpenoids, phenolics (tannins), glycosides and alkaloids. Antimicrobial activity and immune enhancement probably are the two major properties of phytobiotics which are essential for the health and overall well-being of the chicken (Fallah *et al.*, 2013).

    Following are some of the possible mechanism of action of phytobiotics. First by modulating the cell membrane of microbes leading to their membrane disruption and secondly, increasing the hydrophobicity of the microbial species affecting the surface characteristics of microbial cells and thereby affects the pathogenic properties of the microbes. Another is by stimulating the growth of favourable bacteria such as *Lactobacilli* and *Bifidobacteria* in the gut. Phytobiotics act as an immunomodulatory substance and protect the intestinal tissue from microbial attack. The phytobiotics especially those from the group of essential oils have been reported to improve flavour and palatability of feed and may thus improve the feed intake and performance of chickens. Eucalyptus oil, carvacrol, thymol are plant based oils used in broiler production and are known for their effect on *E coli* and *Clostridium* causing necrotic enteritis. Recent developments show use of coated essential oil blend that ensures that the active ingredients remain in stable state during feed processing. Phytogenic compounds show the ability to stimulate the proliferation and growth of absorptive cells in the gastrointestinal tract resulting in greater villus height and deeper crypt.

11. **Polyunsaturated fatty acids:** Polyunsaturated fatty acids include n-3 and n-6 fatty acids are essential for body immunity. Dietary n-3 PUFAs (combination of sunflower oil and palm oil) improved the immune response of birds, as evidenced by the increase in spleen weight, and infectious bronchitis disease (IBD) and ND antibody titres and IL-2 and IFN-c concentrations.

    Study showed that n-3 PUFAs possess antimicrobial activities. Altogether, the biological variations of birds (e.g., strain, sex, age, etc.), type of the essential fatty acids, dietary composition and the ratio between n-3 to n-6 fatty acids in the diet seem to affect the immune response of birds fed PUFAs. Microalgae are unicellular, photosynthetic aquatic plants, introduced to poultry diets mainly as a rich source of n-3 long chain PUFA, including docohexaenoic and eicosapentaenoic acid, but they can also serve as a protein, microelement, vitamin and antioxidant source, as well as a pigmentation agent for skin and egg yolks. Different species of microalgae as *Spirulina, Chlorella* and others proved positive influences on poultry nutrition. Red algal extracts up regulates the expression of genes responsible for establishment of gut ecosystem and prevention of pathogenic colonies.

12. **Water quality:** Good quality water is essential for proper digestion and to create a healthy gut ecosystem as it will help absorb all the essential nutrients. Providing good quality water with adequate quantity is also important for poultry performance so, its physicochemical characteristics should be measured, controlled and improved at the farm level. The pH should be maintained slightly acidic, (5.5-7), because basic water reduces the activity of most digestive enzymes. Lower the pH can help in reducing the bacterial population and also help in protein digestion. Adding an enhanced acidifier will deliver additional performance benefits as well as reducing the level of bacteria in water. Biofilm are complex communities of a matrix of different species of microbial cells and are firmly adhered to surfaces (Xavier and Foster, 2007). Biofilm bacteria are different from their free-living planktonic in terms of growth rate and composition, and show increased level of resistance to disinfectants (Oliveira *et al*., 2010). Water system biofilm can harbor pathogens such as *Campylobacter, Salmonella, Escherichia coli* including avian pathogenic (APEC) strains, *Pseudomonas*; including protozoans, and viruses thus develop the threat of flock to these pathogens (Dou *et al.,* 2016). Birds, particularly chicks, remain vulnerable to microbial challenges from biofilm (Zimmer *et al.,* 2003).

13. **Good management practices:** Managemental conditions like optimum temperature, air velocity, and relative humidity according to the age, production stage, size of the birds and external environmental conditions are important for health, poultry productivity (Kocaman *et al*., 2006) and control of pathogens. With broilers, layers, turkeys, and ducks, environmental stress due to heat or cold, very dry or very humid air, or drafts can alter their feed intake patterns and intestinal motility thereby causing reduced digestion and the ensuing gut problems. All environmental stresses adversely affect the immunological system of birds, upto the extent

that they cannot maintain microbial load inside the GIT and translocation of bacteria to the bloodstream can occur. Lighting patterns may also show impact on feed intake, gut motility and digestion (Olanrewaju *et al.*, 2006).

14. **Effect of Feed Processing on Gut Health:** Finer feed particle size enables optimal nutrient utilization and enhances birds' performance due to increased surface area permitting better action of digestive enzymes. But, there is permissible limit for the fineness of the feed particle size, as very fine particles result in adverse effect on gut causing higher incidences of gizzard dysfunction in poultry. Coarse particle size increases gut acidification which may favor in controlling proliferation of enteric pathogens such as *C. perfringens, Salmonella* and *E. coli.*

    There are many advantages that can be accredited to feed processing, comprising availability of nutrients, destruction of inhibitors and toxins, facilitating use of different ingredients in diet formulations, production of hygienic feed, and reduction of feed wastage. However, the various processing parameters such as particle modification, processing temperature, pressure, duration, and water determine the physical and chemical reactions in and between nutrients as well as the adhesive properties on the feed particle surfaces, the final physicochemical structure and the cleanliness of the feed. These attributes can directly or indirectly influence on the digestive tract ecology and thus animal health, performance, and feed cost.

Other advanced methods for improving gut ecosystem

1. **Microbiota engineering:** Microbiota engineering involves amplifying the innate benefits provided by a commensal bacteria or probiotic via recombinant expression of the therapeutic molecules or functions (Kali, 2015). Subtractive therapies would use targeted antimicrobials, such as bacteriophages and bacteriocins, to selectively remove pathogenic bacteria from the microbiota leaving the beneficial microbes to develop a new microbial community that provides improved gut health and increased birds performance. Supplementation or introduction of bacteriophages would be a valid mechanism for enhancing naturally occurring levels of beneficial bacteria and/or removing harmful bacteria, preventing detrimental establishment of enteric pathogens, and treating diseases.

   Bacteriocins are a class of bacterially produced, ribosomally synthesized peptides with antimicrobial activity that can be narrow or broad in their spectra of activity. Bacteriocins, occupy a precise intestinal commensal bacterial place that can influence competition in the gastrointestinal tract effective enough approach to specifically eliminate intestinal colonization by deleterious bacteria, without major disruption of the indigenous microbiota (Kommineni *et al.*, 2015)

2. **Use of spray dried plasma:** Dried spray plasma can be used in young chicks and is a highly digestible and palatable ingredient. It is prepared from fresh blood collected from healthy animals and subjected to heating to inactivate the microorganisms. It is highly digestible, readily absorbed and thus improve the integrity of gut wall. Dried plasma contain significant amount of antibodies that prevents infection of the gut ecosystem and plays significant role in immune modulation. Studies have revealed outstanding result when used in juvenile chicks with reduced mortality.
3. **nfluence of Climate and Seasonal Changes:** The chicken under intensive breeding needs a scrupulous charge of the conditions mainly the temperature and the relative humidity in the commercial enterprises to optimize the growth of the birds. However, even when regulating the internal factors of the poultry house, external climatic conditions, particularly extreme heat, can negatively affect chicken gut health and productivity (Farag and Alagawany, 2018). Again, many studies reported differences in the gut microbiota profiles of poultry according to geographic location (Pandit *et al.*, 2018)

Conclusion

Intestinal microbiota is considered to be a crucial player in maintaining the health of the host by modulating several physiological functions including nutrition, metabolism, and immunity. The digestive process is strongly linked to gut microbiota; nutrient absorption, feed digestibility, energy harvest and therefore, productivity are influenced by microbiota composition and diversity.

References

Adeola, O. and Cowieson, A.J. 2011. Board-invited review: opportunities and challenges in using exogenous enzymes to improve nonruminant animal production. Journal of Animal Science, 89(10), pp.3189-3218.

Apajalahti J, Kettunen A, Graham H. 2004. Characteristics of the gastrointestinal microbial communities, with special reference to the chicken. Worlds Poultry Science Journal, 60(2):223–32.

Bailey, R A. 2010. Intestinal microbiota and the pathogenesis of dysbacteriosis in broiler chickens. PhD thesis submitted to the University of East Anglia. Institute of Food Research, United Kingdom

Ballou, A.L., Ali, R.A., Mendoza, M.A., Ellis, J.C., Hassan, H.M., Croom, W.J. and Koci, M.D. 2016. Development of the chick microbiome: how early exposure influences future microbial diversity. Frontiers in Veterinary Science, 3, pp 2.

Brisbin, J.T., Gong, J., Parvizi, P. and Sharif, S. 2010. Effects of lactobacilli on cytokine expression by chicken spleen and cecal tonsil cells. Clinical and Vaccine Immunology, 17(9): 1337-1343.

Cherbut, C. 2003. Motor effects of short-chain fatty acids and lactate in the gastrointestinal tract. Proceedings of the Nutrition Society, 62(1): 95-99.

Classen, H. L., Apajalahti, J., Svihus, B. and Choct, M. 2016. The role of the crop in poultry production. Worlds Poultry Science Journal, 72: 459–472.

De Vadder F, Kovatcheva-Datchary P, Goncalves D, Vinera J, Zitoun C, Duchampt A, et al. 2014. Microbiota-generated metabolites promote metabolic benefits via gut-brain neural circuits. Cell, 156(1): 84–96.

Ding, J., Dai, R., Yang, L., He, C., Xu, K., Liu, S., Zhao, W., Xiao, L., Luo, L., Zhang, Y. and Meng, H. 2017. Inheritance and establishment of gut microbiota in chickens. Frontiers in Microbiology, 8: 1967.

Ewing, W.N. and Cole, D.J.A.1994. The living gut: an introduction to micro-organisms in nutrition. Context Publications.

Fallah, R., Kiani, A., Azarfar, A. 2013. A review of the role of five kinds of alternatives to infeed antibiotics in broiler production. Journal of Veterinary Medicine and Animal Health, 5: 317–321.

Farag, M.R. and Alagawany, M., 2018. Physiological alterations of poultry to the high environmental temperature. Journal of Thermal Biology, 76: 101-106.

Hartini, S., Choct, M., Hinch, G., Kocher, A. & Nolan, J.V. 2002. Effects of light intensity during rearing, beak trimming and dietary fibre sources on mortality, egg production and performance of ISA brown laying hens. Journal of Applied Poultry Research, 11: 104–110.

Huyghebaert, G., Ducatelle, R., Van Immerseel, F. 2011. An update on alternatives to antimicrobial growth promoters for broilers. Veterinary Journal, 187: 182–188.

Jha. R. and Berrocoso, J.D. 2015. Dietary fiber utilization and its effects on physiological functions and gut health of swine. Animal, 9(9): 1441–52.

Kabir, S.M.L. 2009. The role of probiotics in the poultry industry. International Journal of Molecular Science, 10: 3531–3546.

Kali, A. 2015. Human microbiome engineering: the future and beyond. Journal of Clinical and Diagnostic Research, 9(9): DE01.

Kers, J.G., Velkers, F.C., Fischer, E.A., Hermes, G.D., Stegeman, J.A. and Smidt, H. 2018. Host and environmental factors affecting the intestinal microbiota in chickens. Frontiers in Microbiology, 9: 235.

Kommineni, S., Bretl, D.J., Lam, V., Chakraboty, R., Hayward, M., Simpson, P., Cao, Y., Bousounios, P., Kristich, C.J., Salzman, N.H. 2015. Bacteriocin production augments niche competition by enterococci in the mammalian gastrointestinal tract. Nature, 576: 719–722.

Mancabelli, L., Ferrario, C., Milani, C., Mangifesta, M., Turroni, F., Duranti, S., Lugli, G.A., Viappiani, A., Ossiprandi, M.C., van Sinderen, D. and Ventura, M. 2016. Insights into the biodiversity of the gut microbiota of broiler chickens. Environmental Microbiology, 18(12): 4727-4738.

Mathlouthi, N., Mallet, S., Saulnier, L., Quemener, B. and Larbier, M. 2002. Effects of xylanase and β-glucanase addition on performance, nutrient digestibility, and physico-chemical conditions in the small intestine contents and caecal microflora of broiler chickens fed a wheat and barley-based diet. Animal Research, 51(05): 395-406.

Murugesan, G.R., Ledoux, D.R., Naehrer, K., Berthiller, F., Applegate, T.J., Grenier, B., Phillips, T.D., Schatzmayr, G. 2015. Prevalence and effects of mycotoxins on poultry health and performance, and recent development in mycotoxin counteracting strategies. Poultry Science, 94: 1298–1315.

Naidu, A.S., Bidlack, W.R. and Clemens, R.A. 1999. Probiotic spectra of lactic acid bacteria (LAB). Critical Reviews in Food Science and Nutrition, 39(1): 13-126.

Nian, F., Guo, Y.M., Ru, Y.J., Li, F.D., Pe′ron, A. 2011. Effect of exogenous xylanase supplementation on the performance, net energy and gut microflora of broiler chickens fed wheat-based diets. Asian-Australian Journal of Animal Science, 24: 400–406.

OECD/FAO. 2017. OECD-FAO Agricultural Outlook 2017–2026; OECD-FAO Agricultural Outlook; OECD: Paris, France, ISBN 9789264275478

Pan, D., and Yu, Z. 2014. Intestinal microbiome of poultry and itsinteraction with host and diet. Gut Microbes, 5: 108–119.

Pandit, R.J., Hinsu, A.T., Patel, N.V., Koringa, P.G., Jakhesara, S.J., Thakkar, J.R., Shah, T.M., Limon, G., Psifidi, A., Guitian, J. and Hume, D.A. 2018. Microbial diversity and community composition of caecal microbiota in commercial and indigenous Indian chickens determined using 16s rDNA amplicon sequencing. Microbiome, 6: 1-13.

Partanen, K.H. and Mroz, Z. 1999. Organic acids for performance enhancement in pig diets. Nutrition Review, 12: 117–145.

Rehman, H. U., W. Vahjen, W. A. Awad, and J. Zentek. 2007. Indigenous bacteria and bacterial metabolic products in the gastrointestinal tract of broiler chickens. Archives of Animal Nutrition, 61: 319–335.

Rinttila, T. and Apajalahti, J. 2013. Intestinal microbiota and metabolites-implications for broiler chicken health and performance. Journal of Applied Poultry Research, 22: 647–658.

Sacranie, A., Svihus, B., Denstadli, V., Moen, B., Iji, P.A. and Choct, M. 2012. The effect of insoluble fiber and intermittent feeding on gizzard development, gut motility, and performance of broiler chickens. Poultry Science, 91(3): 693-700.

Santovito, E., Greco, D., D'Ascanio, V., Marquis, V., Raspoet, R., Logrieco, A.F. and Avantaggiato, G. 2019. Equilibrium isotherm approach to measure the capability of yeast cell wall to adsorb Clostridium perfringens. Foodborne Pathogens and Disease, 16(9): 630-637.

Sarra, P. G., Morelli, L. and Bottazzi, V. 1992. The lactic microflora of fowl. Pages 3–19 in The Lactic Acid Bacteria in Health and Disease. B. J. B. Wood ed. Springer, Boston, MA, USA.

Sekelja, M., Rud, I., Knutsen, S.H., Denstadli, V., Westereng, B., Naes, T. and Rudi, K. 2012. Abrupt temporal fluctuations in the chicken fecal microbiota are explained by its gastrointestinal origin. Applied and Environmental Microbiology, 78(8): 2941-2948.

Sklan, D. 2001. Development of the digestive tract of poultry. World's Poultry Science Journal, 57: 415–427.

Stanley, D., Geier, M.S., Denman, S.E., Haring, V.R., Crowley, T.M., Hughes, R.J. and Moore, R.J. 2013. Identification of chicken intestinal microbiota correlated with the efficiency of energy extraction from feed. Veterinary Microbiology, 164(1-2): 85-92.

Van Immerseel, F., Russell, J.B., Flythe, M.D., Gantois, I., Timbermont, L., Pasmans, F., Haesebrouck, F., Ducatelle, R. 2006. The use of organic acids to combat Salmonella in poultry: a mechanistic explanation of the efficacy. Avian Pathology, 35: 182–188.

Yegani, M. and Korver, D.R. 2008. Factors affecting intestinal health in poultry. Poultry Science, 87: 2052–2063.

Zhu, X.Y., Zhong, T., Pandya, Y. and Joerger, R.D. 2002. 16S rRNA-based analysis of microbiota from the cecum of broiler chickens. Applied and Environmental Microbiology, 68(1): 124-137.

7

Latest Trends in Feed Additives in Chicken Nutrition

Amitav Bhattacharyya and Pankaj Kumar Shukla

Department of Poultry Science, College of Veterinary Science and Animal and Animal Husbandry, DUVASU, Mathura

Introduction

Over the years, antibiotics have been used at sub therapeutic levels for enhancing the production and immunity of birds. The advantages of using antibiotics as feed supplements in terms of improvement of growth and feed efficiency have been well documented. However, the growing concern over the transmission and the proliferation of resistant bacteria via the food chain led to a ban on the use of antibiotic growth promoters (AGP) in livestock within the European Union in 2006.Thus, quest for alternatives to AGP gained momentum in the first decade of this century. There has been emergence of various feed additives like prebiotics, probiotics, organic acids, enzymes, essential oils, fatty acids, phytobiotics etc. Feed additives are used in to elicit the production performance and health of chicken. Further, feed additives are also used to improve the quality of feed and chicken products. In this chapter, the role of important feed additives in chicken shall be briefly discussed.

1. **Probiotics:** 'Probiotic' is a word derived from Greek word 'pro' and 'biotic' meaning 'for life'. Probiotics are live microbial feed supplements, which beneficially affect poultry by improving the intestinal microbial balance. Probiotics may be classified into two major types: viable microbial cultures *viz. Lactobacilli, Streptococci, Bacillus etc* and microbial fermentation products.

Mechanism of action

Several mechanisms have been postulated to explain the mode of action of probiotics. They are as follows:

- Probiotics cause beneficial changes in the gut flora with reduction in population of *E. coli* and thus reduce the release of toxins. Lactobacilli, the most common microbe of probiotics compete with coliforms and pathogenic microorganisms for the site of adherence on the intestinal surface.

- Probiotics like lactobacillus increase lactic acid production with subsequent change in intestinal pH. Lactic acid release in the intestine reduces the pH up to 4.5, which is lethal for pathogens but allow the growth of some strains of Lactobacilli.
- Live yeast culture is capable of releasing phytase for phosphorous digestion, lipase for fat digestion and endotryptase for protein digestion. It triggers the growth of cellulolytic bacteria resulting into digestion of fibre portion of feed. The yeast also facilitates the growth of lactobacillus and ferments the carbohydrate. The fermentation products inactivate the intestinal toxins that reduce the appetite of poultry. Yeasts are also a rich source of vitamin B complex.

Beneficial effects

Use of probiotic in poultry diets improved FCR, carcass quality and immune-competence traits in poultry (Panda *et al.*, 2008, Tiwari *et al.*, 2012, Rajput *et al.*, 2019). It has also been noted that dietary supplementation of probiotics in broilers resulted in a significant reduction on the total serum cholesterol concentration and crop *Escherichia coli* count (Panda *et al.*, 2001). Use of probiotics in layer diets resulted in better hen body weight, egg production, egg weight, egg mass, egg component percentages, egg shell thickness, egg shell weight, feed intake, feed conversion, livability, decrease in meat and blood spots and decreased egg yolk and serum cholesterol (Yakout *et al.*, 2004; Kurtoglu *et al.*, 2004).

2. **Prebiotics:** Prebiotic foods, either as natural components of food or as fermented food have been consumed for centuries. However, in the later 1800s and early 1900, interest in dietary use of prebiotics blossomed. Prebiotic is a non-digestible food ingredient that beneficially affects the host by selectivity stimulating the growth and/or activity of one or limited number of bacteria in the colon, and thus improves host health (Gibson and Roberfroid, 1995). Based on this definition, Russell (1998) formulated the criteria according to which a substance can be a prebiotic. Firstly, prebiotics are always feed ingredients that are not digested by the host, not or little used and/or metabolised as they pass through the upper portion of the intestinal tract, so they can reach the flora of the large intestine. Secondly, they have to be able to serve as a substrate for one or more bacterial species with a potentially beneficial effect on the host. Finally, they have to be able to cause a shift in the microflora that improves the health of the host.

The most important monosaccharide prebiotics are pentoses and hexoses. These monosaccharides can form the basis for enzymatically constructed oligo or polysaccharides. Isomerization products of disaccharides can be used as prebiotics e.g. lactulose (based on lactose). Lactose, lactulose and lactosucrose have prebiotic effects in chickens. The most important polysaccharide prebiotic for chickens is guar gum, produced from the seeds of the guar bean, *Cyamopsis tetragonolobus*.

Another classification is based on the source of origin of prebiotics: natural or synthetic saccharides (Iji and Tivey, 1998). Examples of natural sources are soybeans, oil palm kernels, white lupin, blue lupin, chick pea and black gram. Synthetic oligosaccharides are lactulose, mannan-oligosaccharides and isomalto-oligosaccharides etc.

Mechanism of action

Prebiotics can have a direct effect either by direct binding of pathogens or by increasing the osmotic value in the intestinal lumen. However, their effects are mostly indirect, mediated by metabolites, which are generated by the intestinal flora that uses the prebiotics for their own metabolism. Such metabolites include short-chain fatty acids, lactate, polyamines and bactericins.

Beneficial effects

Prebiotics increase biomass and stool bulking. It increases production of volatile fatty acids. Prebiotics also improves mineral absorption and enhances vitamin-B synthesis. It lowers serum cholesterol. Prebiotics also increase the beneficial bacteria and limit foodborne pathogens in the GIT of chickens (Ricke, 2018; Santovito *et al.*, 2018). Prebiotics have been found to minimize the incidence of ascites (Santos *et al.*, 2005). Prebiotics also lower egg cholesterol (Chen *et al.*, 2005a), increase egg production and feed efficiency of layers (Chen *et al.*, 2005b) and improve eggshell quality (Chen and Chen, 2004). Inclusion of MOS @ 0.5g/kg significantly enhanced serum antibody titre against sheep red blood cells and increased macrophage activity in chickens (Shao *et al.*, 2000). Including MOS in the diets of broilers containing aflatoxins led to significant improvement in titre values against Newcastle disease and infectious bursal disease (Swamy and Devegowda, 1998). MOS has also been found to lower the total egg and serum cholesterol and LDL cholesterol in layers when provided with 1.0 g/kg in the ration (Stanley and Sefton, 1999).

A combination of probiotics and prebiotics is known as synbiotic. This combination could improve the survival of the probiotic organism, because its specific substrate is available for fermentation. Examples of synbiotics are FOS and bifido bacteria, lactilol and lactobacilli.

3. **Enzymes:** Efforts have been made to use unconventional feed ingredients, which have several anti-nutritional factors that adversely affect the performance of poultry. Exogenous feed enzymes improve nutrient digestibility and utilization, thereby mitigating the excreta output and lowering nutrient excretion, particularly excess nitrogen, phosphorus, zinc and copper (Abd El-Hack *et al.*, 2017a, b; Berwanger *et al.*, 2017; Rehman *et al.*, 2017). Enzymes are organic and biological catalysts that can initiate or accelerate biochemical reactions, converting one or more substrate into products. In other words, enzymes are protein molecules that catalyze specific chemical reactions. Several exogenous enzymes are being used in poultry to optimize the production and these have been enlisted in Table 1.

Table 1: Enzymes used in poultry feed

Enzyme	Classification	Production organism	Function
Phytase	Phosphatase	*Aspergillus* sp., *Penicillium* sp., *Phytase canola, Pichia pastoris, d- Aspergillus niger, d-Escherichia coli*	Hydrolyses phytate
Glucose oxidase	Oxidoreductase	*Aspergillus niger*	Degrades glucose to hydrogen peroxide and gluconic acid
Catalase	Oxidoreductase	*Aspergillus niger var., Micrococcus lysodeikticus*	Produces water and oxygen from hydrogen peroxide
Trypsin	Protease	Animal pancreas	Hydrolyzes proteins
Protease	Protease	*Aspergillus niger*, *Aspergillus* sp., *Bacillus* sp.	Hydrolyzes proteins
Pepsin	Protease	Animal stomachs	Hydrolyzes proteins
Papain	Protease	Papaya (*Carica papaya*)	Hydrolyzes proteins
Keratinase	Protease	*Bacillus licheniformis*	Hydrolyzes proteins
Ficain	Protease	*Ficus glabrata*	Hydrolyzes proteins
Bromelain	Protease	Pineapple (*Ananas cosmosus*) stem and fruit	Hydrolyzes proteins
Lipase	Lipase	*Aspergillus niger*, *Candida* sp., *Rhizomucor* sp., *Rhizopus* sp.	Hydrolyze triglycerides, diglycerides and glycerol monoesters
Xylanase	Carbohydrase	*Aspergillus* sp., *Bacillus* sp., *Humicola* sp., *Penicillum* sp., *Trichoderma*	Hydrolyzes xylans
Pullulanase	Carbohydrase	*Bacillus acidopullulyticus*	Hydrolyzes starch

Pectinase	Carbohydrase	*Aspergillus aculeatus*, *Aspergillus niger*, *Rhizopus oryzae*	Breaks down protein
β-Mannanase	Carbohydrase	*Aspergillus niger*, *Bacillus lentus*, *Trichoderma reeseic*	Hydrolyzes β-mannans
Lactase	Carbohydrase	*Aspergillus niger*, *Aspergillus oryzae*, *Candida pseudotropicalis*	Hydrolyzes lactose to glucose and galactose
Invertase	Carbohydrase	*Aspergillus niger*, *Saccharomyces* sp.	Hydrolyzes sucrose to glucose and fructose
Hemicellulase	Carbohydrase	*Aspergillus* sp., *Bacillus* sp., *Humicola* sp., *Trichoderma* sp	Breaks down hemicellulose
Glucoamylase (amylosglucosidase)	Carbohydrase	*Aspergillus niger*, *Aspergillus oryzae*, *Rhizopus niveus*, *Rhizopus oryzae*	Hydrolyzes starch with production of glucose
β-Glucosidase	Carbohydrase	*Aspergillus niger*	Hydrolyzes cellulose degradation products to glucose
β-Glucanase	Carbohydrase	*Aspergillus* sp., *Bacillus* sp.	Hydrolyzes β-glucans
α-Galactosidase	Carbohydrase	*Aspergillus niger*, *Morteirella vinaceae var Saccharomyces* sp.	Hydrolyzes oligosaccharides
Cellulase	Carbohydrase	*Aspergillus niger*	Breaks down cellulose
β-Amylase	Carbohydrase	Barley malt	Hydrolyzes starch with production of maltose
Maltogenic a-amylase	Carbohydrase	*Bacillus subtilis*, *d-Bacillus stearothermophilus*	Hydrolyzes starch with production of maltose
α-Amylase	Carbohydrase	*Aspergillus* sp., *Bacillus* sp., *Rhizopus* sp.	Hydrolyzes starch

(Munir and Maqsood, 2013)

4. **Organic acids:** An organic acid is an organic compound with acidic properties. The most common organic acids are the carboxylic acids, whose acidity is associated with their carboxyl group –COOH. Organic acids are both bacteriostatic and bactericidal.

Mechanism of action

As un-dissociated organic acids are lipophilic, they can cross the cell membrane of Gram negative bacteria, such as Salmonella. Once inside the cell, the higher cytosolic pH causes the acid to dissociate, releasing hydrogen ions, which consequently reduces the intracellular pH. Microbial metabolism is dependent on enzyme activity, which is depressed at lower pH. To restore the balance, the cell is forced to use energy to expel protons out across the membrane via the H+-ATPase pump. Over a period of exposure to an organic acid, this can be sufficient to kill cell. Expelling protons also leads to an accumulation of acid anions in the cell (Lambert and Stratford, 1998), which inhibits intracellular metabolic reactions, including the synthesis of macromolecules and disrupts internal membranes. Lactic acid bacteria are less sensitive to pH differential across the cell membrane and thus remain unaffected. Inhibition of microbial growth by this mode of action has been exploited for thousands of years in food preservation.

Beneficial effects

It has already been reported around four decades back that lactic acid bacteria (LAB) play an important role in absorption of vitamins D and K and formation of soluble salts of calcium and iron in broilers. Recently it has been observed that acidification of drinking water of poultry for the first 7 days of life, when the birds are first placed in the house, is considered critical, because the crop and intestinal microbial morphology would still be under development. Maintenance of low crop pH by LAB in newly hatched chicks and poults is critical. The acidified drinking water provides a second layer of protection to the LAB and helps to be established as crop's normal microbiota. Once the crop's LAB population has been established, the bird can maintain a low crop pH on its own as long as feed is available (Menconi *et al*., 2014 and Dawson, 2009).

The first 3 weeks of life comprise a critical period in chick's life for gut maturation. During this period, healthy birds perform at maximum potential without diverting energy towards immune response processes. It has been observed that pH of gastro intestinal tract (GIT) is reduced by butyric acid supplementation (Leeson *et al.,* 2005). Further, butyric acid may play a role in the development of intestinal epithelium (Rama Rao *et al.,* 2003). Acetic acid improves the heath of chicken due to higher production of pancreatic enzyme, which improves GIT health. Dietary inclusion of acetic acid may improve FCR, bodyweight and carcass yield in broilers (Denli *et al*., 2003; Abdel Fattah *et al*., 2008). Citric acid improves FCR, gut health immunity and live body weight in broilers (Chaveerach *et al.,* 2004; Mendez Albores *et al.,*

2005). Propionic acid has pH reducing property. It also improves gut health, FCR, immunity in broiler chicks at young stage (Dibner and Buttin, 2002).

It has also been reported that organic acid in diet increases hen day egg production and hen house egg production in layers (Chen and Chen, 2004). Level of gamma globulin is increased in broilers with dietary inclusion of organic acids (Rahmani and Speer, 2005).

5. **Essential Oils:** Essentials oils (EOs) also called volatile or ethereal oils are complex aromatic oils typically obtained from plant materials by the process of distillation and possess characteristic odour and are soluble in organic solvents like ether, benzene, acetone, etc. They exist either in volatile or liquid form at the ambient temperature. They are broadly divided into two classes: Terpenes and Phenylpropenes. Terpenes are sub–divided based on the 5–carbon isoprene unit (building block) into mono ($C10H6$), sesqui ($C15H24$) and diterpenes ($C20H32$), while the phenylpropenes consist of 6-carbon aromatic ring having a 3-carbon side chain (C6-C3 compounds).

Mechanism of action

1. Essential oils have antimicrobial activity. Carvacrol and thymol have anticoccidial action against *E. tenella* (Giannenas *et al*., 2003).
2. Essential oils have strong anti-inflammatory activity. Terpenoids and flavonoids suppress the metabolism of inflammatory prostaglandins (Craig, 2001).
3. Essential oils may have the potential for immune modulation. Hanieh *et al.* (2010) suggested that the immunomodulatory effect of garlic may be due to enhanced production of interleukins, tumor necrosis factor (TNF-α) and interferon (INF-γ).
4. Essential oils have antioxidant activity. They protect other biological molecules against oxidation by either donating hydrogen or an electron to free radicals or delocalize the unpaired electron within the aromatic structure (Fernandez-Panchon *et al*., 2008).

Beneficial effects

Among diverse categories of essential oils, carvacrol, thymol and linalool are of immense importance, enriched with specific health strengthening virtues. Dietary essential oil supplementation has a positive effect on the growth performance and immunity in poultry (Gopi *et al*., 2012; Gopi *et al*., 2014; Du *et al*., 2016; Yang *et al*., 2018).

6. **Medium chain and short chain fatty acids:** Medium chain fatty acids (MCFA) are a group of fatty acids with 6 to 12 carbon atoms obtained

from edible fats such as coconut oil and milk fat by lipid fraction separation. Commercial medium chain fatty acid products usually have 8 to 10 carbon atoms. Short chain fatty acids (SCFA) contain up to 4 carbon atoms. MCFAs consist of greater amounts of lauric acid (C12) and smaller amounts of Capra fatty acids (C6, C8, and C10). They are more effectively absorbed and metabolized as compared to saturated long-chain fatty acids.

Mechanism of action

1. Fatty acids are generally inhibitory to microorganisms, but different fatty acids have different minimum inhibitory concentrations, depending on the type of fatty acid, type of microorganism and environmental pH.
2. MCFA has direct and strong antimicrobial effect on Gram+ bacteria. MCFA inhibit growth of pathogens and increase the digestibility that boosts the production and growth of birds. MCFA influence Salmonella virulence gene expression in birds (Van Immerseel *et al*., 2004). Lauric acids disrupt cytoplasm structure of bacterial cells (Shilling *et al*. 2013).
3. Low pH increases the concentration of dissociated SCFA, which can pass into the bacterial cells where the intercellular pH is higher. The higher pH dissociates the SCFA, so intracellular pH decreases and subsequently changes the metabolism of bacterial cell (Deschepper *et al*., 2013).

Beneficial effects

Laying rate, eggshell strength and eggshell thickness were significantly increased by supplementing medium chain monoglyceride at 300 mg/kg body weight (Liu *et al*. 2020). Dietary supplementation of MCFAs at 0.5% increased serum levels of IgM and interleukin 10 and had no significant influence on the serum level of complement 3 as compared to the control group (Shimaa *et al*., 2021). Studies on short chain fatty acids have already been mentioned in the section 'Organic Acids.'

SCFA has a synergestic effect with MCFA when added together as a feed additive in poultry. Combination of organic acids and MCFA significantly reduced clinical symptoms of diseases in artificial necrotic enteritis of broilers (Mathis *et al*., 2005). Further, Del Alamo *et al*. (2007) reported that addition of SCFA and MCFA together in feed of broilers infected with viral malabsorption syndrome enhanced growth and resulted in bigger body weight at the end of the production cycle.

7. **Phytobiotics:** Phytobiotics are plant derivatives that include herbs, plant extracts or spices and have a wide range of activities such as stimulation of feed intake, growth and act as immunomodulators. Most of the phytobiotics are rich in essential oils. The mechanism of action of essential oils has been

discussed in detail in the section 'Essential oils'. In recent years, several studies have been carried out to test the efficacy of phytobiotics on the growth, immunocompetence and production traits in poultry. However, it is beyond the scope of this chapter to discuss all of them. Hence, an attempt has been made to briefly discuss the role of some commonly used phytobiotics in poultry especially chicken.

1. *Curcuma longa (haldi):* Studies have been undertaken on the effect of *Curcuma longa* on the growth and immunocompetence traits in poultry. Sultan (2003) reported that turmeric at a level of 0.5% in the feed enhances overall performance of broiler chickens. Further, Rajput *et al.* (2019) reported that supplementation of 0.5% of turmeric powder resulted in better FCR and significantly higher immunocompetence traits in turkey poults.
2. *Emblica officinalis (Amla):* Fruits of *Emblica officinalis* are rich in vitamin C. However, Bhattacharya *et al.* (1999) had earlier reported that the antioxidant activity of *E. officinalis* may reside in the tannoids of the fruits of the plant, which have vitamin C like properties, rather than vitamin C itself. It has been observed that *Emblica officinalis* strengthened the defence mechanisms against free radical damage induced during stress (Rege *et al.*, 1999). Bhattacharya *et al.* (2000) also concluded that anti-stress activity of *E. officinalis* may be partly due to its tendency to normalize stress-induced perturbations in oxidative free radical scavenging activity as several stress related diseases may be related to accumulation of oxidative free radicals in different tissues. Dietary supplementation of 1% amla pulp powder resulted in better FCR and significantly higher immunocompetence traits in turkey poults (Rajput *et al.* 2019).
3. *Ocimum sanctum (Tulsi):* Tulsi (*Ocimum sanctum*) contains a volatile oil consisting of about 70% eugenols as well as methyl eugenol and caryophyllene. Other constituents with likely pharmacological activity include the triterpenoidursonic acid, rosmarinic acid, alkalids, saponins, flavonoids (including apigenin and luteolin and glycosides thereof), phenylpropane glucosides and tannins. The seeds of tulsi contain affixed oil containing five fatty acids, including about 17% linolenic acid and just over 50% linoleic acid. Lanjewar *et al.* (2008) reported that supplementation of tulsi leaf powder @ 0.5% and 1.0% significantly increased the final body weight and weekly body weight gain in broiler chicken. Further, it was noted that supplementation of tulsi leaf powder @ 1.0% in broiler diet reduced the meat and serum cholesterol with increase in serum HDL–cholesterol. Kumar *et al.* (2019) reported that dietary supplementation of dietary supplementation of 0.5% Tulsi leaf powder resulted in better FCR and immunocompetence traits in commercial broilers.

4. *Hippophae rhamnoides (Sea buckthorn):* Sea buckthorn (SBT) is a naturally growing shrub that is native to eastern Europe and Asia and is found in the high altitudes of Indian Himalayan region. Leaves, stems, tubers, roots of sea buckthorn contain a high content of vitamin C and also carotenoids, polyphenols, flavonoids, tocopherols, alkaloids, chlorophyll derivatives, amino acids, amines and high content of essential oils (Singh *et al.*, 2006). *Hippophae* leaves contain significant amounts of proteins (20.7%), amino acids (0.73% lysine, 0.13% methionine and cystine) minerals (Ca, Mg and K), folic acid, catechins, esterified sterols, triterpenols and isoprenols (Guan *et al.*, 2005; Biswas *et al.*, 2010). Tannins hippophaenins A and B have been isolated from SBT leaf (Kumar *et al.*, 2011). Biswas *et al.* (2010) stated that weight and egg rate of poultry are increased greatly after feeding poultry with leaves, seeds and fruit residues of SBT. Chen *et al.* (2011) observed that 0.5% SBT leaves improved the growth performance in broilers and 1% SBT leaves improved absorption of the calcium and phosphorous and the deposition of calcium. Sharma *et al.* (2018) reported that supplementation of sea buckthorn leaf meal @ 0.5% elicited production performance of turkey poults.

5. *Tinospora cordifolia* (*Giloe):* Giloe is a deciduous climbing shrub. Stem powder of *Tinospora cordifolia* at 0.1% level, when fed to coloured broilers through feed resulted in increase in overall bodyweight gain (Kulkarni *et al.*, 2011). Sharma *et al.* (2018) noted that HA and IgM response to 1% SRBC was comparatively better in the 0.5% giloe leaf meal supplemented group as compared to the control group.

6. *Asparagus racemosus (Shatavari):* Shatavari contains four steroid saponins: Shatavarins 1 to 4. Efforts have been made to study the effect of dietary supplementation of Shatavari root powder on production performance and immunity of chicken (Dahale *et al*., 2014, Yadav *et al*., 2018).

7. *Moringa oleifera (Moringa):* Moringa leaves have been reported to enhance the shelf life of fat containing foods due to the presence of various types of antioxidant compounds such as ascorbic acid, flavonoids, phenolics and carotenoids (Siddhuraju and Becker, 2003). Leaves of moringa tree are preferred for use in animal diets as leaf meal. It has been incorporated in the poultry diet by nutritionists to examine its effects on productive performance of broilers and laying hens (Banjo, 2012; Moreki and Kenaleone, 2014). Patel *et al.* (2019) observed that dietary supplementation of 1% moringa leaf meal resulted in significantly higher humoral immune response in chicken.

8. *Mint:* Mentha also known as mint contains various types of essential oils, such as menthol, mentone, cavone, methyl acetate and piperitone. These essential oils promote biological effects such as antimicrobial growth, anti-oxidation and stimulation of bile acid secretion, growth improvement and ammonia reduction in broilers. Studies have been undertaken on mint leaf meal as dietary supplement in poultry (Ameri *et al.*, 2016; Kumar *et al.*, 2019). It has been found that the supplementation of peppermint in diets has beneficial effects on growth performance, body temperature regulation and internal organ weight (Khempaka *et al.*, 2013; Arab *et al.*, 2016). Dietary supplementation of 0.75% mint leaf meal resulted in better growth performance after 4 weeks of age and significantly higher humoral and cell mediated immune response in coloured chicken (Kumar *et al.*, 2019).

Conclusion

The ban on the use of conventional growth promoters due to development of resistant antibiotic strains, antibiotic residues in humans food chain has reduced their utilization in the diet of poultry. There are several options like prebiotics, probiotics, enzymes, organic acids, phytogenics etc that can be used as growth promoters, though their activity is not at par with antibiotics but, they can be used in the diet of poultry for safe and quality meat production.

References

Abd El-Hack, M.E., Alagawany, M., Laudadio, V., Demauro, R. and Tufarelli, V. 2017b. Dietary inclusion of raw faba bean instead of soybean meal and enzyme supplementation in laying hens: effect on performance and egg quality. Saudi Journal of Biological Sciences, 24: 276-285.

Abd El-Hack, M.E., Chaudhry, M.T., Mahrose, K.M., Noreldin, A., Eman, M. and Algawany, M. 2017a. The efficacy of using exogenous enzymes cocktail on production, egg quality, egg nutrients and blood metabolites of laying hens fed distiller's dried grains with solubles. Journal of Animal Physiology and Animal Nutrition, doi: 10.1111/ jpn.12825.

Abdel-Fattah, S.A., El-Sanhoury, M.H., El-Mednay, N.M. and Abdel-Azeem, F. 2008. Thyroid activity, some blood constituents, organs morphology and performance of broiler chicks fed supplemental organic acids. International Journal of Poultry Science, 7: 215–222.

Ameri, S.A., Samadi, F., Dastar, B. and Zarehdaran, S. 2016. Efficiency of peppermint (Mentha piperita) powder on performance, body temperature and carcass characteristics of broiler chickens in heat stress condition. Iranian Journal of Applied Animal Science, 6(4): 943-950.

Arab Ameri, S., Samadi, F., Dastar, B. and Zerehdaran, S. 2016. Effect of peppermint (Mentha piperita) powder on immune response of broiler chickens in heat stress. Iranian Journal of Applied Animal Science, 6: 435-445.

Banjo, S. 2012. Growth and performance as affected by inclusion of Moringa oleifera leaf meal in broiler chick diet. Journal of Biology, Agriculture and Healthcare, 2(9): 35-38.

Berwanger, E., Nunes, R.V., Pasquetti, T.J., Murakami, A.E., Moraes de Oliveira, T.M., Bayerle, D.F. and Frank, R. 2017. Sunflower cake with or without enzymatic complex for broiler chickens feeding. Asian-Australasian Journal of Animal Sciences, 30: 410-416.

Bhattacharya, A., Chatterjee, A., Ghosal, S. and Bhattacharya, S. K. 1999. Antioxidant activity of active tannoid principles of Emblica officinalis (amla). Indian Journal of Experimental Biology,37: 676-679.

Bhattacharya, A., Ghosal, S. and Bhattacharya, S. K. 2000. Antioxidant activity of tannoid principles of Emblica officinalis (amla) in chronic stress induced changes in rat brain. Indian Journal of Experimental Biology, 38: 877-880.

Biswas, A., Bharti, V. K., Acharya, S., Pawar, D. D. and Singh, S. B. 2010. Sea buckthorn: new feed opportunity for poultry in cold arid Ladakh region of India. World's Poultry Science Journal, 66(04): 707-714.

Chaveerach, P., Keuzenkamp, D.A., Lipman, L.J.A and Van Knapen, F. 2004. Effect of organic acids in drinking water for young broilers on Campylobacter infection, volatile fatty acid production, gut micro flora and histological cell changes. Poultry Science, 83: 330-334.

Chen, X., Zhao, W., Liu, H. N., Su, J., Zhang Z. H. and Li, Y. 2011. Effect of sea buckthorn leaves on growth performance and calcium metabolism in Arbor Acres broilers. Dongbei Nongye Daxue Xuebao, 42: 19-24.

Chen, Y.C. and Chen, T.C. 2004. Mineral utilization in layers as influenced by dietary oligofructose and inulin. International Journal of Poultry Science, 3: 442-445.

Chen, Y.C., Nakthong, C. and Chen T.C. 2005a. Improvement of chicory fructans on egg cholesterol in commercial laying hen. International Journal of Poultry Science, 4: 109-114.

Chen, Y.C., Nakthong, C. and Chen T.C. 2005b. Improvement of laying hen performance by dietary prebiotic chicory oligofructose and inulin. International Journal of Poultry Science, 4: 103-108.

Craig, W.J. Herbal remedies that promote health and prevent disease. In: Watson RR (Ed.). Vegetables, fruits, and herbs in health promotion. CRC Press, Boca Raton, Florina, USA, pp. 179-204.

Dahale, G. S., Wankhede, S. M. and Kale, V. R. 2014. Growth performance, serum biochemical profile and carcass quality of broiler chickens fed diets supplemented with shatavari (Asparagus racemosus) root powder. Indian Journal of Animal Nutrition, 31: 166-171.

Dawson, A. 2009. Effect of enzyme supplementation and acidification of diets on nutrient digestibility and growth performance of broiler chicks. Poultry Science, 88(1): 111–117.

Del Alamo, A.G., Enting, H., De los Mozos, J. and Perez De Ayala, P. 2007. The effect of dietary short and medium chain fatty acids on the performance of broiler chickens. 19th Australian Symposium on Poultry Science, 169-172.

Denli, M., Okan, F. and Celik, K. 2003. Effect of dietary probiotic, organic acid and antibiotic supplementation to diets on broiler performance and carcass yield. Pakistan Journal of Nutrition, 2: 89–91.

Deschepper, K., Gantois, I., Maertens, L. and Van Meenen, E. 2013. A balanced mixture of medium chain fatty acids improves zootechnical performances and slaughter results of broilers: In Proceedings of the 19th European Symposium of Nutrition, PPV 10

Dibner, J.J. and Buttin, P. 2002. Use of organic acid as a model to study the impact of gut microflora on nutrition and metabolism. Journal of Applied Poultry Research, 11: 453-463.

Du, E., Wang, W., Gan, L., Li, Z., Guo, S. and Guo, Y. 2016. Effects of thymol and carvacrol supplementation on intestinal integrity and immune responses of broiler chickens challenged with Clostridium perfringens. Journal of Animal Science and Biotechnology, 7(1):19.

Fernandez-Panchon, M.S., Villano, D., Troncoso, A. M. and Garcia-Parrilla, M. C. 2008. Antioxidant activity of phenolic compounds: from in vitro results to in vivo evidence. Critical Reviews in Food Science and Nutrition, 48(7): 649-671.

Giannenas, I., Florou-Paneri, P., Papazahariadou, M., Christaki, E. and Botsoglou, N.A. 2003. Effect of dietary supplementation with oregano essential oil on performance of broilers after experimental infection with Eimeria tenella. Arch Tierernahr, 57: 99-106.

Gibson, G.R. and Roberfroid, M.B. 1995.Dietary modulation of the human colonic microbiota introducing the concept of prebiotics. Journal of Nutrition, 125: 1401-1412.

Gopi, M., Karthik, K., Manjunathachar, H.V., Tamilmahan, P., Kesavan, M., Dashprakash, M., Balaraju, B.L. and Purushothaman,M.R. 2014. Essential oils as a feed additive in poultry nutrition. Advances in Animal and Veterinary Sciences, 2(1): 1-7.

Gopi, M., Kathirvelan, C., Premchander, D., Vasanthakumar, P., Pangayarselvi, B., Sasikumar, P. and Chandrasekaran, D. 2012. Effect of cinnamon powder (Cinnamomum zeylanicum) supplementation on growth performance of broilers. Commercial and rural poultry production: Novel concepts and strategies to meet growing demand and changing consumer needs. Annual Conference and National Symposium of Indian Poultry Science Association, pp: 35–36.

Guan, T. T. Y., Cenkowski, S. and Hydamaka, A. 2005. Effect of drying on the nutraceutical quality of Sea buckthorn (Hippophae rhamnoides L. ssp. Sinensis) leaves. Journal of Food Science, 70: 514-518.

Hanieh, H., Narabara, K., Piao, M., Gerile, C. and Abe, A. 2010. Modulatory effects of two levels of dietary alliums on immune response and certain immunological variables, following immunization, in White Leghorn chickens. Animal Science Journal, 81: 673- 680.

Iji, P.A., and Tivey, D.R. 1998. Natural and synthetic oligosaccharides in broiler chicken diets. World's Poultry Science Journal, 54: 129-143.

Khempaka, S., Pudpila, U. and Molee, W. 2013. Effect of dried peppermint (Mentha cordifolia) on growth performance, nutrient digestibility, carcass traits, antioxidant properties, and ammonia production in broilers. Journal of Applied Poultry Research, 22: 904-912.

Kulkarni, R. C., Mandal, A. B., Munj, C. P., Dan, A., Saxena, A. and Tyagi, P. K. 2011. Response of coloured broilers to dietary addition of geloi (Tinospora cordifolia) during extreme summer. Indian Journal of Poultry Science, 46(1): 70-74.

Kumar, A., Shukla, P. K. and Bhattacharyya, A. 2020. Effect of graded levels of mint leaf meal on the body weight gain, feed conversion ratio, immune competence traits and meat composition of coloured chicken. International Journal of Livestock Research, 10 (6): 97-103.

Kumar, R., Kumar, G.P., Chaurasia, O.P. and Singh, S.B. 2011. Phytochemical and pharmacological profile of Sea buckthorn oil: A review. Research Journal of Medicinal Plants, 5: 491-499.

Kumar, S., Singh, H.N., Rai, A., Verma, A. and Bhattacharyya, A. 2019. Comparative efficacy of antibiotic and tulsi leaf meal supplement on body weight gain, feed conversion ratio, immunocompetence traits, faecal microbial count and development of digestive organs of commercial broilers. VIPM, Nov 8-9, DUVASU, Mathura, pp-138.

Kurtoglu,V., Kurtoglu. F., Seker, E., Coskun, B., Balevi, T. and Polat, E.S. 2004. Effect of probiotic supplementation on laying hen diets on yield performance and serum and egg yolk cholesterol. Food Additives and Contaminants, 21: 817-823.

Lambert, R.J. & Stratford, M.1998. Weak-acid preservatives: modelling microbial inhibition and response. Journal of Applied Bacteriology, 86: 157-164.

Lanjewar, R. D., Szanzad, A. A., Ramteke, B. N., Ingewar, S. M. and Patankar, R. B. 2008. Effect of dietary supplementation of tulsi (Ocimum sanctum) leaf powder on meat cholesterol and serum lipid profile in broilers. Ildex India.

Leeson, S., Namkung, H., Antongiovanni, M. and Lee, E.H. 2005. Effect of butyric acid on the performance and carcass yield on broiler chickens. Poultry Science, 84: 1418-1422.

Liu, T., Tang, J. and Feng, F.Y. 2020. Medium-chain á-monoglycerides improves productive performance and egg quality in aged hens associated with gut microbiota modulation. Poultry Science, 99: 7122-7132.

Mathis, G.F., Van, Dam, J.T.P., Corujo, Fernández, A. and Hofacre, Cl. 2005. Effect of an organic acids and medium-chain fatty acids containing product in feed on the course of artificial necrotic enteritis infection in broiler chickens. WPSA 15th European Symposium on Poultry Nutrition, Hungary, 25-29.

Menconi, A., Kuttappan, V.A., Hernandez-Velasco, X., et al. 2014. Evaluation of a commercially available organic acid product on body weight loss, carcass yield, and meat quality during preslaughter feed withdrawal in broiler chickens: A poultry welfare and economic perspective. Poultry Science, 93(2): 448–455.

Mendez- Albores, A., Arambula-Villa, G., Loarca-Pina, M.G.F, Castano-Tostado, E., Moreno-Martinez, E. 2005. Safety and efficiency evaluation of aqueous citric acid to degrade β-aflatoxins in maize. Food and Chemical Toxicology, 43: 233-238.

Moreki, J.C. and Kenaleone, G. 2014. Potential use of Moringa oleifera in poultry diets. Global Journal of Animal Scientific Research, 2: 109-115.

Munir, K. and Maqsood, S. 2013. A review on role of exogenous enzyme supplementation in poultry production. Emirates Journal of Food and Agriculture, 25: 66-80.

Panda, A.K., Rao, S.S.R., Raju, M.V.L.N. and Sharma, S.S. 2008. Effect of probiotic (Lactobacillus sporogenes) feeding on egg productuion and quality, yolk cholesterol and humoral immune response of White Leghorn layer breeders. Journal of Science of Food and Agriculture, 88: 43-47.

Panda, A.K., Reddy, M.R. and Praharaj, N.K. 2001. Dietary supplementation of probiotic on growth, serum cholesterol and gut microflora of broilers. Indian Journal of Animal Science, 71: 488-490.

Patel, M. K., Bhattacharyya, A.and Shukla, P. K. 2020. Effect of graded levels of moringa leaf meal on the body weight gain, feed conversion ratio, immune competence traits and meat composition of coloured chicken. International Journal of Livestock Research, 10 (6): 66-72.

Rahmani, H.R. and Speer, W. 2005. Natural additives influence the performance and humoral immunity of broilers. International Journal of Poultry Science, 4: 713-717.

Rajput, J. S., Singh, H.N., Verma, A., Rai, A. and Bhattacharyya, A. 2019. Effect of probiotic and herbal supplements on growth performance, faecal microbial count and immunocompetence traits of turkey poults. Proceedings of Veterinary Internal Preventive Medicine Conference, Nov 8-9, DUVASU, Mathura, pp-139.

Rama Rao, S.V., Panda, A.K., Raju, M.V.L.N., Sunder, G.S. and Praharaj, N.K. 2003. Requirement of calcium for commercial broiler and white leghorn layer at low dietary phosphorous levels. Animal Feed Science and Technology, 106: 199-208.

Rege, N. N., Thatte, U. M. and Dahanukar, S. A. 1999. Adaptogenic properties of six rasayana herbs used in Ayurvedic medicine. Phytotherapy Research, 13: 275-291.

Rehman, Z.U., Kamran, J., Abd El-Hack, M.E., Alagawany, M., Bhatti, S.A., Ahmad, G., Saleem, A., Ullah Z., Yameen, R.M.K. and Ding, C. 2017. Influence of low protein and amino acid diets with different sources of protease on performance, carcasses and nitrogen retention of broiler chickens. Animal Production Science, 58(9): 1625-1631.

Ricke, S. C. 2018. Impact of prebiotics on poultry production and food safety. Yale Journal of Biology and Medicine, 91: 151–159.

Russell, Y.J. 1998. The effect of natural source of non-digestible oligosaccharides on the fecal microflora of the dog and effects on digestion. Friskies R&D Center, Missouri, U.S.A.

Santos, F.S. de los, Farnell, M.B., Tellez, G., Balog, J.M. and Anthony, N.B. 2005. Effect of prebiotic on gut development and ascitis incidence of broilers reared in a hypoxic environment. Poultry Science, 84: 1092-1100.

Santovito, E., Greco, D., Logrieco, A. F., and Avantaggiato, G. 2018. Eubiotics for food security at farm level: yeast cell wall products and their antimicrobial potential against pathogenic bacteria. Foodborne Pathogens and Disease, 15: 531–537.

Shao, L.P., Zhou, L.J., Li, G.P. and Lin, I.P. 2000. Effects of different levels of mannan-oligosaccharides on cellular immune response and gastro-intestinal microecology in chickens. Journal of Fujian Agricultural University, 28: 86-89.

Sharma, A., Shukla, P.K., Bhattacharyya, A., Kumar, U. and Roy, D. 2018. Effect of dietary supplementation of sea buckthorn and giloe leaf meal on the body weight gain, feed conversion ratio, biochemical attributes and meat composition of turkey poults. Veterinary World, 11 (1): 93-98.

Shilling, M., Matt, L., Rubin, E., Visitacion, M.P., Haller, N.A., Grey, S.F. and Woolverton, C.J. 2013. Antimicrobial effects of virgin coconut oil and its medium-chain fatty acids on Clostridium difficile. Journal of Medicinal Food, 16: 1079–1085.

Shimaa, A., Amer, 1., Afaf A-Nasser., Hanan, S., Al-Khalaifah, Dina, M. M., Alsadek, Doaa, M., Abdel, fattah, Elshimaa, M., Roushdy, Wafaa, R. I. A., Sherief, Mohamed, F. M., Farag, Dalia, E., Altohamy, Ahmed, A. A., Abdel-Wareth and Abdallah, E. Metwally. 2021. Effect of dietary medium-chain á-monoglycerides on the growth performance, intestinal histomorphology, amino acid digestibility and broiler chickens' blood biochemical parameters. Animals, 11: 57.

Siddhuraju, P. and Becker, K. 2003. Antioxidant properties of various solvent extracts of total phenolic constituents from three different agro-climatic origins of drumstick tree (Moringa oleifera Lam.). Journal of Agriculture and Food Chemistry, 15: 2144-2155.

Singh, V., Yang, B., Kallio, H., Bala, M., Sawhney, R. C., Gupta, R. K., Morsel, J. T., Lu, R. and Tolkachev, O. N. 2006. Sea buckthorn (Hippophae L.)-A multipurpose wonder plant. Vol. II: Biochemical Pharmacology, 600.

Stanley, V.G. and Sefton, A.E. 1999. Egg and serum cholesterol as influenced by mannanoligosaccharide and aflatoxin. In:Egg nutrition and biotechnology (Ed. Sin, J.S., Nakai, S., Guenter, W.) Walling ford, U.K., CABI Publishing pp. 441-443.

Sultan, S. I. 2003. The effect of turmeric (feed additive) on overall performance of broiler chickens. Indian Journal of Poultry Science, 2: 351-353.

Swamy, H.V.L.N. and Devegowda, G. 1998. Ability of mycosorb to counteract aflatoxicosis in commercial broilers. Indian Journal of Poultry Science, 33: 273-278.

Tiwari, M., Bhattacharyya A. and Singh, H.N. 2012. Effect of probiotic and phytobiotics on feed conversion ratio, carcass quality traits and development of digestive organs of commercial broilers. Journal of Animal Research, 2(1): 53-60.

Van Immerseel, F., De Buck, J., Boyen, F., Bohez, L., Pasmans, F., Volf, J., Sevcik, M., Rychlik, I.,Haesebrouck, F. and Ducatelle R. 2004. Medium-chain fatty acids decrease colonization and invasion through hila suppression shortly after infection of chickens with Salmonella enterica serovar Enteritidis. Applied and Environmental Microbiology, 70(6): 3582-3587.

Yadav, B. K., Shukla, P. K., Bhattacharyya, A., Roy, D., Sharma, A. and Sirohi, R. 2018. Effect of graded levels of shatavari root meal on the body weight, feed conversion ratio, biochemical attributes and immune competence traits of coloured chicken. International Journal of Livestock Research, 8(10): 115-123.

Yakout, H.M., Omara, M. E. Marie, Y. and Hasan, R.A. 2004. Effect of incorporating growth promoters and different dietary protein levels into Mandarah hens layer's diets. Egyptian Poultry Science Journal, 24: 977-994.

Yang, Z., Qi, X. M., Yang, H. M., Dai, H., Xu, C. X. and Wang, Z. Y. 2018. Effects of dietary copper on growth performance, slaughter performance and nutrient content of fecal in growing goslings from 28 to 70 days of Age. Brazilian Journal of Poultry Science, 20(1): 45-52.

8

Enzyme Technology in Poultry Nutrition: Present and Future Scenario

Praveen K. Tyagi, Rokade J. and Monika M.

ICAR-Central Avian Research Institute, Izantnagr-243 122, Uttar Pradesh

Introduction

During last four decade poultry has taken giant step and become corporate sector with double digit growth. Especially in India poultry play pivotal role in fight against malnutrition, unemployment and also contributing in women empowerment. In poultry production the biggest single expense is of feed, which accounting for 70% of total production cost per bird (Kumar *et al*., 2011). So, obviously more Research and Development focus and new innovative technology need to be implemented in poultry nutrition area. Since last 40 years, feed enzymes have played a major part in helping radically to improve the efficiency of meat and egg production by changing the nutritional profile of feed ingredients. Doing this feed enzymes help meet consumer demand for safe, high quality and affordable food. Animals use enzymes to digest the food by using enzyme produced by themselves or by gut microbes. But poultry birds can digest only 75 to 80% feed they eat because of indigestible anti-nutritional factors from feed ingredients. This feed inefficiency cause economical loss to producers along with environmental pollution. Feed enzymes allow poultry to extract more nutrients from the feed and so improve feed efficiency by targeting specific anti-nutrients in certain feed ingredients (Almirall *et al.*, 1995). This quality allows greater flexibility in feed ingredients used for fed formulation. Also enzymes helps is sustainable poultry production by reducing negative effect on environmental because of less production of animal waste.

At the most basic level, feedstuffs consist of protein, starch, fat and fibre. In monogastric animals the fibre component has been considered to be wasted and, in some instances, compounds called Non-starch polysaccharides (NSP) can exert anti-nutritive activity on the animal. The NSP of barley, wheat and rye has been the most intensively investigated. Wheat and rye contain relatively high levels of arabinoxylans or pentosans which can also have a negative effect on broiler performance. Ingestion of NSP by birds results in increased viscosity of the digesta. This increased viscosity reduces the passage rate of the feed leading to overall reductions in consumption and decreased performance, sticky droppings (pasted vents) and dirty eggs (Annison *et al.,* 1991). In order to address NSP viscosity, exogenous enzymes have been used in the feed industry for decades to improve the nutritive value of feedstuffs. Apart from NSP, the increased presence of undigested protein in the gastro-intestinal tract may be also a predisposing factor for microbial challenges. The increased presence of insoluble fibre leads to maintenance energy losses as the bird inefficiently breaks down the anti-nutrients or substrates in this more complex feed with its own enzymes. Exogenous enzyme addition enhances the digestibility and bird's performance, improve manure quality and increase the use of lower cost feed ingredients. The nutrients of the feed stuff can be proficiently utilized with enzyme supplementation. Naturally; the gastrointestinal tract of poultry produces enzymes to aid the digestion of nutrients. However, the birds do not have enough enzymes to digest fibre completely and need some commercial exogenous enzymes in the diets to improve the digestion.

Enzyme is a biological catalyst composed of proteins, amino acids with minerals and vitamins. The advantages of using commercial enzymes in poultry feeds include improved productive performance and feed utilization, minimized environmental pollution due to reduced nutrient of manure (Barletta, 2001). The enzyme uses and its applications in poultry production are as follows.

- Release of phosphorous from phytate hydrolysis
- Elimination of the nutrient encapsulating effect of the cell walls and therefore improved energy and amino acid availabilities
- Solubilization of cell wall non starch polysaccharides (NSP) for more effective hindgut fermentation and improved overall energy utilization
- Hydrolysis of certain types of carbohydrate–protein linkages and therefore improved availability of amino acids
- Elimination of the antinutritive properties of certain dietary NSP by their enzymatic hydrolysis to prebiotic type components which, in turn, may facilitate gut development and health in young chickens.

With this background, in the present chapter we will discuss brief about enzymes, its types and advantages of its application in poultry rearing.

Enzymes

Enzymes are one of the many types of protein in biological systems. Their essential characteristic is to catalyse the rate of a reaction but is not themselves altered by it. They are involved in all anabolic and catabolic pathways of digestion and metabolism. Enzymes tend to be very specific catalysts that act on one or, at most, a limited group of compounds known as substrates. We may also broadly categorize the digestive enzymes as endogenous or exogenous - referring to those produced by the bird's itself and those administered from outside, respectively. For example, pancreatic lipase, which splits fat or lipid into glycerol and fatty acids, is an endogenous enzyme. Those enzymes added to feed as a supplement are exogenous enzymes.

Sources of Enzymes

Enzymes are produced in every living organism from the highest developed animals and plants to the simplest unicellular forms of life, as they are essential for metabolic process. Most of the enzymes currently used in the food and beverage industry are from Aspergillus, but hemicelluloses and celluloses are derived from Trichoderma. Recently, genes encoding for different enzymes, including phytases, β-glucanases, and xylanases, have been cloned and expressed in different commercial systems (microorganisms and plants). It is possible to produce large amounts of cheap enzyme by continually selecting favourable microbes, growing them in advanced fermentation systems and by streamlining the extraction and purification of the enzyme (Wallis, 1996). Microorganisms that generally involved in production of enzymes are; Bacteria (*Bacillus subtilis, Bacillus lentus, Bacillus amyloliquifaciens and Bacillus stearothermophils)*, Fungus *(Triochodermalongi brachiatum, Asperigillus oryzae and Asperigillus niger)* and Yeast *(S. cerevisiae)*.

Table 1: Microbes used in commercial enzyme production (Mulisa Faji Dida, 2016)

Enzyme	Source	Action
α-amylase	*Bacillus subtilis,Bacillus licheniformis, Aspergillus oryzae*	Endo-hydrolysis of α-1, 4- glucosidic Linkages
	Bacillus subtilis, Aspergillus niger, Penicillium emersonii	Degrades β-glucan by cleaving β-1,3 (4) glucosidic linkages
Pectinase	*Aspergillus oryzae, Aspergillus niger, Rhizopu soryzae*	Degrades pectinα-1,4-linked Anhydrogalacuronic acid
Pullulanase	*Klebsiella aerogenes*	Splits the α-1,6-glycosidic linkages

Classification of Enzyme (Dida, 2016)

According to the purpose of application, feed enzymes can be fundamentally divided in to:

1. Enzymes which quantitatively supplement endogenous digestive enzymes of mono gastric animals. *e.g.*, Proteases, lipases, Amylases
2. Enzymes which are not produced by mono-gastric animals *e.g.*, β-glucanases, Pentosanases and Phytases.

Mode of Enzyme Action

Enzyme supplementation improves the nutrients utilization as well as production of the birds.

I. *Reducing the Gut Viscosity*

Viscous cereals' like barley, wheat, rye, oats and triticale contain high proportions of their energy in the form of Non-Starch Polysaccharides. Cereals contain soluble β-glucans, lignin, anti-nutritional factors like phytic acid, cellulose fiber and arabinoxylans (Bedford and Classen, 1992; Choct and Annison, 1992; Bedford and Morgan, 1996). Because of these NSP's ability to bind large amount of water viscosity of gut gets affected. This results in decrease in rate of passage of digesta resulting in limited absorption of nutrients, compromised FCR & increase in the amount of sticky droppings. These problems are overcome by the addition of suitable multi enzyme preparation like β-glucanases and xylanases, because they break down the gel form characteristic of soluble fibers & allows the bird's digestive enzyme to function more efficiently. This improves starch, protein, fat, amino acids and energy digestibility. Reduction in water holding capacity of the gut contents due to enzymes also increases the dry matter content stimulating feed intake. Other benefits like associated with digesta viscosity include reduction in the number of dirty eggs and enhanced egg yolk colour.

II. Effect on Litter Problems

Increase in rate of passage of digesta because of enzyme supplementation leads to reduction in the dry matter outside the body. This reduces on excreta volume and composition due to better protein digestibility (Mulisa Faji Dida, 2016). Reduced viscosity improves nutrient digestion, lower water intake and help to reduce litter problems.

III. Release of Nutrients

Enzymatic de polymerization renders the NSP free releasing nutrients in the gut and it available to the animal. Starch masked by cell structure is released leading to increase in metabolizable energy. Proteins are also released by action of proteases. This release leads to maximum absorption of minerals and results in improvement in nutrient utilization.

IV. Increase in Available Energy

Enzyme supplementation enhances carbohydrate digestibility, reducing gut viscosity, and improving fat utilization. The effect of enzyme supplementation increases dry matter digestibility range from 0.9 (Schutte *et al.,* 1995) to 17% (Bedford *et al*., 1992) in poultry. To increase the available energy content of the diet wheat- and barley-based poultry diets must be supplemented with enzymes. Enzymes like glycanases cleave Non Starch Polysaccharides SPs into smaller polymers, thereby removing their ability to form viscous digesta and enhancing nutrient digestibility. The supplementation of phytase in feed increases utilization of phytate phosphorus & reduce excretion of organic phosphorus (almost by 40%) to the environment.

Diet formulation has become more flexible when differences in feed ingredientquality or animals' digestibility capacity can be controlled by supplementalenzymes. Enzyme supplementation allows greater use of raw materials with lower nutritional value & by-products, such as bran, which are typically rich in fibre.

Table 2: Types of Enzyme Available for Poultry

Plant enzymes	**Microbial enzymes**
Narrow spectrum hydrolyzing enzymes.	Synthetic broad-spectrum hydrolytic enzymes
Less stable in extreme reaction conditions	More stable enzymes on extreme reaction conditions
Standardization not done	Better standardized
Lower yield	Higher yield
Not economical	Economical

The potential enzymes used in poultry feed industry include cellulase (β-glucanases), xylanases and associated enzymes, phytases, proteases, lipases, and galactosidases (Table 2). These enzymes neutralize the effects of the viscous, non-starch polysaccharides in cereals such as barley, wheat, rye, and triticale. These antinutritive carbohydrates are undesirable, as they reduce digestion and absorption of all nutrients in the diet, especially fat and protein. Recently, considerable interest has been shown in the use of phytase as a feed additive, as it not only increases the availability of phosphate in plants but also reduces environmental pollution.

Table 3: Enzymes Used in Poultry Feeds

Enzymes	**Substrate**	**Effect**
β-glucanases	Barley, Oats	Reduction of intestinal digest viscosity Reduction of dirty egg problems
Xylanases	Wheat, Rye, Triticale Rice bran	Reduction of intestinal digest viscosity
β-galactosidases	Grain legumes, Lupins	Removal of a galactosides
Phytases	Plant feedstuffs	Enhanced utilization of plant phosphorus
Proteases	Proteins	
Lipases	Lipids	
Amylases	Starch	

Source: The role of feed enzymes in poultry nutrition, 2011

Benefits of enzymes

- Reduction in digesta viscosity.
- Enhanced digestion and absorption of nutrients especially fat and protein.
- Improved Apparent Metabolizable Energy (AME) value of the diet.
- Increased feed intake, weight gain and feed gain ratio.
- Reduced beak impaction and vent plugging.
- Decreased size of gastrointestinal tract.
- Altered population of microorganisms in gastro intestinal tract.
- Reduced water intake.
- Reduced water content of excreta.
- Reduced production of ammonia from excreta.
- Reduced output of excreta including reduced N and P.

Enzymes in Poultry Nutrition

Consistent increase in the price of feed ingredients has been a major constraint in most of the developing countries. As a consequence, cheaper and non-conventional feed ingredients have to be used which contain higher percentage of Non-Starch Polysaccharides (soluble and insoluble/crude fibre) along with starch. Non-Starch Polysaccharides (NSPs) are polymeric carbohydrates which differ in composition and structure from starch (Morgan *et al.,* 1995) and possess chemical cross linking among them therefore, are not well digested by poultry (Adams and Pough, 1993; Annison, 1993). A part of these NSPs is water-soluble which is notorious for forming a gel like viscous consistency in the intestinal tract (Ward, 1995) thus by reducing gut performance. Predominantly water soluble and viscous arabinoxylans, which belong to pentosan group, are assumed to be the factor responsible. These pentosans also greatly increase the water intake by the birds, which lead to unmanageable litter problems caused by wet and sticky droppings. This deteriorates the hygienic conditions and carcass quality (Dunn, 1996). On the other hand, β-glucans adversely affect all nutrients, especially protein and starch utilization and are known to give rise highly viscous conditions in the small intestine of the chicks (Hasselman and Aman, 1986). Poultry do not produce enzymes for the hydrolysis of Non-Starch Polysaccharide present in the cell wall of the grains and they remain un-hydrolysed. This results in low feed efficiency. Research work has suggested that the negative effects of NSPs can be overcome by dietary modifications including supplementation of diets with suitable exogenous enzyme preparations (Creswell, 1994). Enzymes break down the NSPs, decreases intestinal viscosity and eventually improve the digestibility of nutrients by improving gut performance.

Role of Enzymes in Poultry Nutrition

Poultry do not produce enzymes for the hydrolysis of Non-Starch Polysaccharides present in the cell wall of the grains and they remain un-hydrolyzed. Non-Starch Polysaccharides are polymeric carbohydrates which differ in composition and structure from starch and possess chemical cross linking among them therefore, are not well digested by poultry. A part of these Non-Starch Polysaccharides is watersoluble which is notorious for forming a gel like viscous consistency in the intestinal tract, thus by reducing gut performance. Predominantly water soluble and viscous arabinoxylans, which belong to pentosan group, are assumed to be the factor responsible for wet and sticky droppings. This deteriorates the hygienic conditions and carcass quality. On the other hand, ß-glucans adversely affect all nutrients, especially protein and starch utilization and are known to give rise highly viscous conditions in the small intestine of the chicks. Studies suggested that the negative effects of NSPs can be overcome by dietary modifications including supplementation of diets with suitable exogenous enzyme preparations. Enzymes break down the Non-Starch Polysaccharides, decreases intestinal viscosity and eventually improve the digestibility of nutrients by improving gut performance. Poultry do not produce enzyme for the hydrolyses of these non-starch polysaccharide present in the cell wall of the grains. The production of endogenous enzymes may be a limiting factor due to various reasons depending on the age, health; type of feed, environment etc. Addition of enzymes specific for a given feed formulation will enhance the bioavailability of above feed components. The exogenous enzyme in feed additive can complement to endogenous enzymes in the digestive system during adverse climatic condition and at an early age, to give an increase role of digestion.

As exogenous enzyme promotes better digestibility, which enhances the feed intake,efficiency, growth rate and productivity. Enzymes also act as supplement to the normal digestive enzymes especially during stress condition reduces anti nutritional products like tannins, saponin and goitrogen. Release minerals for assimilation e.g; Ca, Mg, Zn, P etc. Checks chelating of minerals such as Zn, Mn, Fe, Ca, K with phytic acid, less chelation means more mineral availability. Prevents precipitation of penta calcium phosphate and there by improves absorption of calcium and phosphorus. Apart from enhancing digestibility, enzymes have impact on bird's health also, eg. Coccidiosis problems could be prevented by using enzymes. Birds fed a wheat-based diet with and without glycanase supplementation showed vastly different responses to coccidiosis challenge. Growth was depressed by 52.5% in the control group but by only

30.5% in the enzyme group, which also had a much better lesion score. An increase in digesta passage rate and a reduction in excreta moisture are often noted when glycanases are added to poultry diets, which may be detrimental to the life cycle of the organism. It's also used as:

- Improvement in animal hygiene and health.
- Corrects digestive disorders especially when birds are crowded.
- Fattening performance is increased.
- Prevents damages to chicken anaemia agent.
- Checks cellular damages caused by toxins.
- Promotes growth to bones.
- Prevents diarrhoea due to poor fibre digestion.
- Minimizes excreta, water droppings and of ammonia.
- Reduces viscosity and ammonia level in intestine.

Enzymes indirectly yield better quality poultry products by increasing the egg production and hatchability in layers. Egg quality is also maintained. More clean eggs with thick shell is maintained. Improves flock uniformity leading to more consistent sized birds. Improved slaughter results, high carcass weights and better grading. Genetic Potential of birds can be explored enabling them to consume more quality of feed to achieve maximum growth and production.

Enzymes: Role in Least Cost Feed Formulation

An increased precision in least cost feed formulation, hence a more uniform performance of the birds. Enzymes also allow a wide range of ingredients to be used in a diet with a desired outcome. This gives the producer a great deal of flexibility to formulate a nutritionally balanced least-cost diet.

Benefits of Enzymes to Environment have been approved for use in poultry feed because they are natural products of fermentation and therefore pose no threat to the animal or the consumer. Enzymes not only will enable livestock and poultry producers to economically use new feedstuffs, but will also prove to be environmentally friendly, as they reduce the pollution associated with animal production. As well as contributing to improved poultry production, feed enzymes can have a positive impact on the environment. In areas with intensive poultry production, the phosphorus output is often very high, resulting in environmental problems such as eutrophication. This happens because most of the phosphorus contained in typical feedstuffs exists as the plant storage form phytate, which is indigestible for poultry. The phytase enzyme frees the phosphorus in feedstuffs and also achieves the release of other minerals (e.g. Ca, Mg), as well as proteins and amino acids bound to phytate. Thus, by releasing bound phosphorus in feed ingredients, phytase reduces the quantity of inorganic phosphorus needed in diets, makes more phosphorus available for the bird, and decreases the amount excreted into the environment.

Therefore benefits of enzymes to environment include

- Reduction in manure volume: wet excreta leads to dirty eggs and they are not suitable for sale as second-grade eggs. Wet droppings may also cause increased gas production (i.e. ammonia) and fly and rodent population in the shed. Wet dropping can also affect the health of the staff working in the shed.
- Reduced nitrogen and Phosphorus exertion.
- Less environmental waste and therefore less pollution.
- Reduced environmental stress resulting from reduced litter volume.

Future

The world population is forecast to rise from the current 6.7 billion people (2009) to 9.1 billion people by 2050, with most of the growth coming fromdeveloping countries (FAO, 2009d). With over one-third more mouths to feed, the UN Food and Agriculture Organization (FAO) predict that 70% more food will need to be produced by 2050.This is great challenge for animal production industry along with many other challenges like feed ingredients, animalgenetics & disease challenges. In terms of countries offering significant potential for business growth, inthe medium term, markets such as Brazil, Russia, China and India are likely to become increasingly attractive. In China and India, increased economic wealth together with growth in the human population will increase the demand for poultry meat. So by 2050, Indian will be a leading market for enzymes. The future for technologies such as feed enzymes is very bright. Feed enzymes will play a major role in efficiently supporting the growth in animal derived food products needed to feed the world in a safe, affordable and sustainable way.

Conclusion

The competition between humans and animals for feed ingredient & increasing price of poultry feed sources is always a big challenge for poultry industry. This leads to the search for suitable alternatives to use instead of the traditional feed materials. Many non-nutritional substances & sugars found in plant negatively affect poultry performance & also Non-starch polysaccharides (NSP) like components can't be digested. Also ingredients such as maize, soybean and, particularly, grain by-products contain relatively high levels of dietary fibres.

This allows forth option of using the enzyme to improve growth and feed gain or, alternatively, to use it in diets with lowered levels of energy and protein/amino acids, with higher by-product levels, to maintain performance with lower net feed costs.

References

Adams, E.A. and R. Pough. 1993. Non-starch polysaccharides and their digestion in poultry. Feed Compounder, 13: 19-21.

Almirall, M., Francesch, M., Perez-Vendrell, A.M., Brufau, J. and Esteve-Garcia, E. 1995. The differences in intestinal viscosity produced by barley and b-glucanase alter digesta enzyme activities and ileal nutrient digestibility more in broiler chicks than in cocks. The Journal of Nutrition, 125(4): 947-955.

Annison, G. 1993. The role of wheat non-starch polysaccharides in broiler nutrition. Australian Journal of Agricultural Research, 44(3): 405-422.

Annison, G. 1991. Relationship between the levels of soluble nonstarch polysaccharides and the apparent metabolizable energy of wheats assessed in broiler chickens. Journal of Agricultural and Food Chemistry, 39(7): 1252-1256.

Barletta, R.G and Harris, N.B. 2001. Mycobacterium avium subsp. paratuberculosis in veterinary medicine. Clinical Microbiology Reviews, 14(3): 489-512.

Bedford, M.R. 1996. The effect of enzymes on digestion. Journal of Applied Poultry Research, 5: 370-378.

Bedford, M.R. and Classen, H.L. 1992. Reduction of intestinal viscosity through manipulation of dietary rye and pentosanase concentration is effected through changes in the carbohydrate composition of the intestinal aqueous phase and results in improved growth rate and food conversion efficiency of broiler chicks. The Journal of Nutrition, 122(3): 560-569.

Choct, M. and G. Annison. 1990. Anti-nutritive activity of wheat pentosans in broiler diets. British Poultry Science, 30: 811–821.

Creswell, D.C. 1994. Upgrading the nutritional value of grains with the use of enzymes. Technical bulletin, American Soybean Association, 341 Orchard Road No.11-03 Liat Towers, Singapore.

Dida, M.F. 2017. Review paper on enzyme supplementation in poultry ration. International Journal of Bioorganic Chemistry, 1(1): 1-7.

Dunn, N. 1996. Combating the pentosans in cereals. World Poultry, 12(1): 24-25.

Hasselman, K. and P. Aman. 1986. The effect of ßglucanase on the utilization of starch and nitrogen by broiler chicks fed on barley of low or high viscosity. Animal Feed Science and Technology, 15: 83-93.

Kumar, A., Mahajan, S., Dhara, S.K. and Dey, S (Eds.). 2018. Practicability, Scope and Future Prospects of Ethno-botanicals in Minimizing Antibiotic Resistance, Division of Medicine, ICAR-Indian Veterinary Research Institute, Izatnagar, India 170 pp.

Morgan, A.J. and M. R. Bedford. 1995. Advances in the development and application of feed enzymes. Australian Poultry Science Symposium, 7: 109–115.

Mulisa Faji Dida., 2016. Review Paper on Enzyme Supplementation in Poultry Ration. 2016. International Journal of Bioorganic Chemistry, 1(1): 1-7.

Schutte, J.B., de Jong, J. and Langhout, D. J. 1995. Effect of a xylanase enzyme supplementation to wheat-based diets in broiler chicks in relation to dietary factors. Proceedings of the Second European Symposium on Feed Enzymes, Noordwijkerhout, Netherlands, pp. 95–101.

Wallis, I. 1996. Enzymes in poultry Nutrition. Scottish Agricultural Colleges.

Ward, N. 1996. Intestinal viscosity, broiler performance. Poultry Digest, 55: 12-17.

9

Role of Phytase in Poultry Nutrition

H.P. Shrivastava

Ex Principal Scientist and Head PGET, ICAR - Central Avian Research Institute Izatnagar, Bareilly, Uttar Pradesh, India

Introduction

Feeding cost and the price of poultry products have recently increased due to increasing competition between humans and animals for the same feed resources having different valuable nutrients. As you know that like other living creatures, the birds do need several nutrients in their diets to maintain optimum body growth, normal health and maximum production of edible egg and meat. Accordingly the efforts should always be made to feed poultry with a diet adequately balanced with almost all essential nutrients so that they do perform efficiently within a normal physiological form.

Realising the benefits of nutritive enrichment of various feedstuffs for poultry, several processing methods have been attempted in the past to obtain a good amount of easily digestible form of feedstuffs containing more available nutrients. In this direction, the addition or supplementation of enzyme, being proteinand acting asa biological catalyst (biocatalyst) to accelerate chemical reactions and thus converting the substrates into different molecules known as product. The functional impactof enzyme is primarily concerned with utilization of anti-nutrients inherently present invarious feed ingredients. Similarly the phytase which is a digestive enzyme that increases the digestibility of phytate-bound phosphorus (P), which improve the overall availability of dietary P to poultry once they are consuming vegetable based diet. The phytic acid is a highly reactive acidic compound that readily binds mineral cations and this complexed form is known as phytate cations or phytin. Plants such as cereals, grains, oilseeds store phosphorus (P) in a compound known as phytic acid. The stored P over 60% of total P in cereal grains and oil seeds and their by-products in phytin or phytate form which is not available to poultry as they lack in endogenous phytase enzyme which is responsible for making P available after degrading of phytate. In the absence of endogenous phytase enzyme, the unabsorbed phytate-bound P passes through the gastrointestinal tract and elevates its excretion in poultry manure that can lead to environmental problem.

Though the inclusion of microbial phytase in poultry diets has increased remarkably, mainly in response to heightened concerns over utilization of phytate-bound P and also reduction of P pollution in environment, but its limitations should also be not overlooked due to several factors involved such as its cost, inactivation at high temperatures required for pelleting (>80°C), loss of activity during storage and narrow optimum pH range. The capacity of this feed enzyme to release phytate-bound P and reduce P excretion is now well documented. In a simple way we can understand that the phytase is used as a dietary supplement in broiler nutrition to improve P bioavailability. Based on limited studies, it appears that the exogenous or extracellular phytase hydrolyses less than 0.35% of dietary phytate in broilers at ileal level. If so, there is considerable scope to enhance phytate degradation by the introduction of more effective phytase-phytate degrading enzyme or enzyme combination. Phytase is now present in over 60% of monogastric feed and possibly even in higher percentage of poultry diets. Thus it constitutes more than half of all feed enzyme sales throughout the globe. Microbial phytase has been considered to be an effective tool to increase P availability/digestibility from vegetable sources under phytate-P utilization and also to partially or completely replace inorganic P supplementation being of higher cost P sources such as dicalcium phosphate (DCP) and bone meal. Phytase initiates the phosphate hydrolysis from phytate and produce myo-inositol and inorganic phosphate by catalysing the stepwise removal of the phosphate group.

Chemical state of phytate

Commercial poultry feed is composed of cereal grains, grain by-products, vegetable proteins such as oil seed meals, animal proteins, mineral and vitamin mixtures. Majority of vegetable feed ingredients contain inherently one or other anti-nutrients or anti-nutritive substances or deleterious (toxic substances) principles and most of them can be destroyed during processing prior to use in poultry feeds.

The phytic acid is a unique natural substance, but anti-nutritional constituent of plant derived feeds. The phytic acid, discovered in 1903 is a six-fold dihydrogenphosphate ester of inositol or inositol polyphosphate or myo-inositol hexakisphosphate. Its chemical formula is $C_6H_{18}O_{24}P_6$. Chemically six phosphate molecules are bound in one phytic acid molecule. When phytic acid from plant source is consumed, it binds to other minerals to create insoluble compound such as phytate. It has received considerable attention due to its effects on mineral absorption. The phytic acid impairs the absorption of calcium (Ca), copper (Cu), iron (Fe), magnesium (Mg), manganese (Mn), phosphorus (P) and zinc (Zn) and may cause mineral deficiencies. Therefore, it is often referred to as an anti-nutrient. The phytate-bound P or phytin P carries a considerable importance in poultry nutrition as plant feedstuffs do contain phytic acid to store 70-80% of total P.

Availability of phytate

Among the common feed stuffs, maize, rice, rice bran and sesame meal have the highest level of phytate. Investigations have revealed that the concentration of phytate in poultry rations ranges from 2.5 to 4g/kg. About 2/3 of the total P present in plant feed ingredients is in phytate or phytin form being non available to birds. Each phytic acid molecule contains about 28% P. The poultry have limited capability to utilize phytate P. Capability of the poultry to utilize phytate P ranges from 0-50%. Bioavailability of P in maize and soybean meal for poultry ranges from 10-30%. Low availability of phytate-P in poultry results in two problems: a) There is a need to add inorganic P supplements to diets and b) Excretion of large amounts of P into the nature which is responsible for environmental pollution.

One molecule of phytic acid binds with 3 to 6 molecules of Ca to form insoluble complex at the pH of small intestine. Excess Ca in the diet leads to the formation of Ca phytate complexes which are highly insoluble and poorly digested. Zn forms the most insoluble salt with phyticacid; therefore Zn is a limiting mineral in high phytate diets as it forms a highly insoluble complex at pH 6.4, which is the pH of the upper intestine, where most mineral absorption occurs.

Degradation of phytate

Hydrolysis of phytate of plants occurs through various processing effects or by an action of enzyme known as phytase which hydrolyses phytate phytic acid to inositol and inorganic P, leading to improved P utilization. In poultry nutrition, the P is one of the essential major minerals for bone development and egg shell deposition is non-available to poultry if it is present in phytate form in vegetable ingredients.

A phytase (myo-inositol hexakisphosphate phosphohydrolase) is a type of phosphatase enzyme that catalyzes the process of hydrolysis of phytic acid (myo-inositol hexakisphosphate) which is an indigestible and organic form of P found in many plant feedstuffs especially in grains and oil seeds. Consequent upon hydrolysis of phytate a usable form of inorganic P is released. The phytases have been found to occur in animals, plants, fungi and bacteria, but the phytase enzyme is not present in poultry intestine. Therefore, the addition of phytase enzyme in poultry diets is very much required as it can hydrolyse phytate-bound P of plant feedstuffs and increases the availability of P for various functions concerning bone development and egg production.

Sources of phytase

A phytase (myo-inositol hexakisphosphate phosphohydrolase) is any type of phosphatase enzyme that catalyzes the hydrolysis of phytic acid (myo-hexakisphosphate) an indigestible, organic form of P that is found in many plant tissues, especially grains and oilseeds and releases a usable P, while phytases have been found to occur in animals, plants, fungi and bacteria. Phytase is used as an animal feed supplement often in pig and poultry to enhance the nutritive value of plant material by liberation of inorganic phosphate from phytic acid (myo-hexakisphosphate). Phytase enzymes are capable of removing the phosphates from phytate. Phytases are a cost effective alternative to ensure animals to obtain adequate available P from the plant based diets, because they can turn the plant phytate into a very valuable resource of P. Monogastric animals including poultry lack sufficient endogenous phystase (a digestive enzyme releaseing P through phytate degradation) in their gastrointestinal tracts and are unable to utilize the phytates once they eat plant feedstuffs. Therefore adding extra exogenous phystases to the diet increases phytate breakdown and consequent utilization of plant P. If more P is available naturally then less of this substance has to be added to the diet, but this situation may not arise in poultry if they consume P from vegetable feeds and the phytin-P may not be made available to the birds. This greatly reduces the feed costs. If P in the diet is utilized more efficiently, then less of this substance is excreted. This reduces the impact of livestock production on the environment. Phytase is produced by bacteria found in the gut of ruminant animals (cattle and sheep) making it possible for them to use the phytic acid or phytate found in grains as a source of P. Non-ruminants (monogastric animals) like human beings, dogs, pigs and poultry do not produce phytase.

Phytase is widely distributed in plants, animals and microbes. Intestinal phytase found in digestive secretions and phytase produced by endogenous microbes in the digestive tract of ruminants are not concerned with poultry. Broadly, the commercially available phytase enzymes can be derived from plants, animals and microorganisms. Phytase enzymes have been isolated and characterized from a number of plant sources such as maize, rape seed, rice, rye, soybean and wheat.

Bacteria and fungi comprise the most important sources of microbial phytase. Among yeasts *Aspergillus ficuum*, *Aspergillus fumigatus*, *Aspergillus niger*, *Bacillus subtilis*, *Citrobacter braaki*, *Escherichia coli*, *Penicillium funiculosum*, *Peniophora lycii*, *Saccharomyces cerevisiae* and *Schwanniomyces occidentalis* are commonly used strains for commercial production of phytases.

Though, the first plant for phytase production was found in 1907 from rice bran and in 1908 from an animal (calf's liver and blood). In 1962, began the first attempt at commercializing phytases for animal feed nutrition for enhancing purposes when International Minerals & Chemicals (IMC) studied over 2000 microorganisms to find the most suitable ones for phytase production. *Aspergillus (ficuum) niger* fungal strain NRRL 3135 (ATCC 66876) was identified as a promising candidate as it was able to produce large amounts of extracellular phytases but the organism's efficiency was not enough for commercialization.

In 1991 BASF began to sell the first commercial phytase produced in *Aspergillus niger* under the trademark Natuphos which was used to increase the nutrient content of animal feed. In 1999 *Escherichia coli* bacterial phytases were identified as being more effective than *Aspergillus niger* fungal phytases. Subsequently, this led to the animal feed use of this new generation of bacterial phytases which were superior to fungal phytases in many aspects.

Four distinct classes of phytase have been characterized in the literature: histidine acid phosphatases (HAPS), beta-propeller phytases (BPPs), purple acid phosphatases (PAPs), and most recently, protein tyrosine phosphatase-like phytases (PTP-like phytases).

Use of exogenous or extracellular phytase enzyme is a new concept in the composite poultry feed industry in India. Liberation of P bound as phytate in all vegetable type raw materials to lower feed cost by reducing the amount of inorganic P added to the diet and having a degradation of phytic acid known as anti-nutritional factor. Dicalcium phosphate (DCP) is used in the animal feed as Ca and P minerals. Phytase can be used to replace DCP in animal feed possibly to the level of 50 to 60%. There are several commercial products dealing with phytase enzymes to be used in poultry feed are available in the country and their details including price can be obtained from https://dir.indiamart.com/impcat/phytase.html. Several companies such as AB Vista, Adisseo, BASF, Biotech Pvt Ltd, Bioven Ingredients, Dimitech International LLP, DuPont, Mitushi Biopharma, Novozymes/DSM, Rossari Biotech Ltd., Ulytreze Enzymes Pvt Ltd, are engaged in phytase enzyme production.

Action of phytase enzyme

Microbial phytase hydrolyses phytate and releases Ca, P and trace minerals. One phytase unit (FTU, FYT, PTU) is the amount of phytase that releases 1 mol inorganic P per minute from an excess of sodium phytate at 37^{0}C and pH 5.5. 500 FYT/kg feed releases 0.12% P from phytate. Phytase enzymes are commercially available and are being used in poultry rations.

Phytase is produced endogenously by bacteria found in the gut of ruminant animals (cattle, sheep) making it possible for them to use this enzyme to degrade phytate or phytic acid bound P. Non-ruminants (monogastric animals) like human beings, dogs, pigs, birds, etc. do not produce phytase. Research in the field of animal nutrition has put forth the idea of supplementing feed with phytase enzyme so as to make available to the animal phytate-bound nutrients like Ca and P minerals, carbohydrates, amino acids and proteins.

Phytase is used as an animal feed supplement-often in poultry and swine- to enhance the nutritive value of plant material by liberation of inorganic phosphate from phytic acid (myo-inositol hexakisphosphate). Phytase can be purified from transgenicmicrobes and has been produced recently in transgenic canola, alfalfa and rice plants.

Crop and proventriculus are the main sites of phytase activity in poultry. In chickens, 69 to 86 per cent microbial phytase activity is observed in the crop and 31 to 38% in the proventriculus. No phytase activity was detected in the small intestine.

The improvement in nitrogen retention, protein and amino acid utilization by dietary phytase supplementation is relatively small and highly variable. The efficacy of supplemental phytase is affected by atleast three dietary factors: Ca:P ratio, cholecalciferol and organic acids. High levels of dietary Ca and/ or wide Ca:P ratio reduced the availability of phytic acid-bound P even in the presence of high levels of phytase.

Nutritional benefits of phytase

a) **General Benefits:** In poultry, feed is accounting up to 70% of total production cost. Consistent increase in the price of feed ingredients has been a major constraint in most of the developing countries like India. As a consequence, cheaper and non-conventional feed ingredients have to be used which contain higher percentage of starch and non starch polysaccharides (NSP) constituting major part of dietary fiber. Adequate research findings on use of exogenous microbial phytase enzymes in poultry diets have revealed several benefits such as:

- Improves growth rate productivity and maximum profit.
- Ensures better growth, production and feed conversion ratio.
- Improves fertility, hatchability and embryonic development.
- Improves egg shell quality and reduces broken eggs.
- Improves bone strength and meat quality.
- Improves immune function and gut health.
- Reduces sickness and prevents disease occurrence.
- Reduces inflammation, stress and improved drug efficacy.

- Helps in utilization of other nutrients.
- Reduces air, soil and water pollution from poultry waste.

b) **Specific Benefits:** Several studies indicate that the supplementation of exogenous microbial phytase increases body weight gain, feed intake, feed efficiency and overall growth performance in broiler chickens. The improvement in growth performance in chickens fed with phytase may be due to increased bioavailability of P by phytase, increase in feed intake and feed efficiency, increase in utilization of inositol etc. In layer rations, the supplementation of phytase is very effective in replacing inorganic P by releasing more P through enzymic actions. It can be explained in a more common way that the phytase supplementation in low P diet improves bioavailability of phytate phosphorus resulting an increase in feed intake, egg production, egg weight and egg shell thickness.

Main aim of using microbial phytase is to release of P from plant derived feed ingredients. Supplemental phytase increases the P availability from 20 to 40%, decreases the P excretion by 50% and also improves serum inorganic P concentration in broilers. The amount of phytate P released by microbial phytase depends on:

1. Concentration of phytate in the diet
2. Concentration and source of the added phytase. Supplementation of phytase @ 500FYT/Kg to low P diet increased P retention by 12.4% similarly supplementation of phytase @ 800 FYT/Kg to wheat-sorghum-soy based diet increased availability of P by 40.3 % (low), 58.9 % (medium) 44.1% (high) phytate phosphorus diet.
3. Supplementation of microbial phytase increases the availability of Ca in broiler chicks.
4. Retention Ca increases as the level of phytase increases in the diet and decreases as the ratio of Ca: P becomes wider in the diet. Phytase increases tibia or toe ash in broilers, this may be due to increased bioavailability of phosphorus and Ca by phytase.
5. Addition of vitamin D_3 along with phytase increases the utilization of phytate.
6. Phytase hydrolyses the phytic acid and releases variable amount of bound minerals.
7. Supplementation of microbial phytase increases the retention of Zn from 27.6% to 34.7%.
8. Phytase improves Zn utilization by reducing Zn excretion in broilers and there by reduces requirement of Zn in broiler diet.

9. Phytase increases the retention of Cu from 2.46% to 5.4% in broilers fed low P diet and improves utilization of Mn in broiler chicks.

Economics of phytase supplementation

The use of feed enzymes in poultry feed has gained more acceptance by producers over the past few years in India. The use of feed enzymes in poultry feed allows producers to benefit from advances in enzyme technology in today's competitive and challenging market. Enzyme supplements are used widely in poultry diets in an attempt to improve nutrient utilization, the health and welfare, product quality and to reduce pollution as well as to increase the choice and content of ingredients. It is well established that the poultry diets supplemented with microbial phytase result in an improved growth performance and increased digestibility and availability of phytate bound Ca, Cu, Fe, Mg, Mn, P, Zn.

The efficacy of supplemental microbial phytase depends on its rate of inclusion, dietary Ca and P ratio, vitamin D_3, nature of diet, age and genotype of birds. Thus microbial phytase can be used to exploit the inherent nutritional potential of feedstuffs for more economic and environmentall friendly poultry production.

Dietary P is one of the costliest item in poultry feed. Replacement of inorganic P by available organic P as released only after degradation of phytic acid or phytate-bound P by supplemental exogenous phytase enzyme leads to more economic poultry production. Supplementation of exogenous phytase @ 25g/100 kg in corn-soy-wheat bran based diets without DCP reduced the feed cost. Supplementation of broiler diets with phytase @ 30 gm /100kg of feed without DCP resulted in increase in net income by 9.47%. In an experiment the phytase supplementation has significantly increased growth rate and improved production index regardless of the level of olive cake (OC) in broiler feed. In addition phytase supplementation significantly increased plasma inorganic P of broiler fed different levels of OC and economic efficiency of broilers fed 10% OC. Phytase supplementation to 10% OC diets yields the highest return over cost and economic efficiency. Multi enzyme preparation improves bird's performance in following ways:

1. Improves amino acids, energy, fat, protein and starch digestibility.
2. Reduces the water holding capacity of the gut contents thus increasing the dry matter content stimulating feed intake.
3. Reduces the dry matter outside the body thus has marked impact on excreta volume and composition.

4. Pro-Maxyl of ABTL is an enzyme containing phytase and a combination of mannase, protease and xylanase enzymes and has brought favourable feedbacks after using this enzyme product in broiler and layer farms @ 50 gms/100 kg feed showing improved egg and meat production performance and feed utilization.

Conclusion

Like other living creatures, the birds do need several nutrients in their diets to maintain optimum body growth, normal health and maximum production of edible egg and meat. Among various major minerals, P plays a vital role in bone development, egg production and egg shell quality. About 2/3 of total P is present in phytin form and bound with phytic acid forming a complex compound known as phytate in vegetable based poultry diet. Phytate-bound P utilization by poultry varies from 0-50% depending upon the source of phytate, age of birds, and dietary levels of Ca and vitamin D_3.Phytase has the capacity to counteract the anti-nutritional effects of phytate by hydrolyzing the phytic acid to inositol and inorganic P. Supplementation of exogenous microbial phytase along with feed ingredients improves the growth performance and retention of Ca, Cu & P, when fed to poultry. Phytase also increases the apparent metabolizable energy (AME) and ileal digestibility of protein and amino acids. Therefore, supplemental exogenous microbial phytase can be used in poultry ration to increase phytic acid degradation and the availability of plant P can have major benefits for poultry producers. With the result an increase in the growth performance, digestibility of nutrients and reduction in feed cost by replacing expensive inorganic P source such as DCP have been concerned with benefits of phytase supplementation.

References

Al-Harthi, M.A., Attia, Y.A., El-Shafey, A.S. and Elgandy, M.F. 2020. Impact of phytase on improving the utilisation of pelleted broiler diets containing olive by-products. Italian Journal of Animal Science 19(1):310-318. https://doi.org/10.1080/1828051x.2020.1740896.

Daniel, J.D., Manas, N.H.A., Azlee, N.I.W., Eyahmalay, J., Yahaya, S.A., Malek, R.A., Siwapiragam, V., Sukumawati, D., and Enhasy, H.E. 2018. Current and future applications of phytases in poultry industry: A critical review. Journal of Advances in Vet Bioscience and Techniques, 3(3):65-74. http://doi.org/10.31797/vetbio.455687.

Lei, X.G. and Stahl, C. H. 2000. Nutritional benefits of phytase and dietary determinants of its efficacy. Journal of Applied Animal Research 17(1):97-112. https://doi.org/10.1080/0971 2119.2000.9706294.

Phytase.en.m.wikipedia.org.

Phytase at best price in India. https://dir.indiamart.com/impcat/phytase.html.

Ravindran, V., Bryden, W.L and Kornegay, E.T. 1995. Phytates: occurrence, bioavailability and implications in poultry nutrition. Poultry and Avian Biology Review 6(2):125 – 143.https:// agris.fao.org/agris-search/search.do?recordID=GB9620706.

Sannamani, P., Venkata Reddy, J K and Rengarajan, K. 2019. Role of phytic acid and phytase in poultry nutrition. Poultry Punch, May 24. poultrypunch.com https://en.wikipedia.org/wiki/Phytase.

Selle, P.H. and Ravindran, V. 2007. Microbial phytase in poultry nutrition. Animal Feed Science and Technology. 135(1-2):1-41. https://doi.org/10.1016/j.ani.feedsci 2006.06.010.

Singh, P. K. 2008. Significance of phytic acid and supplemental phytase in chicken nutrition: a review. World's Poultry Science Journal 64(4):553-580. https://doi.org/10.1017/S0043933908000202.

10

Exploration of Natural Additives in Poultry Production

D. Uma Maheswari, N. Elanchezhian, R. Suresh and George Dominic

Department of Animal Nutrition, Rajiv Gandhi Institute of Veterinary Education and Research, Puducherry

Feed additives

Feed additives may be defined as those substances that are added in livestock feeds to improve quality, digestibility and utilisation of feeds. It is also aimed at production improved quality of livestock produce, performance and health of the livestock and birds.

Classification of Additives

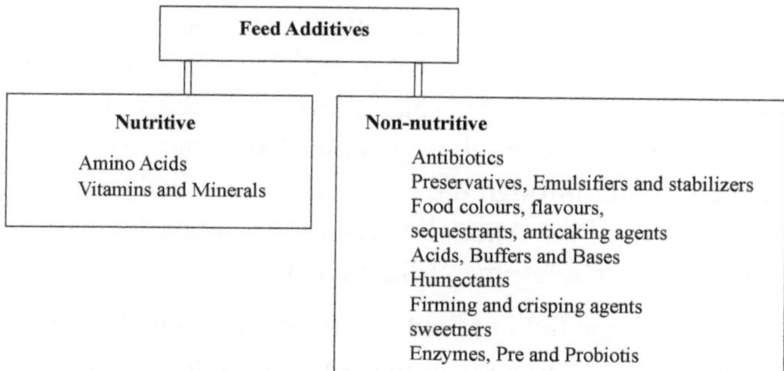

Fig. 1: Broad classification of feed additives

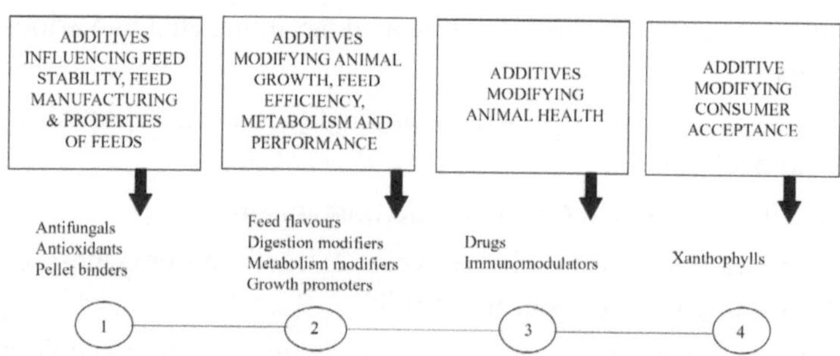

Fig. 2: Classification based on mode of action

Feed additives have been used since decades in animal feeds for enhancing production in terms of meat, milk, etc. However, the present decade has seen an enormous change in the use of feed additives. The old school of thought of additives in terms of categories such as Improving the palatability of feeds, Improving digestion and absorption, Improving the metabolism and utilisation still holds good. But, now the scenario has turned to one major area wherein animal health, growth and performance is seen on par with human health and weighted with the economics of return from animal products. The scale of profit for farmers in terms of animal products is balanced with consumer preference and health. Over the last two decades, a major change has taken place in the feed industry mainly towards all-natural production. An intensive pressure from the consumer groups towards the usage of hormones, antibiotics and any growth promoter or therapeutic agents in animal feeds or anything that are considered to be non-natural has now changed the trend of additives in animal feeds and their inclusion.

The earlier use of hormonal additives and BST, though found to be highly beneficial is linked with the safety of the consumer. The same applies to the antibiotic growth promoters. The hormones though have a positive effect the more important factor involved is how it affects milk consumption. The non-natural additive image in the health-conscious market has led to the withdrawal of these additives in animal production. In the case of antibiotic growth promoters, the development of resistance in pathogens and transfer of the resistance to other bacteria via R-plasmids has led to controlled and limited use of antibiotics in animal feeds. The regulatory bodies have come to force to ensure the safety of the consumer through the judicious use of feed additives. It has become a profound duty of the Animal Nutrition and Feed Industry to cater the consumer natural and wholesome milk, meat and egg.

The advent of biotechnology in the field of feed additives has opened vistas of natural additives in animal feeds. The wide arena wherein biotechnology has its hold is:

- Amino acid production *viz.* lysine, glutamic acid, arginine, etc., by various microorganisms
- Peptides and their isolates with known metabolic function *viz.* metabolites from lactic acid bacteria.
- Production of vitamins via GRAS listed microorganisms
- Flavours of varying ranges from cheese, yeast extract with enzymes and bacteria and also functional protein from milk
- Colour from yeast strains which are reputed to contain up to 5% colour compounds

- Trace mineral nutrition and metabolism in terms of increased bioavailability
- Lactic acid bacteria and its inclusion in diets
- Exogenous enzyme production and its application
- Production of transgenic animals with improved rate of gain
- Anti mould or toxin inhibitor
- Improved hindgut fermentation with selective stimulation of certain bacteria
- Environmental control
- Electrolyte balance
- Iron metabolism through the use of transferrin as supplemental iron transport
- New ingredients-Production of microbial proteins as new feed sources in animal feeding (e.g. single cell protein, yeast protein).
- Designer ingredients-Nutritional enhancement (e.g. high-oil maize, high-methionine lupins) or reduction in the level of anti-nutritive components in common feed ingredients (e.g. low-phytate maize).

Nutritive Feed additves in Poultry feeds

The common nutritive feed additives in poultry comprise the use of amino acids, minerals and vitamins. The nutritive additves encompasses the need for improved amino acid balance, reduced feed cost, replacement of normal protein resources with high protein newer ingredients and improved performance in poultry due to improved health.

1. **Ideal Proteins:** The concept of adding commercial lysine to diets has markedly reduced the feed cost and also improved the balance of critical amino acids in animal feed in addition to increasing productivity. The threat of limiting amino acid from the second and third amino acids in line is now alleviated by the biotechnology intervention in the preparation of these amino acids. However, the latest trend is to feed the amino acids or design them in the form of di, tri, and tetrapeptides since most of the amino acids are absorbed in their peptide forms. When fed as peptides we stand to gain more from their biological action and more weightage is there for their nutritional importance. This also raises the importance of feeding amino acids as peptide mineral complexes.
2. **Protein rich feed additives:** Algae are another form of protein additive in poultry feeding. Algae may be obtained from natural sources or cultivated in artificial ponds, e.g. phototrophic microalgae. The most popular algae

is spirulina. Spirulina (*Arthrospira platensis*) belongs to unicellular microalgae living in natural or artificial water reservoirs. Tests proved that adding microalgae to fodder in poultry feeding increase content of unsaturated fatty acids (NNKT) and carotenoids in egg yolks. The best results were noted in a group of 10% additive of algae in which the biggest growth of body mass, decrease of fat content in blood and liver were noted, as compared to control group.

Azolla is another fresh water fern found in tropical and subtropical countries which is now used as a protein source in the feed of broilers and back yard poultry. Azolla contains 25-30% total protein in addition to being a rich source minerals, chlorophyll, carotinoids, amino acids, vitamins etc. It is also a potential source of nitrogen and is a potential feed ingredient for livestock.Basak *et.al* (2002) concluded from their studies that azolla can be safely included at 5% level in the diet of broilers .However, azolla is much preferred in backyard poultry farming for a economical returns. Bidya Shankar Sinha *et al.*(2018) opined that fresh Azolla is a good feed supplement for reducing the feed cost and highest Benefit Cost ratio in backyard poultry. Usually 100 gram per bird per day may be fed for the better body weight gain as well as more number of egg production thereby for more profit.

A new concept of feeding insect and fly protein is now under study in Asia, Africa and Latin America.Nutritonists looking for new unique protein source are considering the insect meal from larvae of insects and house fly on productivity and development of microbiome in birds.However the concerns on the production cost of the insect meal and its biosafety is under scrutiny of the scientists and may require more time before it is recommended in livestock and poultry feeding.

3. **Boron based amino acids:** Next to carbon, boron has the property to form simple compounds with hydrogen. The structure in its simplest form as boron hydride is similar to methane and is sensitive to hydrolysis in water as boric acid. The recent advance in science has overcome this sensitivity and has come out with boron biomolecules that cross membrane barriers much more easily than their carbon counterparts. One such example is boroglycerine which possesses anticancer and anti-bacterial effects.

Trace minerals and their role as additives

1. **Chromium in animal nutrition:** Chromium as organic chromium has emerged as one of the vital elements in animal nutrition in the recent past. While talking about the element one should be aware that chromium as trivalent chromium is the one with potential use as an additive and

not the hexavalent one from industrial settings. The biological function of chromium is attributed to its association with insulin or as a glucose tolerance factor which potentiates the action of insulin. Recent studies have proven dietary chromium is necessary for normal insulin sensitivity in peripheral tissues in addition to preserving normal pancreatic beta-cell sensitivity /insulin production. The organic form of chromium is preferred over its inorganic counterpart for easier negation to certain dietary precursors and conversion to bioactive forms. Thus Cr as proteinates, trinicotinate, Cr yeast or amino acid chelated Cr are preferred over the inorganic form of chromium in animal feeds. Inorganic chromium sources are poorly absorbed as compared to organic chelated chromium. Most available supplemental sources are chromium picolinate and chromium nicotinate.

Chromium has been added as a stress protectant. Chromium supplementation to high yielding dairy cows during transition period improves feed intake and milk production during early lactation. Further, it also improves reproductive performance, cell-mediated and humoral-immune responses. It has been established in mice that chromium is protectant against stress-related losses of several trace elements like zinc, copper, iron and manganese. Chromium is an important factor since it is related with normal insulin action. Important implications of chromium as an additive exist in animal welfare as an anti-stress agent and in terms of improving animal health and immunity.

2. **Role of selenium (Se) in animal nutrition:** Selenium and its importance in animal nutrition was established when certain deficiencies were reported in early fifties which were initially considered due to an unknown factor and was later correlated to Selenium. The most common deficiency being muscular dystrophy in livestock and poultry. The compromised immune status in animals is another complication in Se deficiency. Swine dysentery, mastitis, infertility and reduced growth rate are some of the cases reported due to Se deficiency. Biochemically Se is *correlated* with the enzyme glutathione peroxidase and the level of vitamin E. In order to prevent deficiencies that could occur due to Se improving soil content through fertilization with selenium salt or supplementation of inorganic or organic form has been suggested. However, it was noticed that the organic form of supplementation was more beneficial than inorganic. Some of the methods suggested for the supplementation were through selenium yeast. Through this method one can achieve their goal as follows:

- Organic selenium compounds do not have peroxidative effects of selenite
- When fed as selenium yeast it has the same effect as of selenoprotein

- Tissue incorporation of Se was high
- Body protein mobilization and selenium homeostasis was better
- Glutathione peroxidase activity however was not influenced by the source of selenium and remained unaltered.

3. **Zinc proteinates in animal feed:** The role of chelated minerals in immune status is well established in animal nutrition. Nutritional factors related to immune status include protein/energy level, trace minerals and vitamins in animal feeds. The role of trace minerals in monogastric nutrition is well established. Zinc is attributed as the 2nd most abundant among trace minerals and serve as an integral part of over 300 enzymes regarding their structure or metabolic and catalytic activity (Sahraei *et al.*, 2013). It has its share in many important functions such as an antioxidant. Many hormones such as somatomedin, testosterone, osteocalcin, thyroid hormone, growth hormone, insulin require zinc for their proper secretion and functioning (Salim *et al.*, 2012). Being an important component of nucleic acids synthesis, cell division calcified matrix, it is also responsible to maintain integrity of epithelial tissues, keratin generation and bone metabolism. Moreover, it plays a key role in synthesis of proteins, catalytic and structural regulation of different enzymes, protein, fat and carbohydrate metabolism and some immune functions as well. Organically complexed zinc has higher bioavailability than it is in organic form and proves to be more useful for birds (Salim *et al.*, 2011). Zinc is reported to interact with vitamins during heat stress and improves antioxidative effect.

4. **Copper:** Copper (Cu) is a micronutrient involved in many physiological processes and immunity, and it is necessary for optimal health and growth of poultry. Cu is involved in both humoral (facilitates antibody production) and cell-mediated immunity (assists in eliminating invading bacteria). It shows immune stimulating action and supports maintaining appropriate microbiological balance in the digestive tract (Makarski *et al.*, 2014). Thus, it has been used in poultry production as a nutritional supplement due to its microbiological activities and the ability to increase body weight (Wang *et al.*, 2008). Copper as a feed additive has a helpful effect on the body weight gain (BWG), feed conversion ratio (FCR) and modification of the bacterial microflora in the gut.

Vitamins

Antioxidants are the foundation of immunity and health. Vitamin A, E and C are capable of reacting with free radicals, thereby reducing their amounts and preventing lipid peroxidation in the birds. Micro minerals (Zn, Se) are not directly capable of preventing or reducing ROS formation. However, they are essential cofactors for those enzymes which have the attribute of reacting with free radicals.

Ferdous *et al.* (2018) stated that vitamins may be used with drinking water to get good results in BWG, hematological indices and biochemical profiles without any harmful effects on broiler chickens. Vitamins may improve the development of the intestinal mucosa and protect enterocytes from proapoptotic oxidant stress (Hassanpour *et al.*, 2016). The proper ratios of the fat-soluble vitamins and the combination of the four vitamins – A, D, E and C, as a vitamin emulsion positively affected the performance of broiler chicks (Kamalzadeh *et al.,* 2009). In summary, vitamins improve the physiological and health status of birds.

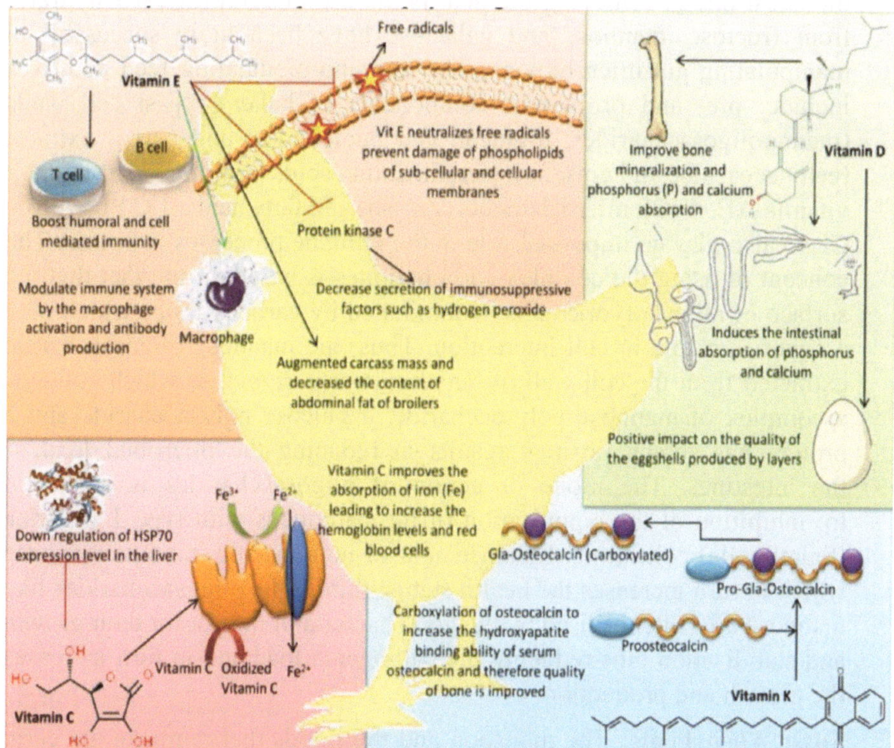

Fig. 3: Beneficial effects of different vitamins on poultry health (Alagawany et al., 2020)

Non-nutritive feed additives

The non-nutritive feed additives included in the feed depending on species, types of feed, and market. These include natural or synthetic pigmenters to enhance egg yolk and broiler skin color (e.g., carophyll, lutein, zeaxanthin), mold inhibitors to prevent mold growth (e.g., organic acids), mycotoxin binders that bind to the mycotoxins and prevent them from being absorbed, coccidiostats to prevent coccidiosis (protozoan infection in poultry), immune modulators and pellet binders to reduce feed dust and help pellets adhere better.

1. **Immune modulators:** Immune modulators are in the diet of animals in an aim to control intestinal pathogens which is of an immense challenge to livestock producers. The effect of immunomodulators is through their direct action on the cells of the immune system that ensure an immune response. Modification of the process of determined immune reactions in this way increases the organism resistance to viral, bacterial and parasite infections. The category of additives in the form of antibiotics, acidifiers in feed and water and, competitive exclusion of pathogens through probiotics are some of the modes applied successfully for the purpose. However, the latest one in achieving the goal is the use of complex carbohydrates from fructose, mannose and galactose have been more successful in manipulating gut microbiology. The immuno-modulating feed additives include: pre- and probiotics, components of baker's yeast cell walls (mannooligosaccharides, ß-glucan and nucleotides) and herbal extracts (echinacea, aloe and ginseng). Certain amino acids (arginine, methionine), vitamins (E, A, C), microelements (Zn, Sn) and fatty acids (LC PUFA n-3, CLA) also play an important role in the immune processes in poultry.The concept of using the complex carbohydrates is based on the fact that the surface of all eukaryotic cells is dominated by carbohydrates which play a significant role in cell interaction. Thus, the mannose oligosaccharide extracted from the cell wall of *Saccharomyces cerevicae* which contains a complex of mannose polysaccharide, a glucose polysaccharide and a protein has shown positive results in reducing the microbial load of the intestines. The mode of action of oligosaccharides is attributed to: inhibition of the colonisation of the pathogens with type 1 fimbriae (Salmonella) coliformis. Enhancement of non-specific immune response which in turn increases the health status: thirdly the oligosaccharides like mannose are better utilised by the good bacteria of the gut for their growth and stabilisation thus reducing the pathogenic load and in turn increases the growth and production.

2. **Toxin Absorbents:** The monsoon and the floods that rampage the earth have been a major concern of the nutritionists and feed manufacturers who face the monster in name moulds and the toxins that they produce which can lead to both economic loss and mortality to the livestock and poultry. Of these toxins the fusarium and aflatoxin are more imminent and needs a proper control to avoid loss in swine and poultry industry. The use of yeast in alleviating these problems in addition to the commercial toxin binders likes aluminum silicate and methionine which has now caught the trend as additives in the animal feed industry.

Additives in poultry nutrition

To run an economically profitable poultry farm one has to think in terms of efficient production and returns. The efficiency of production narrows down to feeding and management. As feed cost forms the major (70%) input for any farmer his return is dependent on feed efficiency. This is where the feed additives come in hand for effective feed conversion efficiency. The role of the additives in poultry nutrition is varied. In addition to growth promoter the additives are also aimed at production of final products according to the consumer preference, thus widening their role in production of designer meat and egg.

Examples of some Feed additives that are widely used in Poultry nutrition

1. Antimicrobials- To suppress the growth of harmful bacteria and promote the establishment of a desirable gut flora balance (e.g. antibiotics)
2. Crystalline amino acids- To increase dietary supply of specific amino acid and improve protein balance in diet formulations.
3. Feed enzymes- To improve availability of nutrients (energy, amino acids, phosphorus etc) in feed ingredients by reducing the negative effects of anti-nutritive components (e.g. microbial phytases acting on phytate, xylanases acting on arabinoxylans in wheat).

Gut ecosystem enhancers

1. Probiotics promote the establishment of a desirable gut ecosystem through the proliferation of beneficial species (e.g. direct-fed microbials).
2. Prebiotics competitively exclude harmful organisms and promote the establishment of a desirable gut ecosystem (e.g. mannan oligosaccharides).

Recent trends in additives

Additives in feed and water are the common practices in poultry industry. The classification, kind and scope of application of feed additives are viewed in line with consumer demand. However, there are many challenges that need to be overcome by adopting suitable strategies to produce a profitable poultry market without compromising the consumer health. The present era of additives in poultry production is emphasised on natural additives which are the alternative to antibiotic growth promoters. A broad classification of additves now preferred over AGF is listed in Table 1.

With the FDA defining its norms in additives in animal feeds many earlier trends of using antibiotics and hormones are now not in vogue. How to keep with the productivity and to provide a wholesome meat and milk and animal produce to the consumers globally many novel additives have entered the market under the canopy of "Natural Additives". The use of "Neutraceuticals" the substance that may be considered a food or part of a food and provides medical or health benefits, encompassing, prevention and treatment of diseases are also considered under the feed additives umbrella.

Table 1: Newer Additives in Poultry Feeds-An alternative to antibiotic growth Promoters (AGPs)

Alternatives to AGPs	Active ingredients	Basic functions	Effects on broiler
Probiotics	*Bacillus subtilis, Enterococcus faecium Lactobacillus acidophilus, Bacilluslicheniformis, Bifidobacterium bifidum*	Appetite and digestion stimulant, antioxidant	• Increased body weight and FCR. • Improved absorptive surface of duodenum and ileum. • Increase nutrient retention
Prebiotics	Fructo-oligosaccharides (FOS), Inulin, galacto-oligosaccharides (GOS), Trans-galacto oligo-saccharides	Digestion, stimulant	• Increased growth performance • Stimulation of metabolic activity in intestine
Organic acids	Citric acid, Ascorbic acid Propionic acid and sodium bentonite, Butyrate	Digestion, stimulant, increased feed effciency	• Increased body weight • Improved ileal nutrient digestibility, cell proliferation, epithelial and villi height
Amino acids and enzymes	Phytase, lysins	Digestion, stimulant	• Improved growth performance
Phytogenic feed additives	Pepper	Digestion, stymulant	No effect on live performance
	Garlic	Digestion, stimulant, Antiseptic	Higher body weight
	Ginger	Gastric stymulant	No effects on performance
	Rosemary	Digestion, stimulant, antiseptic,antioxidant	Improved live weight and feed effciency
	Thyme		No significant effect on BW/FCR
	Mint	Appetite, digestion, stimulant, antiseptic	Decreased serum total cholesterol, triglycerides, and low-density lipoprotein concentration

Nanoparticles (NPs)	Silver NPs, Selenium NPs, Copper NPs, Metal NPs such as zinc oxide, zirconium dioxide, and platinum Zn-bearing zeolite, clinoptilolite, NPs Nanosuspensions of clay minerals	Digestion, Stimulant	Increased body weight and FCR

(Makala, 2021)

Natural additives

Over the last two decades emphasis is on the use of natural additives like enzymes, which aid in biochemical functions and gastrointestinal development. In addition to this more attention has been focused on the use of probiotics, prebiotics, yeast culture and acidifiers in the swine and poultry industry.

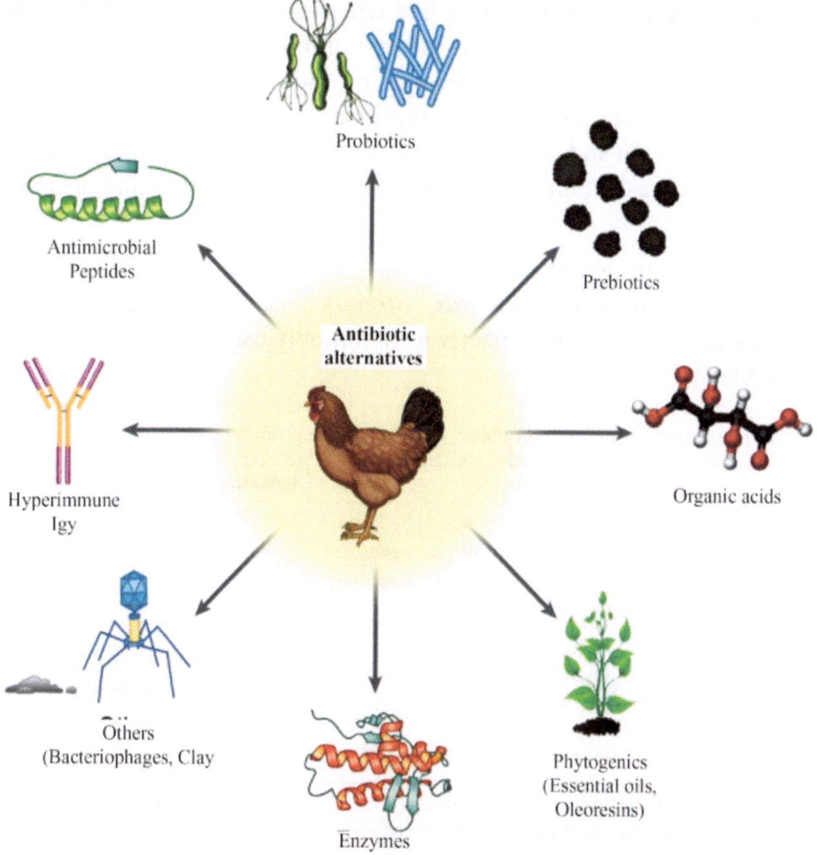

Fig. 4: Alternatives to Antibiotic Growth Promoters in Poultry Feed (Gadde *et al.*, 2017)

1. **Probiotics:** Several studies have proved that the addition of live organisms like *L. acidophilus* and *S. faecium* have helped in maintaining gut health by 'competitive inhibition of pathogenic bacteria (Chapman, J.D. 1989). This in turn aids in improved gut health, prevention of disease, improved absorption and have utilization of nutrients by the animals and thus its improved production. This method is an alternative to antibiotic growth promoters and does not have any residual effect to the consumer. Probiotic supplementation is an alternative to AGP and is much more beneficial. The effect of probiotics is based on: (1) modification of the intestinal microbiota, (2) stimulation of the immune system, (3) reduction in inflammatory reactions, (4) prevention of pathogen colonization, (5) enhancement of growth performance, (6) alteration of the ileal digestibility and total tract apparent digestibility coefficient, and (7) decrease in ammonia and urea excretion. The use of probiotics in poultry nutrition has increased over the years, The selection of the strain is dependant on its protective efficacy,mode of action and when a combination of strains are used it is based on the synergistic effect exhibited on the host . The basic criteria for selection of strain depends on the tolerance of the microbe in the gut mucosa, competitive inhibition or exclusion of pathogenic strains from the gut and survival in manufacturing, transportation, storage, application processes, and their ability to maintain viability and desirable characteristics.

The common microorganisms used as probitic are *Bifidobacterium*, *Lactococcus*, *Lactobacillus*, *Bacillus*, *Streptococcus,* and yeast such as *Candida.* Some of the beneficial bacteria commnonly used in poultry feeds are listed in Table 2.

Table 2: Summary of the beneficial probiotic species used in poultry production

Strain	Characteristics	Benefits
Bacillus amyloliquefaciens	Root-colonizing biocontrol bacteria used to fight plant root pathogens in agriculture, aquaculture, and hydroponics.	Enhances gut health and growth performance.
Bacillus coagulans	Bacteria exhibit the characteristics of both genera Lactobacillus and Bacillus.	Improve growth performance and gut histomorphology.
Bacillus licheniformis	Bacteria commonly found in soil.	Prevents necrotic enteritis and enhances growth performance.
Bacillus subtilis	Bacteria found in soil and the gastrointestinal tract of ruminants and humans.	Enhances laying performance and helps the immune system and gut health.

Bifidobacterium animalis	Bacteria found in the large intestines of most mammals.	Helps the immune system, gut physiology, and health.
Bifidobacterium bifidum	Bacteria that is one of the most common probiotic bacteria that can be found in the body of mammals.	Helps the immune system and gut health.
Lactobacillus acidophilus	Bacteria found in the human and animal gastrointestinal tract and mouth.	Enhances gut health and growth performance.
Lactobacillus bulgaricus	Bacteria found in the gastrointestinal tract of mammals and naturally fermented products.	Enhances growth performance and improves immune functions.
Lactobacillus bifermentans	Bacteria found in the human and animal gastrointestinal tract.	Enhances growth performance and digestive health.
Lactobacillus fermentum	Bacteria found in fermenting animal and plant material.	Enhances growth performance, gut histomorphology, and immune functions.
Lactobacillus salivarius	Bacteria found in the human and animal gastrointestinal tract.	Improves laying performance and enhances gut histomorphology.
Lactobacillus sanfranciscensis	Heterofermentative bacteria closely related or normally present in sour dough.	Enhances growth performance.
Lactobacillus reuteri	Bacteria that naturally inhabits the gut of mammals and birds.	Enhances growth performance, gut histomorphology, immune system, and gut health.
Pediococcus acidilactici	Bacteria found in fermented vegetables, fermented dairy products, and meat.	Improves laying performance and modulates the gut microbiota.
Propionibacterium acidipropionici	Found in dairy products and the environment.	Contributes to the better development of gut mucosa.
Saccharomyces cerevisiae	A species of yeast found primarily on ripe fruits such as grapes.	Enhances growth performance and improves laying performance.
Streptococcus faecium	Bacteria inhabiting the gastrointestinal tracts of humans and other mammals.	Improves immune functions.

(Rajesh *et al.*, 2020)

2. **Prebiotics:** The effect of nutrition on health and immunity is a lifelong relationship. The food provides nutrition, which aids in growth and provides building blocks of the immune system. The nutrients specifically complex carbohydrates play a major role in disease prevention and immune-boosting of the animals. This has sparked the interest of nutritionists and feed manufacturers globally to explore the complex carbohydrates in animal feed as additives. Carbohydrates were initially

thought to be the source of energy alone due to the simplified structure of the monosaccharide. But unlike two amino acids which can form one dipeptide, two identical monosaccharides can form 11 distinct disaccharides which explain the human blood groups and the immunity of humans against bacterial infections caused by K99 *E.coli* in livestock. This explains the role of complex carbohydrates in animal health. The most common example is the mannan oligosaccharide (MOS). MOS is a glucose polysaccharide from the yeast cell wall and as an adsorber of enteric pathogens and immune modulator. The bacterial attachment in the intestines occurs through lectins which are specific for sugars such as galactose, fucose however the lectins specific for intestinal pathogens is predominated by mannose. Thus MOS adsorbs these pathogens preventing their colonization in the gut and removes from the gut. The addition of mannose oligosaccharides in the diet of the poultry proved to be beneficial by bringing about a marked decrease in *Salmonlla typhimurium* and its colonization in the caecum. Similar to this the MOS is also found to inhibit the proliferation of the *Escherichia coli* in the gut by binding to the lectins and preventing the proliferation. The oligosaccharides particularly the mannose oligosaccharide have adjuvant and antigen properties which stimulate the liver to produce mannose-binding protein which in turn influences the immune system. This mannose-binding protein binds to the capsule of bacteria and triggers the complement cascade. As an immune modulator, the glucomannoprotein also has a role wherein upon administration in laboratory animals it triggered an immediate decrease in properdin levels followed by an increase. Properdin is known to be an important component of the alternate pathway for complement fixation which explains the increased effect glucomannoprotein on the bactericidal activity of the animal sera. Thus the prebiotics are known to control pathogens by preventing their proliferation, and support the growth of beneficial bacteria and, aid in improved immune activity.

Acidifiers in Animal Nutrition

Acidifiers have been in use as an alternative to antibiotics since the late 90s. Organic acidifiers like formic acid, acetic acid and their salts were used to promote gut health and production in swine. Organic acidification using fumaric and malic acids was studied in broilers and it was observed that the acidification of the broiler diets were beneficial rather than acidification via water. Improved gut health through reduced microbial load was noticed along with a marked difference in the length of the intestinal villi suggestive of increased absorption of the nutrients resulting in improved growth rate. However, the combined use of lactobacillus and yeast culture with acidification of water, have shown improved performance with a notable decrease in mortality rate (Uma Maheswari, 2017).

3. **Enzymes in Animal Nutrition:** Grains play a major role in animal feed as energy sources. However, their use is limited to few choices like maize, wheat and rice when compared to other grains like barley, oats or rye. The initial reason attributed for this was their fiber content. This school of thought is now outdated and the most recent pointer is the nature of bonding in the sugars in feed, like beta-glucans in barley for example. For decades the use of enzymes in beverages was practiced, but the application of the enzymes in animal feeds has been brought to limelight only with the advent of biotechnology. The methodology for extraction enzymes from of microbes have been standardized making it easier for the feed manufacturers and nutritionist to incorporate substrate-specific enzymes for using economic ingredients without compromising their nutrient values. The application of the exogenous enzymes in animal diet has improved their digestion and performance both in healthy young ones and sick animals or animals under stress.

Successful modes of enzyme supplementation

- Aids in nutrient availability by removing or destroying the anti-nutritional factors like beta-glucanase (barley), pentosans (wheat) and phytic acid
- Complements with the endogenous digestivity of animals
- Improves absorption rate of some nutrients from the gut
- Increases the energy value of low nutritive ingredients
- Reduces pollutive effect of the animal excreta
- Helps in combatting specific processing problems

Enzymes applied in Feeds

- Enzymes addition in the diets of animals has resulted in potential benefits to farmers. The use of enzymes in monogastric diets have particularly been effective than the ruminants. Some of the examples of enzymes added are:
- Lipase to improve the energy availability from fats in broilers and swine finishers.
- Beta-glucanase has increased the use of barley in monogastric diets replacing maize. The use of the enzyme has reduced the wet litter problem and has positively improved the performance.
- Pentonase for wheat-based diets.
- Phosphatase has reduced the use of inorganic phosphorus and improved the phosphors availability from plant sources. The problem of erosion due to increased phosphorus in the faeces of animals has reduced considerably due to the enzyme usage which addresses the pollution problems.

- Enzyme addition has paved the way to the inclusion of wastes like feather meal which is a rich source of protein that is normally wasted under normal conditions.

Enzyme addition has gained momentum in ruminant diets wherein exogenous fibrolytic enzymes are added as predigester before feeding the animals for improved digestion and utilization. The main drawback here is the danger of inactivation of the enzymes due to the ruminal pH. Due to the high returns enzyme addition is gaining fast momentum in animal feeding.

Enzyme supplementation to improve nutrient utilization

Enzymes are proteins that facilitate specific chemical reactions and work on specifi c substrates. The enzymes widely used by the industry are the non-starch polysaccharidases (NSPases) that cleave the non-starch polysaccharides (NSP) in viscous cereals (wheat, barley and triticale) and microbial phytases that target the phytate-complexes in plant ingredients (Ravindran & Son, 2011; Pirgozliev & Bedford, 2013). The presence of arabinoxylans in cerals like whet and rye and the mixedlinked beta-D-glucans in barley are the challenges faced by nutritionists. The presence of these result in decreased availability of nutriens, increased digesta viscosity and reduced performance of the birds. In particular, soluble viscous NSPs depress the digestibility of protein, starch and fat in broiler diets, an effect which is easily overcome through use of the appropriate enzyme (Bedford, 2006; Whiting *et al.*, 2017). There is no vertebrate animal that produces enzymes capable of hydrolysing the NSP in diets. Dietary NSPases can break the bonds between sugar units of NSP and signifi cantly reduce the gut content viscosity. Lower gut viscosity will lead to a more complete digestion and absorption of nutrients, reduced microbial proliferation and improved gut health (Pirgozliev *et al.*, 2010; 2015a; Abdulla *et al.*, 2017). The NSP degrading enzymes can also produce some oligosaccharides that may act as prebiotics in the gut of poultry (Masey O'Neill *et al.*, 2014). Dietary NSPases can also improve the hepatic antioxidant capacity of broilers (Pirgozliev *et al.*, 2015b). Approximately 600 to 700 g/kg of the plant-P is present as phytate. Phytic acid (myo-inositol hexakis-dihydrogenphosphate, IP6) is a polyanionic molecule with 6 phosphate groups and is capable of forming insoluble complexes with divalent cations, starch and protein, reducing their availability for poultry (Selle & Ravindran, 2007). The benefits of using dietary phytases are not restricted to the improvement of mineral retention but may improve performance and energy and amino acid availability (Selle & Ravindran, 2007; Pirgozliev *et al.*, 2011). Research by Karadas *et al.* (2010) also found that dietary phytase can improve the hepatic antioxidant capacity of broilers.

Exogenous protease supplementation is gaining in popularity in animal nutrition with beneficial effects on growth performance, nutrient digestibility and endogenous enzyme secretion. In addition, report by Olukosi *et al.* (2015) found that though protease by itself improved nutrient utilization and increased solubilization of NSP components, at the lower dose, a combination of xylanase, amylase, and protease produced effects greater than those of protease alone. Tannase enzyme was recently supplemented to broiler feed in order to improve feeding value of diets containing field beans (Abdulla *et al.*, 2016 a,b). Although results were promising, further research is warranted to study the effectiveness of tannase supplementation in poultry diet formulations by dose response trials with purified tannase preparation.

Table 3: Potential Enzyme Substrates

Antinutrient	Where found	Problem	Enzyme
Arabinoxylans	Cell wall of plant based ingredients	Resistant to digestion, reduce nutrient digestibility, viscosity	xylanase
Cellulose	Plant ingredients	Insoluble & resistant to digestion	cellulase
Oligosaccharides	Soybean meal	Resistant to digestion	α-galactosidase
Starch	Cereals, Cereal by products	Structural resistance	amylase
Phytate	All plant based ingredients	Binds P and other cations, increases endogenous loss	phytase
β-Glucans	Cell wall of cereals such as barley and oats	Soluble form causes viscosity	β-glucanase
Mannans	Soybean meal, Yeast cell walls	Resistant to digestion	β-mannanase
Protein	Corn, Milo, Vegetable meals	Resistant protein to digestion; storage proteins	protease

Source:

Table 4: List of common enzymes, substrates and their effects

<table>
<tr><th>Enzyme</th><th>Substrate</th><th>Functions</th><th>Total benifits</th></tr>
<tr><td>Phytase</td><td>Phytate</td><td>Release phosphorous stored in phytate</td><td rowspan="8">1. Improve FCR
2. Improve litter quality
3. Greater uniformity
4. Reduce feed costs
5. Use cheaper feeds
6. Reduce DCP use & costs
7. Reduce Phosphorous excreation
8. Reduce the mortality
9. Improve overall performance of birds</td></tr>
<tr><td>Protease</td><td>Protien</td><td>Improve protein digestibility</td></tr>
<tr><td>Pectinase</td><td>NSP</td><td>Break down indigestible pectin. Reduce digestive viscosity</td></tr>
<tr><td>Xylanase</td><td>NSP</td><td>Break down fibre</td></tr>
<tr><td>Celluase</td><td>NSP</td><td>Break down fibre</td></tr>
<tr><td>β-Glucanase</td><td>NSP</td><td>Break down fibre</td></tr>
<tr><td>α- Amylase</td><td>Starch</td><td>Improve starch digestibility</td></tr>
<tr><td>Lipase</td><td>Fat</td><td>Improve fat absorption</td></tr>
</table>

Source: (www.glamac.com, 2018)

Role of Yeast as a Feed additive in animals

Yeast cultures have been used for a long as a safe and wholesome additive in human and animal feeds. The array of additives is higher in monogastrics than in ruminants. Yeast and its derived products are recognized as potential feed additives because of their beneficial impacts on poultry. Particularly, yeast exhibited positive effects on the humoral immunity by increasing serum immunoglobulin (Ig) A levels. Moreover, yeast and its products showed immune adjuvant-like properties that helped the broiler chicken to develop faster and stronger innate immune response under pathogenic challenges. Use of yeast and its products as prebiotic/probiotic improves the gut architecture mainly by improving the gut development and gut microbiome, reduction in colonization of pathogens through competitive exclusion, binding of toxins and enhancing digestion and absorption of nutrients. These unique properties of yeast and yeast products enhance animal welfare and productivity; warrant them to be used as a promising feed additive (Bilal, 2021).

4. **Phytobiotics:** Phytobiotics are plant-derived natural bioactive compounds, they are added in the diet to improve animal performance and well-being. Phytobiotcs are plant secondary metabolites (terpenoids, polyphenols, glycosides, essential oils and alkaloids), extracted from various plant sources, such as herbs (roots, leaves and bark) and spices. Much attention is given to phytobiotics due to the ban of antibiotic growth promoters. Further, phytobiotics have wide range of activities, such as improvement of palatability, increment of enzyme activity in the intestinal tract, enhancement of nutrient utilization, increased cell turnover and barrier function, improved antioxidant protection, enhanced antimicrobial activity and immune status. Further, some phytogenic compounds promote intestinal mucus production.Plant extracts have also been used to rediuce noxious ammonia gas production. One such example is use of the dessert plant Yucca scidigera which has been proven to buffer and reduce ammonia (Lyons, 1994).

Table 5: Effect of different herbs on the physiological functions and performance of Poultry

Plant	Used part/ material	Active component	Beneficial effect
Cinnamon (*Cinnamomum zeylanicum*)	bark, leaves/ cinnamon oil	Cinnamaldehyde eugenol, phenolic and polyphenolic substances	Improves appetite and digestion; enhances antioxidant status; antimicrobial and blood purifying activity; alleviation of adverse effects of environmental stress; chemopreventive effect
Garlic (*Allium sativum*)	crushed bulbs	Allicin, ajoene, allyldisulfide, vinyldithiin, phytosterols, mucilages, pectins, flavonoids	Improves immunity by increasing the titer of antibodies, stimulating the activity of lysozyme and increases the phagocytic activity of macrophages; chemopreventive effect, antiseptic and alleviate adverse effect of environmental stress; improves digestion and the blood lipid profile; improves growth and FCR
Coneflower (*Echinacea purpurea*)	leaves root/ dried herb, water and alcohol extracts, root	Polysaccharides, flavonoids, polyphenolic acids –mainly chlorogenic acid and caffeic acid, alkylamides, polyacetylenes	Immunomodulatory - stimulates phagocytic activity of macrophages, increases the activity of lysozyme, increases the titer of antibodies; antimicrobial, antitumor, antidiabetic, and antioxidant, digestion stimulant, improves of growth and FCR
Moringa (*Moringa oleifera*)	leaves/ extracts	Chlorogenic acid, caffeicacid, ascorbic acid, flavonoids, phenolics and carotenoids	Improves egg production and decreases FCR; alleviates adverse effect of environmental stress and antioxidant activity
Pappermint (*Mentha piperita*)	leaves/ powder	Menthol, terpenes	Enhances appetite and stimulate of digestion; causes decrease of FCR; it works antiseptic; improves in the laying performance, quality and freshness of eggs, and an color or the chemical composition of yolk

Turmeric (*Curcuma longa*)	rhizome/ powder	Curcuminoids, turmerones,	Improves the blood lipid profile; improves digestion - choleretic, increases appetite; action antioxidative; anticarcinogenic; antihepatotoxic and immunomodulatory-stimulates the production of interferon; chemopreventive effect
Aloe vera (*Aloe barbadensis*)	Leaves/water extracts, powder, gel powder	Anthraquinones polisaccharides (mainly icemannan) vitamins, enzymes, salicylic acid, anthraquinones and lignin, aminoacids	Immunomodulation - stimulates the activity of granulocytes and granulocytic enzymes (myeloperoxidase, peroxidase), increases the titer of antibodies; alleviate adverse effect of environmental stress; action antidiabetic, and antioxidant-decreasing the lipid peroxidation and increasing the antioxidant status; stimulation of digestion - improve absorption of nutrients from the intestine, improve of intestinal microflora; improve of performance and FCR; increasing and providing protection to the vital phisiological organ like liver and kidney
Ginger (*Zingiber officinale*)	Roots/ extracted basic oil	Monoterpenes and sesquiterpenes	Improves body weight gain due to stimulation of digestive enzymes and improvement of overall digestion, inhibits the growth of harmful bacteria in the intestinal tract due to antimicrobial activity lead to assimilation of nutrients, improves carcass traits, decreases abdominal fat; immunomodulation-increases the activity of lysozyme; chemopreventive effect

(Krauze, 2021)

Table 6: Effect of different herbs on the biochemical components of poultry blood

Plant	Used part/ material	Active component	Beneficial effect
Cinnamon (*Cinnamomum zeylanicum*)	Bark, leaves/	Cinnamon oil cinnamaldehyde, eugenol, phenolic and polyphenolic substances	Increase the proportion of HDL cholesterol, reduction of total cholesterol and triacylglycerols level, decrease lactate dehydrogenase, creatine kinase and β-hydroxybutyrate dehydrogenase activity, normalize the activity of aminotransferases
Garlic (*Allium sativum*)	crushed bulbs	Allicin, ajoene, allyldisulfide, vinyldithiin, phytosterols, mucilages, pectins, flavonoids	Increase of HDL content, decrease of total cholesterol and triacylglycerols level,
Coneflower (*Echinacea purpurea*)	leaves root/ dried herb, water and alcohol extracts	Polysaccharides, flavonoids, polyphenolic acids -mainly chlorogenic acid and caffeic acid, alkylamides, polyacetylenes	Increase of HDL content, decrease of total cholesterol and triacylglycerols level
Lavender (*Lavandula angustifolia*)	Whole plant, oil	Hydrocarbons, alcohols, ketones, esters, aldehydes, oxides, and ethers coumarins and organic acids	Beneficially effects on lipids' digestion and absorption due enhance the synthesis and excretion of bile acids in the liver, it could improve the lipids' digestion and absorption, decrease of total cholesterol
Pappermint (*Mentha piperita*)	Leaves/powder	Menthol, terpenes	Decrease of total cholesterol, triacylglycerols, LDL and glucose level, increase of HDL level,
Nettle (*Urtica dioica*)	Leaves, root/ water extracts	Organic acids carotenoids flavonoids tannins organic compounds, phytoestrogens, sterols, fatty acids	Improves serum lipid profile, decrease of triglycerides and total cholesterol in the blood;

Ginger (*Zingiber officinale*)	Roots/ extracted basic oil	Monoterpenes and sesquiterpenes	Improves serum lipid profile, decreases of triglycerides and total cholesterol serum features, total protein, globulin and antioxidant enzymes were elevated
Oregano (*Origanum vulgare*)	Leaves/oil	Terpenoids: carvacrol and thymol, polyphenols	Increase of HDL content, decrease of total cholesterol and triacylglycerols level, oxidative stability of the produced meat
Shinyprivet (*Ligustrum lucidum*)	Bark, twigs, flowers / water decoctions	Nuzenide, oleuropein, oleanolic acid, betulin	Decrease levels of cholesterol, LDL cholesterol, triglycerides and alanine aminotransferase activity, increased blood serum level of HDL

(Krauze, 2021)

5. **Nutraceuticals:** The term "Nutraceutical" was coined by combining the terms "Nutrition" and "Pharmaceutical" in 1989. According to the North American Veterinary Nutraceutical Council (NAVNC), a nutraceutical is "a substance produced in purified or extracted from which, when administered orally to patients, aims to provide them the necessary elements for their structure and normal function to better their health and well-being."

   "Nutraceutical" is any substance that may be considered a food or part of a food and provides medical or health benefits, encompassing, prevention and treatment of diseases.

   In general the poultry rations are aimed at higher feed conversion using natural feed stuffs. The amino acids in terms of first limitng amino acids are given importance in balancing comercial rations. However, research points out that a threonine the third limiting amino acid also has a major role in meat production with higher protein turnover. The feeding of amino acids like lysine, methionine, threonine and trytophan along with vitamina and minerals as synthetic supplements is more beneficial. This sort of refined neutracueticals in poultry feeding is known to produce better results in terms of digestion, absorbtion, utilisation, metabolism and beneficial health effects in consumers

Amino acids as nutraceuticals

A study conducted on one day old Cobb male broilers illustrated that dietary supplementation of amino acid chelated trace mineral helped in diminishing levels of circulatory and intestinal heat shock protein 70 (HSP70) and proinflammatory cytokine gene expression in heat-stressed broiler chickens. This observation indicates that amino acid chelated trace minerals in the diet can improve gut health by lowering the effect of heat stress (Baxter *et al.,* 2020). There are evidences that amino acid metabolism is affected by health status of birds as shown in some recent studies on challenge vs. non challenge conditions (Chrystal *et al.,* 2020; Hilliar *et al.,* 2020). Diseases like necroticenteritis affect digestion, absorption and metabolism of amino acids. Low protein diet did not affect predisposition to necrotic enteritis but feeding a standard diet or diet with additional amino acid content can mitigate this disease (Hilliar *et al.,* 2020). Amino acid supplementation favor cecal butyric acid and total short-chain fatty acids production and support growth, development, feed conversion efficiency and improve immunity (Chrystal *et al.,* 2020; Hilliar *et al.,* 2020).

Table 7: Summary of the implications and beneficial effects of different amino acids, vitamins and minerals as nutraceuticals in poultry.

Nutraceutical type and dose	Poultry species	Implication/Conclusion
Amino acids		
Trp, Ile, His, Val, Leu, Arg, Gly and Phe	Male broilers	Adding the essential amino acid mixtures to the low CP diets improved the performance, but did not completely overcome the adverse effects of the low CP diets
Threonine (0.4, 0.5, 0.6, 0.7, 0.8, 0.9, 1.0 and 1.1%)	Ross 308 males	Gut functionality like microvilli height, epithelia thickness and crypt depth was improved with even higher levels of dietary standardized ileal digestible threonine level
Arginine (2% L-arginine)	Broilers	Arginine increases specific immune response against Infectious Bursal Disease
Threonine, valine and tryptophan	Laying Japanese Quails	Reducing the CP level in a diet supplemented with crystalline amino acids is a valuable strategy for decreasing feeding cost and mitigating ammonia emission
Threonine and methionine	Broilers	Performance and immune system were improved at higher dietary threonine and methionine levels
Threonine (0.0 (control group), 0.25, 0.50, 0.75 and 1.00 g/kg diet)	Broilers	Adding threonine in the diet may promote the growth of immune organs, encourage the antibodies synthesis and mitigate the immune stress caused by Newcastle disease Virus or *E. coli* challenge

Arginine (0%, 0.45%, 0.90%, 1.35%, and 1.80% Arg)	Broiler	The addition of arginine in the diet could improve the growth performance of broiler chickens at 42 days of age
Lysine and methionine	Male broiler	There are positive effects on meat yield and growth performance in response to supplemental amino acids in diets from 21 to 41 days of age
L-Methionine (8 g/kg diet)	Rabbits	Reduced detrimental impacts of aflatoxinB1 on growth, immune and antioxidant status
Three levels of MetþCys (74%, 77% and 80%) of digestible lysine	Broiler chickens	DL-Met and L-Met are equally effective as a source of methionine for broiler
Threonine (0, 300, 600 and 900 mg/ kg diet)	Broiler chickens	A significant improvement was observed in performance indices of birds fed diet enriched with threonine compared with the control
Threonine, arginine and glutamine	Broiler chickens	May help to minimize over-activation of the innate immune system, which is the most expensive in terms of energy and nutrients, as well as improve the intestinal microbiota
Apparent and standardized ileal amino acid digestibility	Broiler chickens	Increasing dietary levels of highly digestible amino acids may help compensate for malabsorption through the stages of intestinal challenge
Methionine (a control (0.49% methionine) or a deficient (0.28%)	Cobb500 broiler male parent	A methionine deficiency affects essential amino acid digestibility and cysteine, but not the methionine digestibility. The alterations in digestibility are reflected in the expression of mRNA of amino acid transporters across different tissues
Threonine (100, 110, and 120% of NRC recommendation)	Mixed sex broilers (Ross-308)	Use of threonine, above NRC requirements, resulted in a better growth rate, feed utilization and carcass quality, gut health, increased ileal digestibility of amino acids and protein, and immunity
Threonine (i.e., 100%, 110% and 120% of Ross recommendations)	Broiler chickens	An improvement in feed intake through the grower period and an improvement in body weight (BW) throughout the grower and overall period, whereas a better feed conversion ratio through the starter period in birds fed 10% extra threonine in comparison with the control diet

Threonine (100% NRC specification, 100, 110, 120 and 130% threonine of Vencobb-400 strain specification)	Broiler chickens (Vencobb-400)	The immune organs weight was improved with threonine supplementation.
3.0 g threonine/kg feed	Male chicks	The level of intestinal cytokines in lipopolysaccharide challenged chickens was reduced by threonine addition
Vitamins		
Vitamin E	Broiler chickens	Improvement of the immune response and antioxidants concentration in the liver
2 g α-tocopherol acetate/kg feed	Broilers	Increase in carcass mass and decrease in the abdominal fat of broilers
Vitamin E	Broiler chickens	A significant influence on the chicken meat quality by reducing juice drip and increasing WHC of meat
Vitamin A (16,000 IU/kg feed)	Hy-sex	Improvement of productivity performance parameters
Vitamin C (200 mg/kg feed)	Broiler chickens	Protection against the risk of high density by improved final BW, reduction of mortality and downregulation of HSP70 expression level in the liver
Vitamin C (200 mg/kg feed)	Commercial broilers	Improvement of the immunity of broilers
Vitamin A (0, 8,000 and 16,000 IU/kg diet) and vitamin E (0, 250 and 500 mg/kg diet)	Bovans Brown laying hens	Both vitamins play a role in alleviating the harmful impacts of high ambient temperature. Use of 16,000 IU vitamin A with 500 mg vitamin E /kg diet is preferable for obtaining better production of birds exposed to heat stress
Vitamin E (0, 250 mg/kg diet)	Growing Japanese quail	Useful in partly alleviating the adverse impacts of cadmium
Vitamin E	Laying hens	Prevents unsaturated lipid oxidation within cells, therefore protecting the cell membrane from oxidative damage induced by ROS
Vitamin E (200 mg/kg feed)	Male chickens	Enhanced semen quality traits, including the spermatozoa count and motility, and reduced the dead spermatozoa, under heat stress conditions
Vitamin E (100 mg/kg feed)	Poultry ganders	Improved ejaculate volumes, percentages of viable sperm and sperm concentrations and lowered percentages of spermatids

Control with additional 3,000 or 9,000 IU25-hydroxyvitamin D3/kg feed, 3,000 or 9,000 IU vitamin D3/kg feed, 3,000 or 9,000 IU vitamin D2/kg feed	Lohmann white laying hens	Irrespective of forms, the apparent total tract digestibility of calcium was higher in diets enriched with vitamin D. The apparent total tract digestibility of phosphorus was higher in 3,000 IU/kg of vitamin D2 compared to the other treatments. The utilization of calcium and phosphorus by laying birds can be enhanced by the addition of different sources of vitamin D in rations
Minerals		
Ca (3.0, 3.5, 4.0, and 4.5%) and 25OHD3 (0, 69, and 138 lg/ kg feed)	Lohmann LSL-lite layers	Use high levels of calcium and 25OHD3 improved bone strength and decreased risks related to morbidity, leg weakness and mortalities
Copper sulfate (200 mg/kg feed)	Broiler	Useful influence on the growth rate
150 mg copper sulfate/kg feed	Broiler chicks	Improved live BW gain that may be the result of the significant decline in the total pathogenic bacteria the gut
Copper(8.77 and 11.6 mg/ kg feed)	Goslings	Improved growth and carcass yield from 28 to 70 days of age
12 mg Mn (inorganic or organic)/kg feed	Broiler	It was sufficient to provide optimum broiler performance
Zn-Met (25, 50, 75 or 100 mg Zn-Met/kg diet)	Hisex Brown laying hens	Increased Zn status and reduced blood triglyceride, LDL-cholesterol & resulted in improving antioxidant capacity
Chromium propionate with inclusion levels of 0, 200, 400, 800 and 1600 ppb.	Male ROSS-308 broilers	Better performance and weight gain may be achieved if chromium is added in broiler diets at the rate of 400 ppb
Selenium (0, 0.25, 0.50 mg/ kg feed)	Bovans laying hens	Hemoglobin and lymphocytes were increased with increasing dietary Se level in layer reared under heat stress conditions
Selenium	Poultry males	Plays an important role in semen quality and is related to the high proportion of polyunsaturated fatty acids in avian semen and its susceptibility to lipid peroxidation
Organic Se	Cockerel	Dietary supplementation of organic Se in the cockerel's diet increased (more than double) Se concentration in the semen; have a beneficial effect on the antioxidant defense in various tissues including sperm

Selenium (0.3 mg Se/kg feed)	Male chickens	Use of Se in the diet of male chickens increased the activity of GSH-Px in the liver, testes, spermatozoa and seminal plasma
Organic Se (0.3 mg/kg feed)	Male chickens	Under high ambient temperature (33-36 C in poultry farm), use of organic Se in the cockerel diets improved the GSH-Px activity and semen quality (motility and sperm count) and reduced the dead sperms count in a dose-dependent manner
Organic Se (0.3 mg/kg feed)	Male chickens	Enhanced semen quality traits, including the spermatozoa count and motility, and reduced the dead spermatozoa, under heat stress conditions
Selenium (0.3 mg/kg feed)	Poultry ganders	Improved ejaculate volumes, percentages of viable sperm and sperm and lowered percentages of spermatids
0, 0.5, 1.0 or 2.0 mg Se (sodium selenite) /kg diet	Hy-Line roosters	The highest activity of GSH-Px and lowest content of MDA in blood and testis was recorded in the treatment of 0.5 mg/kg
Dietary Se deficiency (0.033 mg of Se/kg feed) in comparison with the control	Hy-line cockerels	Exerts harmful impacts on reproductive organs and the extrinsic and intrinsic pathways and the upstream regulators, like Bcl-2 and p53 are all involved in Se deficiency induced testicular apoptosis
0.15 mg Se/kg feed from sodium selenite, Se-enriched yeast (Se-yeast) or SeMet	Broiler breeders	Apart from sodium selenite, Se-yeast or SeMet increased the activity of thioredoxinreductase-1 in the kidney and liver of breeders and their offspring, but not the activity of GSH-Px1
Se 0.13 mg/kg feed with 0.4 mg Se in the form of sodium selenite (SS) or Se-yeast/kg feed for 9 months	Hy-Line Brown	Increased Se content of the e.g., g from 5.1 mg in the basal diet group to 14.4 and 22.7 mg, in SS or Se-yeast, respectively
Organic selenium (0.5 mg/kg diet)	Poultry breeders	A reduction in mortality with selenium supplementation; increase in e.g., egg production, hatchability, and percentage of settable eggs
Organic selenium (2 vitamin E levels (30 and 120 mg/kg feed) and two selenium sources (sodium selenite and zinc-L-selenomethionine).	Broiler breeder	Promoted heavier hatchling weight until e.g., production egg peak (33 weeks), but did not influence hatchling quality

25 or 75 mg ZnO/kg diet	Laying hens (Hisex Brown)	Dietary zinc addition up to 75 mg/kg used as an effective supplement to improve antioxidant ability and zinc status in laying hens

(Alagawany *et al.*, 2021)

Conclusion

The use of probiotics and prebiotics are based on the strain and dose which is a major limitation in their inclusion as feed additives. The use of enzymes is limited by high manufacturing cost and susceptibility to environment. Though the inclusion of phytobiotics and essential oils are more favourable more indepth study is required in this area. Inspite of these few limiting factors the advantages in biosafety of additives and economic returns from the birds overweigh. Therefore, it may be concluded that the use of these newer additives can be safely included for the benefit of the producer and the consumer alike.

Future trends of some biotechnological applications with potential in animal nutrition

Modification of gut microbes- To genetically modify microorganisms naturally present in the gut to enhance their capacity for defined functions or add new functions (e.g. rumen microbes to improve cellulose digestion).

Introduction of new gut microbes-To introduce new species or strains of microorganisms into the gut.

Bioactive peptides- Improved growth and efficiency (e.g. growth hormone-releasing peptides), improved gut function, immunomodulation, antibacterial properties.

Antimicrobial replacers Antimicrobial enzymes (e.g. lysozyme), delivery of specific antibodies via spray-dried plasma and egg products.

Transgenesis-To modify nutrient metabolism and improve growth efficiency by transfer of genes.

References

Abdulla J., Rose, S. P., Mackenzie, A. M., Ivanova, S. G., Staykova, G. P. and Pirgozliev, V. 2016b. Nutritional value of raw and micronised fi eld beans (Vicia faba L. var. minor) with and without enzyme supplementation containing tannase for growing chickens. Archives of Animal Nutrition, 70(5):350- 363.

Abdulla, J., Rose, S. P., Mackenzie, A. M., and Pirgozliev, V. 2017. Feeding value of fi eld beans (Vicia faba L. var. minor) with and without enzyme containing tannase, pectinase and xylanase activities for broilers. Archives of Animal Nutrition, 71:150-164.

Abdulla, J., Rose, S. P., Mackenzie, A. M., Mirza, W. and Pirgozliev, V. 2016a. Exogenous tannase improves feeding value of diet containing fi eld beans (Vicia faba) when fed to broilers. British Poultry Science, 57: 246-250.

Alagawany, M., Elnesr, S.S., Farag, M.R., Tiwari, R., Yatoo, M.I., Karthik, K., Michalak, I. and Dhama, K., 2021. Nutritional significance of amino acids, vitamins and minerals as nutraceuticals in poultry production and health–a comprehensive review. Veterinary Quarterly, 41(1):1-29.

Baxter, M.F., Greene, E.S., Kidd, M.T., Tellez-Isaias, G., Orlowski, S. and Dridi, S. 2020. Water amino acid-chelated trace mineral supplementation decreases circulating and intestinal HSP70 and proinflammatory cytokine gene expression in heat-stressed broiler chickens. Journal of Animal Science, 98(3), p.skaa049.

Bedford, M. R. 2006. Effect of non-starch polysaccharidases on avian gastrointestinal function. In: Perry GC, editor. Avian gut function in health and disease. Oxfordshire (UK), Carfax Publishing Company, 159-170.

Bilal, R.M., Hassan, F.U., Saeed, M., Rafeeq, M., Zahra, N., Fraz, A., Saeed, S., Khan, M.A., Mahgoub, H.A., Farag, M.R. and Alagawany, M. 2021. Role of yeast and yeast-derived products as feed additives in broiler nutrition. Animal Biotechnology, pp.1-10.

Brethour, J. R. 2019. Ionophores: New findings on performance, bloat, and acidosis. Beef Cattle Science Handbook, 680-686. doi:10.1201/9780429045189-89

Chapman, J. D. 1989. Probiotics, Acidifiers, and Yeast culture: A place for natural additives in Pig and Poultry Production Animal Feeds. Biological Additives, University of Sydney (Ed.). University of Sydney, Post Graduate Committee in Veterinary Science, Sydney South, NSW, Australia, ISBN: 9780909973674, pp: 63-78.

Chrystal PV, Moss AF, Khoddami A, Naranjo VD, Selle PH, Liu SY. 2020. Effects of reduced crude protein levels, dietary electrolyte balance, and energy density on the performance of broiler chickens offered maize-based diets with evaluations of starch, protein, and amino acid metabolism. Poultry Science, 99(3):1421–1431

Dawson, K. A. 1994. Successful Application of Defined Yeast Culture Preparations in Animal Production. Asia –Pacific Lecture Tour, pp: 1-20.

Ferdous, Z., Aktaruzzaman, M., Rahman, M.M. and Howlader, M.M.R. 2018. Effects of multivitamins and enzymes on growth performance and hematological parameters of broilers at Meherpur in Bangladesh. Journal of Dairy Veterinary Science, 5(5), p.555674.

Fuller, R. 1992. History and development of probiotics. In Probiotics (pp. 1-8). Springer, Dordrecht

Hassanpour, H., Bahadoran, S. and Borjian, N. 2016. Vitamin E improves morphology and absorptive surface of small intestine in broiler chickens reared at high altitude. Poultry Science Journal, 4(1), pp:19-26.

Hilliar, M., Keerqin, C., Girish, C.K., Barekatain, R., Wu, S.B. and Swick, R.A. 2020. Reducing protein and supplementing crystalline amino acids, to alter dietary amino acid profiles in birds challenged for subclinical necrotic enteritis. Poultry Science, 99(4):2048-2060.

Jha, R., Das, R., Oak, S. and Mishra, P. 2020. Probiotics (direct-fed microbials) in poultry nutrition and their effects on nutrient utilization, growth and laying performance, and gut health: A systematic review. Animals, 10(10):1863.

Kamalzadeh, A., Ila, N. and Heydarnejad, O. 2009. Effects of emulsified vitamins on broiler performance. World Journal of Zoology, 4(1):42-46.

Krauze, M., 2021. Phytobiotics, a natural growth promoter for poultry. Advanced Studies in the 21st Century Animal Nutrition, pp.1-21.

Lyons, T. P. 1994. Biotechnology in the feed industry and Beyond. Asia –Pacific Lecture Tour, pp: 21-30.

Maka³a, H. 2021. Impact of Selected Feed Additives in Broiler Nutrition on Breeding and the Meat Quality Features. Advanced Studies in the 21st Century Animal Nutrition, 16, p.1.

Makarski, B., Gortat, M., Lechowski, J., Zukiewicz-Sobczak, W., Sobczak, P. and Zawislak, K. 2014. Impact of copper (Cu) at the dose of 50 mg on haematological and biochemical blood parameters in turkeys, and level of Cu accumulation in the selected tissues as a source of information on product safety for consumers. Annals of Agricultural and Environmental Medicine, 21(3).

Masey O'Neill, H.V., Smith, J.A. and Bedford, M.R., 2014. Multicarbohydrase enzymes for non-ruminants. Asian-Australasian journal of animal sciences, 27(2): 290-301.

Mowat, D. N. 1994. Organic Chromium in Animal Nutrition. Asia –Pacific Lecture Tour, pp: 31-44.

Newman, K. 1994. Mannan-Oligosaccharides: Natural Polymers with Significant Impact on the Gastrointestinal Microflora and the Immune System. In: Lyons, T.P. and Jacques, K.A., Eds., Biotechnology in the Feed Industry. Proceeding of Alltech's Tenth Annual Symposium, Nottingham University Press, Nottingham, 167-175.

Olukosi, O. A., Beeson, L. A., Englyst, K. and Romero, L. F. 2015. Effects of exogenous proteases without or with carbohydrases on nutrient digestibility and disappearance of non starch polysaccharides in broiler chickens. Poultry Science, 94(11):2662–2669

Pearce Lyons. C. 1989. Applications for Biotechnology in the Feed Industry: The way forward. Animal Feeds. Biological Addittives, Proceeedings, No.119. pp: 1-18.

Pehrson, B. G. 1994. Selenium in Nutrition with special references to the biopotency of organic and inorganic selenium compounds. Asia –Pacific Lecture Tour, pp: 145-64.

Pirgozliev, V. and Bedford, M. R. 2013. Energy utilisation and growth performance of chicken fed diets containing graded levels of supplementary bacterial phytase. British Journal of Nutrition, 109: 248–253.

Pirgozliev, V., Bedford, M. R., Acamovic, T., Mares, P. and Allimehr, M. 2011. The effects of supplementary bacterial phytase on dietary energy and total tract amino acid digestibility when fed to young chickens. British Poultry Science, 52: 245- 254.

Pirgozliev, V., Bedford, M. R., and Acamovic, T. 2010. The effect of dietary xylanase on energy, amino acid and mineral metabolism and egg production and quality in laying hens. British Poultry Science, 51:639-647.

Pirgozliev, V., Karadas, F., Rose, S. P., Beccaccia, A., Mirza, M. W. and Amerah, A. M. 2015b. Dietary xylanase increases hepatic vitamin E concentration of chickens fed wheat based diet. Journal of Animals and Feed Sciences, 24: 80-84.

Pirgozliev, V., Rose, S. P., Pellny, T., Amerah, A.M., Wickramasinghe, M., Ulker, M., Rakszegi, M., Bedo, Z., Shewry, P. R. and Lovegrove, A. 2015a. Energy utilization and growth performance of chickens fed novel wheat inbred lines selected for different pentosan levels with and without xylanase supplementation. Poultry Science, 94: 232–239

Pirgozliev, V., Rose, S.P. and Ivanova, S. 2019. Feed additives in poultry nutrition. Bulgarian Journal of Agricultural Science, 25(1), pp.8-11.

Ravindran, V. and Son, J.H. 2011. Feed enzyme technology: present status and future developments. Recent patents on food, nutrition & agriculture, 3(2), pp.102-109. Retrieved from https://edis.ifas.ufl.edu/pdffiles/AN/AN28500.pdf

Selle, P. H. and Ravindran, V. 2007. Microbial phytase in poultry nutrition. Animal Feed Science and Technology, 135:1-41

Sinha, B.S., Kumar, S. and Chudhary, G.K. 2018. Use of fresh Azolla as dietary supplementation in backyard poultry. International Journal of Current Microbiology and Applied Science, Special Issue, 7, pp:1358-1361.

Spain, J. 1994. Tissue integrity: A Key defense Against mastitis infection: The Role zinc proteinates and a theory for mode of action. Asia-Pacific Lecture Tour, pp: 65-72.

Uma Maheswari, D. 2017. Organic Acidifiers in Broiler diets. ISBN 10: 3330025425 / ISBN 13: 9783330025424. Published by LAP Lambert Academic Publishing.

Wenk, C. 1994. Practical uses of Enzymes in Poultry diets. Asia-Pacific Lecture Tour. pp: 173-84.

Whiting, L.M., Pirgozliev, V., Rose, S. P., Wilson, J., Amerah, A. M., Ivanova, S. G., Staykova, G. P., Oluwatosin, O. O. and Oso, A. O. 2017. Nutrient availability of different batches of wheat distillers dried grains with solubles with and without exogenous enzymes for broiler chickens. Poultry Science, 96:574–580

Williams, P.E.V. 1989. Understanding the Biochemical Mode of Action of Yeast Culture. In: Animal Feeds: Biological Additives, University of Sydney (Ed.). University of Sydney, Post Graduate Committee in Veterinary Science, Sydney South, NSW, Australia, ISBN: 9780909973674, pp: 79-101.

11

Early Chick Nutrition

S. Adil, Manzoor A. Wani, I.U. Sheikh and M.T. Banday

Division of Livestock Production and Management, Faculty of Veterinary Science and Animal Husbandry, Shuhama, Alusteng, Srinagar, Sher-e-Kashmir University of Agricultural Sciences and Technology of Kashmir, Jammu & Kashmir, India

Introduction

The poultry industry is under pressure to produce safe and good quality meat in the welfare conditions. Many areas such as genetics, biosecurity, and immunoprophylaxis were improved, and hatchery is one of the areas in which welfare could be improved for better production output. Under commercial hatched conditions, poults hatch over a 36 to 48 hour period (called hatching window) and after additional processing are transported to the farm. Hatch window is the time gap from first chick hatched to last chick hatched (Noiva *et al*., 2014). This causes early hatched chicks to be deprived of feed for longer duration (Kadam *et al.*, 2013). Sexing, vaccination, packaging and transportation to farm are other hatchery and management operations responsible for delay in feeding. The scientists showed that starving in this period is very unfavorable and leads to depressing growth with short and long-term effects (Halevy *et al.,* 2000; Bigot *et al.,* 2003) and had lasting negative effects on broiler performance (Tarvid, 1992; Batal and Parsons, 2002; Prabakar *et al.,* 2016). Some scientists confirmed that early posthatch nutrition plays a positive role in muscle development in turkey poults and chicken broilers (Uni and Ferket, 2004). In turkeys, early feeding was found to result in higher body weight, as well as greater breast meat yield at market age (Noy and Sklan,1999), that is, myoblast hyperplasia, which forms new nuclei from muscle progenitor satellite cells (also termed adult myoblasts) in muscle fibers (Velleman *et al.,* 2016). However, there is a limited time window in early life when activated satellite cells can donate nuclei to existing cells that increase muscle potential (Batal and Parsons, 2002). Once this period of donation ends, the main method to increase muscle mass is by increasing the cytoplasm (Prabakar *et al.,* 2016). It was also shown that feeding during the post-hatch period in broilers enhanced satellite cell proliferation and therefore skeletal muscle growth. Studies by Halevy *et al*., 2000, indicated that the immediate post-hatch period (48 h post-hatch) is the most important time to program mature breast muscle size at market age. Delayed access to feed decreases mitotic activity of satellite cells, which negatively influences muscle development (Mozdziak *et al.,* 2002). New technologies such as the Hatch Care system provide newborn chicks with food, fresh water, and light right from the hatch, improving their welfare from the start of their life. It is assumed that the early nutrition, available during the hatching process, is a response to the individual's needs.

In general, time between hatching and placement can range up to 36 h; however, chicks are frequently transported to far off places, and may take up to 72 hours (Fairchild *et al*., 2006). Extended periods of time between hatching and first access to feed have negative impacts on bird performance (Juul-Madsen *et al.,* 2004). The magnitude of the effect is directly proportional to the duration of Delay in feed access (Jabbar *et al.,* 2018).

Role of yolk sac

Towards end of incubation, residual yolk is internalized into abdominal cavity and is sole nutrient source until exogenous feed replaces it (Noble and Ogunyemi, 1989). During immediate post hatch period, yolk is used for maintenance of the bird (Anthony *et al.,* 1989). Yolk nutrients rapidly diminish and are almost depleted by third day post-hatch (Romanoff, 1990). Nutrients in residual yolk are supposed to support chick during fasting period. However, they represent an insufficient contribution for both maintenance and growth of chicks (Bigot *et al.,* 2003). The residual yolk contains approximately 2/3 fat and 1/3 protein. Birds have been created in such a way that if bird has access to feed, fat in residual yolk supply energy and proteins are used for building up the body, and for functional development. If there is no feed available, bird still uses fat from residual yolk as energy, but it has to use the protein in yolk for energy as well. Thus, bird will have less protein for early development. If we want to maximise the potential of bird, we have to avoid the situation that bird uses protein from residual yolk for energy, which means we have to feed the bird as soon as possible (Meijerhof, 2010).

Effects of delayed feeding

Effect on growth of birds

The loss in body weight as per hours of delay in feeding has been summarized in Table 1.

Loss of BW	Delay in feeding	Reference
10% in meat type chicks	48-h	Pinchasov and Noy, 1993
15% in meat type chicks	52-h	Teixeira *et al.*, 2009
12.4% in Egg type chicks	36-h	Shinde *et al.*, 2015
6.3% lower market wt. in meat type chicks	36-h	Tamboli *et al.*, 2018

Effect of delayed feeding on gut

Gastro intestinal tract (GIT) is most rapidly developing organ in later stage of incubation and plays critical role in early stages of chick growth. GIT makes up to 1% of weight of 18 day-old embryo and reaching 3.5% at hatch (Uni *et al.*, 2003). Delayed feeding negatively affects the development and function of GIT of chicks. Post-hatch feed restriction had deleterious effects on small intestine development:

- Lowered relative wt. of intestinal tract
- Reduced intestinal villi ht. and density
- Reduced no. of goblet cells per villus
- Reduced surface area for absorption

(Shinde *et al.*, 2015; Marina *et al.*, 2019)

Other effects of delayed feeding

Gut-associated lymphoid tissue (GALT) activity was significantly delayed during first 2 weeks of life in broiler chicks following delayed access to feed (Shira *et al.*, 2005). Delayed feeding caused lower weight of lymphoid organs and reduced lymphocyte proliferation (Van de Ven *et al.*, 2013). Geyra *et al.* (2001) reported adverse effects of delayed feeding on secretion of vital digestive enzymes. Wang *et al.* (2014) reported that delay in feed access caused adverse effects on liver and muscle glycogen content.

Remedial measures

1. **In-ovo feeding (IOF):** This technique was developed by Uni and Ferket (2003). IOF is a method of supplementing exogenous nutrients into the egg to enhance egg nutrition and post-hatch growth. Modern broilers are selected for higher growth rate and increased muscle size, leading to an increased requirement of chicken embryos for nutrients. Chick embryo solely relies upon egg nutrients, so sufficient nutrients in egg enable a good starting for hatching chicks. Studies have indicated that nutrient reserves in egg may be insufficient to fully support embryonic development (Dibner

et al., 1998). As size of embryo increases, yolk content gradually becomes diminished; therefore, to avoid nutrient deficiency, IOF technology can be a good alternative. The administration of digestible nutrients into the amnion of embryos can bring:

- An improvement in bird quality
- Increased glycogen reserves
- Fast development of digestive tract
- Superior skeletal health
- Better muscle growth rate
- Higher body weight gain
- Improved feed conversion
- Enhanced immune function
- Reduced post-hatch mortality and morbidity

(Peebles, 2018)

2. ***In-ovo* site and timing of inoculation:** The amniotic fluid is considered as most effective site for injection (Kucharska-Gaca *et al.,* 2017). The best time for IOF has been reported as when embryonated eggs are transferred from setter to hatcher at 18 days of incubation (Salahi *et al.,* 2011).

3. **Early post-hatch nutrition:** After hatch, hatched chicks need quick transit from dependence on the yolk to exogenous nutrients for rapid development of digestive organs and proper growth (Sklan, 2001). Nutrient supply from yolk sac is not enough to support rapid growth of newly hatched chick. So early feeding is important to improve growth of birds (Gonzales *et al.,* 2003). During hatching process, energy loss occurs which leads to reduction in glycogen content, therefore, early provision of nutrients is important (John *et al.,* 1988). The first week after hatch counts for approx 20% of lifespan of modern broilers, emphasizing the imp of this period for subsequent performance. Early nutrient supply to chicks is essential:

- To increase the intestinal mechanical activity
- Stimulate yolk utilization
- Faster GIT development
- Greater assimilation of feed
- Development of immunity and
- Overall growth performance

i. ***Effect of Early Feeding on Yolk utilization:*** Residual yolk is used up more quickly in chicks having immediate feed access than those fasted for first 48 h (Juul-Madsen *et al*., 2004). Noy and Sklan (2001) observed that passage of yolk content to intestinal tract is higher when bird is fed as compared when it is fasted. Anti-peristaltic movement, which moves yolk from yolk stalk to duodenum after hatching, appears to be stimulated by presence of feed in the gut (Panda and Reddy, 2007).

ii. ***Effect of Early Feeding on Development of GI:*** Growth of chicken is directly linked to digestion and absorption of nutrients, which is a result of morphological and functional development of small intestine (Jha *et al*., 2019). Early intake of external feed after hatching is associated with rapid development of organs and GI tract (Yegani & Korver, 2008). Maturation and development of GI tract was higher in early fed chicks compared to feed withheld chicks, as reflected by

- Higher intestinal length
- Increased relative spleen and liver weights

(Van de Ven *et al*., 2013)

iii. ***Effect of Early Feeding on Enzyme secretion:*** Because of early access to feed, total digestive enzyme activity tends to increase during early post-hatch period because of rapid increase in weight of pancreas and intestines (Panda *et al*., 2006). In early feed accessed birds, intestinal & pancreatic enzymatic activities increased and were correlated with higher body weights (Sklan and Noy, 2000). Early feeding of chicks resulted in improved intestinal mucosal function compared with fasted chicks (Uni and Sklan, 1998).

iv. ***Effect of Early Feeding on Immune system:*** Early feeding cause's rapid onset of GALT function which plays a significant role in avian immune system (Bar *et al*., 2005). Feed provides nutrients essential for growth and development of lymphoid organs and Immune system (particularly mucosal immune system) (Tamboli *et al*., 2017). Direct feed access facilitates immunological development by faster formation of commensal microbial population affecting mucus dynamics and immune cellular dev. (such as goblet cells) in gut ((Dibner *et al*., 2008).

v. ***Effect of Early Feeding on Growth and Muscle Development:*** Chicken weight at 6 weeks of age has linear relationship with their weight in the first week (Saki, 2005). Immediate access to feed increased BW until 3 wk of age (Sklan *et al*., 2000) and upto market age in broilers (Vieira *et al*., 1999). Early dietary nutrient intake improved BW & breast meat yield compared to chicks held in hatchery trays for 34 and 48 h (Noy and

Sklan, 1999). Attributed to the fact that nutrients have role in activation of satellite cells and thereby development of skeletal muscles (Halvey *et al.*, 2000).

Conclusion

With increase in productivity and highly feed efficient birds, nutritional demand of embryos and early aged chicks has changed over decades. Since, length of time to market progressively has decreased, so immediate post-hatch period represents a proportion of total production time of a bird. In-ovo feeding of several types of nutrients seems to be a promising strategy to promote weight, health and livability of hatched chicks. Early nutrition programming at hatcheries is latest and successful method to prepare chicks with healthy gut, favorable microbiota, improved immunity and overall growth performance. The potential benefits of intervention would be profound if both practices are combined (IOF and Early post-hatch feeding). Further research is required to fine-tune IOF technique for application at commercial scale to understand how early nutrition affects specific genes responsible for performance, intestinal development and overall health-related traits in chicken. Keeping in view the beneficial impacts, early post-hatch nutrition must be made mandatory for commercial hatcheries.

References

Anthony, N.B., Dunnington, E.A. and Siegel, P.B. 1989. Embryo growth of normal and dwarf chickens from lines selected for high and low body weight. Archives fur Geflügelkunde, 53: 116-122.

Augusto, M.A., Santos, T.G., Campos, E.J., Chiarini-Garcia, H. and de Almeida, F.R.C.L. 2019. Effects of Incubation Period and Fasting Time on the Duodenum Morphology from One-Day-Old Commercial Broiler Chicks: An Histomorphometrical Study.

Bhanja, S.K., Goel, A., Pandey, N., Mehra, M., Majumdar, S. and Mandal, A.B. 2015. In ovo carbohydrate supplementation modulates growth and immunityrelated genes in broiler chickens. Journal of animal physiology and animal nutrition, 99(1), pp.163-173.

Bhanja, S.K., Sudhagar, M., Goel, A., Pandey, N., Mehra, M., Agarwal, S.K. and Mandal, A. 2014. Differential expression of growth and immunity related genes influenced by in ovo supplementation of amino acids in broiler chickens. Czech Journal of Animal Science, 59(9): 399-408.

Bigot, K., Mignon, G.S., Picard, M. and Tesseraud, S. 2003. Effects of delayed feed intake on body, intestine and muscle development in neonate broilers. Poultry Science, 82: 781-788.

Dibner, J.J., Knight, C.D., Kitchell, M.L., Atwell, C.A., Downs, A.C. and Ivey, F.J. 1998. Early feeding and development of the immune system in neonatal poultry. Journal of Applied Poultry Research, 7(4): 425-436.

Geyra, A., Uni, Z. and Sklan, D. 2001. Enterocyte dynamics and mucosal development in the post-hatch chick. Poultry Science, 80: 776-782.

Gonzales, E., Kondo, N., Saldanha, E.S.P.B., Loddi, M.M., Careghi, C. and Decuypere, E. 2003. Performance andphysiological parameters of broiler chickens subjected to fasted on the neonatal period. Poultry Science, 82: 1250-1256.

Halevy, O., Geyra, A., Barak, M., Uni, Z. and Sklan, D. 2000. Early posthatch starvation decreases satellite cell proliferation and skeletal muscle growth in chicks. The Journal of Nutrition, 130(4): 858-864.

John, T.M., George, J.C. and Moran, J.R. 1988. Metabolic changes in pectoral muscle and liver of turkey embryos in relation to hatching: Influence of glucose and antibiotic-treatment of eggs. Poultry Science, 67: 463-469.

Juul-Madsen, H.R., Su, G. and Sorensen, P. 2004. Influence of early or late start of first feeding on growth & immune phenotype of broilers. British Poultry Science, 45: 210-222.

Kadam, M.M., Barekatain, M.R., K Bhanja, S. and Iji, P.A. 2013. Prospects of in ovo feeding and nutrient supplementation for poultry: The science and commercial applications-A review. Journal of the Science of Food and Agriculture, 93(15):3654-3661.

Noble, R.C. and Ogunyemi, D. 1989. Lipid changes in the residual yolk and liver of the chick immediately after hatching. Biological Neonate, 56: 228-236.

Noy, Y. and D. Sklan. 1999. Different types of early feeding and performance in chicks and poults. Journal of applied poultry research, 8:16–24.

Noy, Y. and D. Sklan. 2001. Yolk and exogenous feed utilization in the posthatch chick. Poultry Science, 80:1490–1495.

Panda, A.K. and Reddy, M.R. 2007. Boosting the chicks immune system through early chick nutrition. Poultry Internaional, 47: 22-26.

Peebles, E.D. 2018. In ovo applications in poultry: a review. Poultry Science, 97:1–17.

Pinchasov, Y. and Noy, Y. 1993. Comparison of post-hatch holding time and subsequent early performance of broiler chicks and turkey poults. British Poultry Science, 34: 111-120.

Saki, A.A. 2005. Effect of post-hatch feeding on broiler performance. International Journal of Poultry Science, 4: 4-6.

Shira, E.B., Sklan, D. and Friedman, A. 2005. Impaired immune responses in broiler hatchling hindgut following delayed access to feed. Veterinary immunology and immunopathology, 105(1-2): 33-45.

Shira, E.B., Sklan, D. and Friedman, A. 2005. Impaired immune responses in broiler hatchling hindgut following delayed access to feed. Veterinary immunology and immunopathology, 105(1-2): 33-45.

Sklan, D. 2001. Development of the digestive tract of poultry. Worlds Poultry Science Journal, 57: 415-428.

Sklan, D. and Noy, Y. 2000. Hydrolysis and absorption in the small intestines of post hatch chicks. Poultry Science, 79: 1306-1310.

Smirnov, A., Tako, E., Ferket, P.R. and Uni, Z. 2006. Mucin gene expression and mucin content in the chicken intestinal goblet cells are affected by in ovo feeding of carbohydrates. Poultry science, 85(4): 669-673.

Sobolewska, A., Bogucka, J., Dankowiakowska, A., Elminowska-Wenda, G., Stadnicka, K. and Bednarczyk, M. 2017. The impact of synbiotic administration through in ovo technology on the microstructure of a broiler chicken small intestine tissue on the 1st and 42nd day of rearing. Journal of animal science and biotechnology, 8(1): 1-8.

Uni, Z. and Ferket, P. R. 2004. Methods for early nutrition and their potential. World's Poultry Science Journal, 60: 103– 113.

Uni, Z. and Ferket, R.P. 2004. Methods for early nutrition and their potential. World's Poultry Science Journal, 60(1): 101-111.

Uni, Z., and Ferket, P. R. 2003. enhancement of development of oviparous species by in ovo feeding. U.S. Patent 6,592,878. YissumResearchDevelopment Co. of Hebrew University and North Carolina State University Raleigh, N. C.

Uni, Z., Tako, E., Gal-Garber, O. and Sklan, D. 2003. Morphological, molecular, and functional changes in the chicken small intestine of the late-term embryo. Poultry Science, 82: 1747–1754.

Vieira, S. L. and E. T. Jr. Moran. 1999. Effects of delayed placement and used litter on broiler yields. Journal of applied poultry research, 8: 75-81.

Yegani, M. and Korver, D. R. 2008. Factor affecting intestinal health in poultry. Poultry Science, 87: 2052–2063.

12

Aflatoxins- Hazard to Poultry Production

Y.A. Beigh, Haidar Ali Ahmad, M.T. Banday, S. Adil and Z. Haq

Faculty of Veterinary Science and Animal Husbandry, Shuhama, Alusteng Srinagar Sher-e-Kashmir University of Agricultural Sciences and Technology of Kashmir Jammu & Kashmir, India

Introduction

The term 'mycotoxin' coined in 1962 in the aftermath of death of about 1,00,000 turkey poults in London, due to "Turkey X disease" in 1960, linked to a peanut meal contaminated with aflatoxins. Now, about 300 to 400 toxic fungal metabolites have been identified as mycotoxins, of which some are capable of inflicting deleterious effects to animal and avian health. The most commonly affected feedstuffs are cereals (maize, sorghum, barley, wheat, and rice meal), oilseeds (groundnuts) and oilseed meals (cottonseed meal). There are three major genera of fungi that produce mycotoxins: *Aspergilius*, *Fusarium* and *Penicillium* (Bennett and Klich, 2003). Among these, the *Aspergillus* species are of much concern as they are responsible for the production of aflatoxins, the most potent fungal toxin causing aflatoxicoses that have detrimental effects on living beings (Barret, 2000).

Mycotoxicoses tend to be a major problem in the tropics where high humidity and temperature creates optimal conditions for mould growth. When environmental conditions are conducive to fungal growth, mycotoxin contamination of grains may start in the field, and can also take place during processing and storage of harvested products. The moisture content of the harvested product and the ambient temperature are principal determinants of fungal contamination and mycotoxin production. Some fungi, such as *Fusarium* spp., normally infest grains before harvest; others, such as *Penicillium* spp., invade after harvest, while *Aspergillus* spp. can grow both before and after harvest. However, the presence of fungi does not necessarily indicate contamination with mycotoxins.

Different mycotoxins affect in different ways. Some are cancer-causing toxins (e.g., aflatoxin B1, ochratoxin A, fumonisin B1) and some are oestrogenic (zearalenones). Some affect the nervous system (fumonisin B1), while others affect the kidneys (ochratoxins) or suppress the immune system (aflatoxin B1, ochratoxin A, and T-2 toxin). Depending on the degree of contamination, these effects will eventually have negative impacts on performance. It is often difficult to diagnose the effects of a mycotoxin because they are not necessarily unique to a given mycotoxin, but may be shared by others or magnified by interactions with others. Many fungal species are also capable of producing several mycotoxins. Co-contamination of feed samples with multiple mycotoxins, which has serious consequences for both feed safety and animal performance.

The financial impact of mycotoxicoses can be of immense magnitude. These toxins have the capacity not only to impair animal performance due to reduced growth rates, illness or even death, but also to affect humans through toxic residues that can be deposited in animal tissues. Depending on the degree of contamination, mycotoxins or their metabolites may get deposited in meat, visceral organs and eggs. Their concentration in animal products is considerably lower than the levels present in the feed consumed by the animals, and will not cause acute toxicity in humans, but residues of carcinogenic mycotoxins, such as aflatoxins and ochratoxin A, can affect human health. In most cases, however, the principal source of mycotoxins for humans is contaminated cereals and legumes rather than animal products.

As per the FAO reports, about 25% of the world's agricultural produce is contaminated with mycotoxins of which aflatoxins contribute significantly. Aflatoxin development in stored grains has constantly hampered the availability of good quality feed ingredients. Contaminated crops are sometimes diverted into animal and poultry feed causing considerable health and economic implications. The financial impact of mycotoxins is especially on the poultry industry (Beg *et al*., 2006). Aflatoxins cause enormous economic losses to poultry industry by decreasing immunity in flocks and enhancing susceptibility to various infections, decreased egg and meat production, decreased feed consumption, loss of weight gain & nutritional interactions (Jand *et al*., 2005).

Aflatoxins

Currently, there are about 20 known aflatoxins but most of these are metabolites that are formed endogenously in animals by major toxins of *A. flavus* and *A. parasiticus* viz. aflatoxin B1, B2, G1, G2, M1 and M2 ('B' and 'G' denotes blue fluorescence and green fluorescence, and 'M' is due to its presence in milk). Aflatoxin is hepatotoxic, mutagenic and carcinogenic fungal toxin which is capable of producing diseases in farm animals as well as poultry.

The toxic effects of aflatoxins are largely due to their different chemical structures and acute effects require high amounts to be consumed. The symptoms depend on the type of toxin, the amount and duration of the exposure, age, health status and poorly understood synergistic effects involving genetics, dietary status, and interactions with other toxic insults (Bennett and Klich, 2003).

Types of aflatoxins and their metabolism

Aflatoxins are family of related bisfurano-coumarin compounds produced mainly by at least three species of *Aspergillus* namely *A. flavus*, *A. parasiticus* and *A. nominus* (Bennett and Klich, 2003). These are mainly classified in four groups, viz., B1, B2, G1 and G2 (Yiannikouris and Jouany, 2002). Aflatoxins B2 and G2 are the di-hydro derivatives of the parent compound, while M1 and M2 are the hydroxylated metabolites of aflatoxins B1 and B2, respectively excreted in milk and designated as 'M' or milk toxin and are produced when ruminants ingest feed contaminated with B1 and B2 toxins. Of all the types, B1 is the most predominant and the most toxic one. Two more aflatoxin metabolites viz. P1 and Q1 have also been identified to occur in liver or urine of mammals. Aflatoxin B2a, G2a and aspertoxin have also been reported but their pathogenic potential is not fully understood.

Aflatoxins on ingestion are absorbed in small intestines, and they get accumulated in liver and muscles, liver being the principal organ affected. Hepatocytes metabolize these toxins and convert into various metabolites. The 2-hydroxylation of aflatoxin B1 (AFB1) is the common biotransformation in all animal species yielding a comparatively non-toxic metabolite designated as aflatoxin B2a, and G1 on 2-hydroxylation gets transformed into G2a. In liver of birds, aflatoxin B1 and B2 are reduced to aflatoxicol and dihydroaflatoxicol, respectively. In liver, AFB1 irreversibly binds to protein and form adducts such as aflatoxin B1-lysine in albumin.

Effects of aflatoxicosis

The general effects of aflatoxicosis in animals include decreased feed utilization and efficiency leading to poor weight gain, liver and kidney damage, gastrointestinal dysfunction, embryonic death, teratogenicity, carcinogenesis, suppressed immune functions, reduced productivity, anaemia, jaundice and death (Pier, 1992). In birds, immune-suppression, reduced growth and egg production are often noticed (Yaroshenko *et al.*, 2003). Acute liver damage, induction of tumors and immune-toxicities are of much concern (Bennet and Klich, 2003). High level of aflatoxin exposure produces alteration in digestion, absorption and metabolism of nutrients. Chronic or subclinical exposure does not lead to visible signs but leads to carcinogenesis.

High doses of aflatoxins may also result in severe hepatocellular necrosis and prolonged low dosages result in reduced growth rate and hepatomegaly (Bennett and Klich, 2003). It inhibits the DNA-dependent RNA synthesis in nucleus resulting into inhibition of protein synthesis, which results in reduced production of essential metabolic enzymes and structural proteins for growth (Fung and Clark, 2004).

i. ***Nutritional interference***: Chronic aflatoxin exposure has major effects on nutritional status in livestock. In poultry, a drop in feed conversion efficiency and decreased growth rates are consistent signs of chronic aflatoxin exposure and the toxin has been a factor modulating the rate of recovery from protein malnutrition (Bennett and Klich, 2003). Aflatoxin modifies vitamin A nutrition in poultry (Tyczkowski and Hamilton, 1987). Liver vitamin A decreases with increasing concentrations of aflatoxins in female broiler chicks (Reddy *et al.*, 1989). In broilers, the vitamin D concentration is also affected by aflatoxin in the diet. Aflatoxin have been found to reduce plasma 25-hydroxy vitamin D and 1,25- di-hydroxy vitamin D concentrations (Glahn *et al.*, 1991). Zinc and selenium are essential for healthy immune systems, also get affected by aflatoxin in the diet (Hegazy and Adachi, 2000).

ii. ***Carcinogenesis:*** Aflatoxins can induce mutagenesis by alkylation of nuclear DNA, leading to carcinogenesis and teratogenesis. The reaction with DNA occurs with guanine in the codon of tumor suppressor gene p53 where the G to T transversion occurs (Hussain *et al.*, 2007). The International Agency for Research on Cancer (IARC) defines aflatoxin as a Class-I carcinogen, regulated levels being 20 ppb in grains and 0.5 ppb in milk in the United States and 4 ppb in foods and agricultural commodities in many European countries (Henry *et al.*, 1999). Aflatoxin B1 is one of the most potent hepato-carcinogenic substances known and no animal species is immune to its acute toxic effects. The active metabolite of AFB1, the 8, 9-epoxide is a potent carcinogen and named as "proximal carcinogen". It is extremely reactive, and induces chromosomal aberrations and cell toxicity. Aflatoxin G1 is an active carcinogen but aflatoxins B2 and G2 are very less carcinogenic.

iii. ***Immuno-suppression:*** AFB1 is able to induce thymic aplasia, reduce T-lymphocyte function and number and suppress phagocytic and complement activity (Kataria *et al.*, 2005). Aflatoxin impairs the humoral and cellular immune functions thus reducing the primary and secondary immune responses (Fernandez *et al.*, 2000). AFB1 is also known to have immunosuppressive effects on NK cell activity (Methenitou *et al.*, 2001). Impairment of cellular function by aflatoxins seems to be due to its effects on the production of lymphokines (Han *et al.*, 1999). AFB1 have a marked impact on phagocytosis by adversely modulating cytokines produced by the phagocytes (Cusumano *et al.*, 1996). AFB1 also suppress the levels of IL-1, IL-6 and TNF (Dugyala and Sharma, 1996). The percentage of active lymphocytes significantly decreases in chicks due to AFB1 (Ghosh *et al.*, 1990). In birds, development of bursa is affected in chicks during aflatoxin exposure (Verma *et al.*, 2004). Aflatoxins also impair the function of macrophages in avian species (Mohiuddin *et al.*, 1986). In poultry, dietary aflatoxin exposure reduced antibody titers to vaccines for Newcastle disease, Marek's disease and infectious bursal disease (Anjum, 1994).

Manifestation of aflatoxicosis in poultry

Aflatoxins generally affect growing livestock. Dietary levels of aflatoxin (in ppb) generally tolerated are =50 in chicks, =100 in adult chicken, =50 in weaner pigs, =200 in finishing pigs, <100 in calves, and <300 in adult cattle (Ramdell and Eaton, 1990). Avian species are variably sensitive to chronic aflatoxicosis and the intake occurs *via* mycotoxin contaminated feeds. Turkey poults and ducklings are the most sensitive (Lozano and Diaz, 2006). Aflatoxins are highly immunosuppressive and increase the susceptibility of birds to many infectious agents (Dalvi, 1986). The productive performance of birds is also drastically affected (Yaroshenko *et al.*, 2003). Aflatoxicosis in chickens is manifested as lethargy, loss of appetite, decreased feed consumption and growth rate, diarrhoea, ophisthotonus, spasms of neck muscles, arched back and death with legs stretched posteriorly (Borisova *et al.*, 1990). Due to immunosuppressive damage of thymus and bursa of Fabricius, birds become susceptible to infections and fail to induce protective antibody titres (Jand *et al.*, 2005). In layers, there is drop in egg production and poor hatchability (Jand *et al.*, 2005). Acute aflatoxicosis cause sudden death with enlarged mottled liver and extensive bile duct proliferation while chronic exposure of aflatoxins may result in low mortality reduced growth rate, pale firm liver and pale enlarged kidneys (Asuzu and Shetty, 1986). There is congestion of myocardium, catarrhal inflammation of intestines, distension of pericardial sac and haemorrhages in pancreas and serous membranes (Espada *et al.*, 1992). The gross pathological lesions include enlarged liver with pale necrotic lesions and distended gall bladder (Jand e*t al.*, 2005). In chronic cases, cirrhosis of liver is more marked and birds may have gelatinous transudate subcutaneously. Accumulation of fat in liver may also be seen in birds died due to aflatoxicosis (Fukal *et al.*, 1988). In kidneys, there is thickening of capillary basement membrane in glomeruli, ischemia, swollen tubules and multiple and diffuse haemorrhages in parenchyma (Glahn *et al.*, 1991).

In turkeys, the clinical signs and lesions include ruffled feathers, diarrhoea, ataxia, opisthotonus, convulsions, swollen feet, keratoconjunctivitis and generalized edema (Fazal *et al.*, 1980). The immune system of poults is highly compromised during aflatoxicosis (Quist *et al.*, 2000). The liver becomes edematous and orange tinted in acute cases while in chronic condition liver becomes pale, and shrunken. Gross lesions in poults are subcutaneous haemorrhages, enlargement of kidneys, catarrhal enteritis, impaction and distension of gizzard and myocardial congestion.

The characteristic signs of aflatoxicosis in ducks and ducklings include inappetence, poor growth rate, ataxia, opisthotonus, convulsions and subcutaneous haemorrhages in legs and feet (Meissner, 1983). Gross lesions include pale enlarged liver with hyperplastic nodules and pale and swollen kidneys with petechial haemorrhages. Aflatoxicosis augments the hepatotoxicity in birds infected with duck hepatitis virus (Uchida *et al.*, 1988).

Methods of controlling or decontaminating mycotoxins

In general, mycotoxins are relatively stable compounds that are not destroyed by processing of feed, and may even be concentrated by screening. Feeds contaminated with mycotoxins in excess of established levels should not be fed to animals producing eggs or meat for human consumption. It is not easy to prevent mycotoxins in the environment. Prevention of the contamination of agricultural commodities by fungi and their mycotoxins can be divided into the following three levels.

i. *Primary prevention:* The best pre- or post-harvest strategy to use in a particular year depends on the climatic conditions of that year. Unfortunately, avoiding weather that favours fungal infection is beyond human control. Nonetheless, understanding the environmental factors that promote infection, growth and toxin production is the first step in minimizing mycotoxins in feeds. Several practices may help to maintain conditions that are unfavourable for fungal growth: i) development of fungal-resistant crop varieties; ii) control of on-field infection with fungicides; iii) scheduling of harvests in the period suitable for the region; and iv) lowering the moisture content of the feedstuff after harvest and during storage.
ii. *Secondary prevention:* This level of prevention is required when the fungi are already in the feedstuff. The fungi should be eliminated or their growth stopped to prevent further deterioration and mycotoxin contamination. The following measures may be useful: i) protecting stored products from conditions that favour continuing fungal growth; ii) using mould inhibitors (such as organic acids) against fungal growth; iii) storing commodity at low temperatures, where economically possible; iv) stopping the growth of infested fungi by re-drying the products; and v) removing contaminated material.
iii. *Tertiary prevention:* When the product is heavily infested by toxic fungi, primary and secondary prevention are no longer feasible. If the mycotoxin levels are known, it may be possible to dilute the contaminated material

and produce a final blended feed that contains less than the critical level of the specific mycotoxin. Such blending of feeds to reduce mycotoxin concentrations is officially permitted, with restrictions in several countries. A number of additives are available for use in practical diets to remove or detoxify mycotoxins and reduce their negative effects on animals. These additives fall into two categories: mycotoxin binders, which bind and adsorb the mycotoxins and prevent their absorption in the gut; and mycotoxin deactivators, which deactivate specific mycotoxins. The effects of some mycotoxins (aflatoxin, ochratoxin and fumonisin) can be effectively reduced by the inclusion of appropriate adsorbent-type binders, while others (trichothecenes and zearaleone) can be removed only by deactivation. Common mycotoxin binders include hydrated sodium calcium aluminosilicate, esterified yeast-wall polysaccharides, and clays such as zeolites and bentonites. Different sorbents have differing affinities for specific mycotoxins. However, there is a risk that non-specific adsorbing agents may prevent the uptake of micronutrients in the gut. Some effective mycotoxin deactivators that are now available act by enzymatic degradation or biotransformation of mycotoxins.

Anti-caking agents covalently bind aflatoxins and diminish aflatoxin uptake, prevent acute aflatoxicosis and reduces aflatoxin residues in animal products. Preservatives and anti-fungal agents, such as propionic acid and mould inhibitors like hydroxyquinoline and gentian violet may be somewhat effective in reducing aflatoxin formation (Rao, 1995). The UV irradiation and gamma-rays (5-10 Mrad) have been reported to stop growth of molds in feeds (Park, 1993).

Modified gluco-mannans, derivative of yeast cell wall are beneficial in binding to higher levels of aflatoxins at a lower inclusion rate (Murthy and Devegowda, 2004). *Saccharomyces cerevisiae* and lactic acid bacteria are effective biological detoxifying agents (Shetty and Jespersen, 2006). Adding methionine to broiler diet improves the weight gains and reduces the adverse effects of AFB1 by increasing liver glutathione levels (Beers *et al.*, 1992). Feeding of extra vitamin A and K decreases the detrimental effects of aflatoxins (Verma *et al.*, 2001). Antioxidant compounds like selenium, chlorophyll and its derivatives, and medicinal herbs and plant extracts also reduces the toxic effects of aflatoxins (Galvano *et al.*, 2001). Spice oils such as clove and cinnamon oil inhibits the growth of *Aspergillus* species (Juglal *et al.*, 2002).

Conclusion

The impact of mycotoxicoses can be of immense magnitude and toxins produced have the capacity not only to impair animal performance due to reduced growth rates, illness or even death, but also to affect humans through toxic residues that can be deposited in animal tissues. Depending on the degree of contamination, mycotoxins or their metabolites may get deposited in meat, visceral organs and eggs. Their concentration in animal products is considerably lower than the levels present in the feed consumed by the animals, and will not cause acute toxicity in humans, but residues of carcinogenic mycotoxins, such as aflatoxins and ochratoxin A, can affect human health. Hence, the ingredients utilized for feed formulation need to checked properly, stored under proper conditions to rule out all the possibility of fungal growth.

References

Anjum, A.D. 1994. Outbreak of infectious bursal disease in vaccinated chickens due to aflatoxicosis. Indian Veterinary Journal (India), 71: 322-324.

Asuzu, I.U. and Shetty, S.N. 1986. Acute aflatoxicosis in broiler chicken in Nsukka, Nigeria. Tropical veterinarian, 4: 79-80.

Beers, K.W., Nejad, H. and Bottje, W.G. 1992. Aflatoxin and glutathione in domestic fowl (Gallus domesticus)—I. Glutathione elevation and attenuation by high dietary methionine. Comparative Biochemistry and Physiology Part C: Comparative Pharmacology, 101(2): 239-244.

Beg, M.U., Al-Mutairi, M., Beg, K.R., Al-Mazeedi, H.M., Ali, L.N. and Saeed, T. 2006. Mycotoxins in poultry feed in Kuwait. Archives of environmental contamination and toxicology, 50: 594-602.

Bennett, J.W. 2003. Klich. M. Mycotoxins. Clinical Microbiology Reviews, 16(3): 497-516.

Borisova, L., Tacheva, T., Duparinova, M., Belemezov, P., Chavdarova, S., Tikhova, D. and Gerova, M. 1990. Study on the effect of mycotoxins on broiler chickens. I. Aflatoxin B1. Veterinarna Sbirka, 88(7-8): 13-16.

Cusumano, V., Rossano, F., Merendino, R.A., Arena, A., Costa, G.B., Mancuso, G., Baroni, A. and Losi, E. 1996. Immunobiological activities of mould products: functional impairment of human monocytes exposed to aflatoxin B1. Research in microbiology, 147(5): 385-391.

Dalvi, R.R. 1986. An overview of aflatoxicosis of poultry: Its characteristics, prevention and reduction. Veterinary research communications, 10(1): 429-443.

Dugyala, R.R. and Sharma, R.P. 1996. The effect of aflatoxin B1 on cytokine mRNA and corresponding protein levels in peritoneal macrophages and splenic lymphocytes. International journal of immunopharmacology, 18(10): 599-608.

Espada, Y., Domingo, M., Gomez, J. and Calvo, M.A. 1992. Pathological lesions following an experimental intoxication with aflatoxin B1 in broiler chickens. Research in Veterinary Science, 53(3): 275-279.

Fazal, T.M.A., Wyatt, R.D. and Waibel, P.E. 1980. Biochemical and physiological changes in turkey poults during aflatoxicosis and effect of vitamin-electrolyte therapy on performance of turkeys. Poultry Science, 59(7).

Fernandez, A., Hernandez, M., Verde, M.T. and Sanz, M. 2000. Effect of aflatoxin on performance, hematology, and clinical immunology in lambs. Canadian Journal of Veterinary Research, 64(1): 53.

Fukal, L., Haisl, K., Soya, Z. and Reisnerova, H. 1988. Histopathological findings and changes in the aflatoxin and lipid concentrations in the liver of laying hens during acute experimental aflatoxicosis. Veterinarne Medicina, 33: 495-502.

Fung, F. and Clark, R.F. 2004. Health effects of mycotoxins: a toxicological overview. Journal of Toxicology: Clinical Toxicology, 42(2): 217-234.

Galvano, F., Piva, A., Ritieni, A. and Galvano, G. 2001. Dietary strategies to counteract the effects of mycotoxins: a review. Journal of food protection, 64(1): 120-131.

Ghosh, R.C., Chauhan, H.V.S. and Roy, S. 1990. Immunosuppression in broilers under experimental aflatoxicosis. British Veterinary Journal, 146(5): 457-462.

Glahn, R.P., Beers, K.W., Bottje, W.G., Wideman Jr, R.F., Huff, W.E. and Thomas, W. 1991. Aflatoxicosis alters avian renal function, calcium, and vitamin D metabolism. Journal of toxicology and environmental health, 34(3): 309-321.

Han, S.H., Jeon, Y.J., Yea, S.S. and Yang, K.H. 1999. Suppression of the interleukin-2 gene expression by aflatoxin B1 is mediated through the down-regulation of the NF-AT and AP-1 transcription factors. Toxicology letters, 108(1):1-10.

Hegazy, S. M. and Adachi, Y. 2000. Comparison of the effects of dietary selenium, zinc, and selenium and zinc supplementation on growth and immune response between chick groups that were inoculated with Salmonella and aflatoxin or Salmonella. Poultry Science, 79: 331-335.

Henry, S. H., Bosch, F. X., Troxell, T. C. and Bolger, P. M. 1999. Reducing liver cancer global control of aflatoxin. Science, 286: 2453-2454

Hussain, S. P., Schwank, J., Staib, F., Wang, X. W. and Harris, C. C. 2007. TP53 mutations and hepatocellular carcinoma: insights into the etiology and pathogenesis of liver cancer. Oncogene, 26(15): 2166-2176.

Jand, S. K., Kaur, P. and Sharma, N. S. 2005. Mycoses and mycotoxicosis in poultry: A review. Indian Journal of Animal Science, 75(4): 465-476

Juglal, S., Govinden, R. and Odhav, B. 2002. Spice oils for the control of co-occurring mycotoxin-producing fungi. Journal of Food Protection, 65(4): 683-687.

Kataria, J. M., Dhama, K. and Mahendran, M. 2005. Mycotoxicosis in poultry: Immunosuppressive effects and remedial measures for its control. National Seminar-2005, SRDDL, IAH&VB, Bangalore. Souvenir. pp. 25-28.

Lozano, M. C. and Diaz, G. J. 2006. Microsomal and cytosolic biotransformation of aflatoxin B1 in four poultry species. British Poultry Science, 47(6): 734-741.

Meissner, O. H. T. 1983. Effects of contamination of diets with aflatoxin on growing ducks and chickens. Tropical Animal Health Production, 15: 161-168

Methenitou, G., Maravelias, C., Athanaselis, S., Dona, A. and Koutselinis, A. 2001. Immunomodulative effects of aflatoxins and selenium on human natural killer cells. Vet Human Toxicology, 43(4): 232-234.

Mohiuddin, S. M., Reddv, M. V., Reddy, M. M. and Ramakrishna, K. 1986. Studies on phagocyte activity and haematological changes in aflatoxicosis in poultry. Indian Veterinary Journal, 63: 442-445.

Murthy, T. N. K. and Devegowda, G. 2004. Efficacy of modified glucomannan (Mycosorb) to adsorb aflatoxin B1 in gut conditions of broiler chickens. In: 22nd World Poultry Congress. Istanbul, Turkey, pp: 471.

Park D L. 1993. Perspectives on mycotoxin decontamination procedures. Food Addit. Contam., 10(1 & 2): 49-60.

Pier, A. C. 1992. Major biological consequences of aflatoxicosis in animal production. Journal of Animal Science, 70(12): 3964-3967.

Quist, C.F., Bounous, D.I., Kilburn, J.V., Nettles, V.F. and Wyatt, R.D. 2000. The effect of dietary aflatoxin on wild turkey poults. Journal of Wildlife Diseases, 36(3): 436-444.

Ramdell, H. S. and Eaton, D. L. 1990. Species susceptibility to Aflatoxin B1 carcinogenesis. Cancer Research, 50: 615-620.

Rao, V. N. 1995. Emerging trends in combating aflatoxicosis in animals with special reference to chickens. In: Advances in Animal Health and Production. Chauhan R S Sharma P C Rakesh Kumar, Sharma R and Mahipal S K (eds.). pp. 277-280.

Reddy, K. V., Rao, P. V. and Reddy, V. R. 1989. Effect of aflatoxin on the performance of broiler chicks fed diets supplemented with vitamin A. Indian Journal of Animal Science, 59: 140-144.

Shetty, P. H. and Jespersen. L. 2006. Saccharomyces cerevisiae and lactic acid bacteria as potential Mycotoxin decontaminating agents. Trends in Food Science Technology 17(2): 48-55.

Tyczkowski, J. K. and Hamilton, P. B. 1987. Altered metabolism of carotenoids during aflatoxicosis in young chickens. Poultry Science, 66: 1184-1188.

Uchida T., Suzuki, K., Esumi, M., Arii, M. and Shikata, T. 1988. Influence of aflatoxin B1 intoxication on duck livers with duck hepatitis B virus infection. Cancer Research, 48: 1559-1565.

Verma, J., Johri, T. S., Swain, B. K. and Ameena, S. 2004. Effect of graded levels of aflatoxin, ochratoxin and their combinations on the performance and immune response of broilers. British Poultry Science, 45(4): 512-518.

Verma, R. J., Shukla, R. S. and Mehta, D. N. 2001. Amelioration of cytotoxic effects of aflatoxin by vitamin A: an in vitro study on erythrocytes. Toxicology *In Vitro*, 15: 39-42.

Yaroshenko, F., Dvosrska, J. and Surai, P. 2003. Mycotoxins in poultry production: problems and solutions. Poultry International, pp: 12-16.

Yiannikouris, A. and Jouany, J. P. 2002. Mycotoxins in feeds and their fate in animals: A review. Animal Research, 51: 81-99.

13

Mycotoxicological Challenges in Poultry

Krishnamurthy T.N. and G. Devegowda [*]

Associate Professor and Head, Department of Livestock Production Management Veterinary College, Shivamogga, Karnataka

[*] *Professor Emeritus, University of Agricultural Sciences, GKVK, Bangalore*

Introduction

There has been a steady increase in the poultry meat and egg production globally during the past few decades. Though the high biological value of eggs and poultry meat have resulted in an increasing demand for these two products, growing awareness for food quality and safety are becoming increasingly significant in determining the market value of such products. The importance of mycotoxins as one of the major detractor of poultry productivity and also of product quality, hence, becomes more relevant now than ever.

According to the United Nation's Food and Agriculture Organization (FAO), approximately 25% of world's grain supply is contaminated with mycotoxins. The greatest economic impact of mycotoxin contamination is felt by crop and poultry producers, as well as food and feed producers (CAST, 2003). The economic losses caused by mycotoxins in poultry run up to several hundred million dollars annually worldwide. The adverse effects of mycotoxin contaminated diets consumed by poultry on productive performance of the birds range from the undetectable to devastating by way of reduced egg production in layers and breeders, and growth depression in broilers, turkeys, ducks etc.

The threat of mycotoxins has been described as early as the Second World War (II) when the soldiers from the Russian army suffered severe dermal necrosis, hemorrhages and destruction of bone marrow after eating mouldy grains (*Fusarium* contaminated). However, it was not until 1960, when the entire turkey population of Britain was decimated in a fatal liver disease called "Turkey X Disease", that the scientific community recognized the negative effects associated with mycotoxins. British agriculture officials later traced the source of the outbreak to aflatoxin in a shipment of peanut (groundnut) meal that originated from Brazil.

Mycotoxins of importance in poultry are mainly produced by the fungi genera *Aspergillus, Fusarium* and *Penicillia,* at the pre-harvest, harvest and in storage or during feed processing whenever conditions are favorable. No region of the world escapes these silent killers and their negative impact on poultry productivity and human health is enormous (Devegowda, 2002).

Geographical distribution of mycotoxins

At the First Food and Agricultural Organization (FAO) - World Health Organization (WHO) - United Nations Environment Programme (UNEP) Conference on mycotoxins in 1977, a review was presented on the occurrence of mycotoxins in various commodities throughout the world. Only seven mycotoxins were reported to occur significantly in naturally contaminated foods and feeds: aflatoxins, ochratoxin A, patulin, zearalenone, trichothecenes, citrinin and penicillic acid (Jelinek *et al.,* 1989). The occurrence of mycotoxins in nature is considered a global problem. However, in certain geographical areas of the world, some mycotoxins are produced more readily than others. In colder, more temperate, regions such as Canada, the Northern U.S. and most of the European countries, aflatoxins are not considered to be a major problem except in imported feedstuffs grown in warmer southern climates. Economically, in these regions the most important mycotoxins are deoxynivalenol (=vomitoxin) (DON), zearalenone (ZEA), ochratoxin A (OTA), diacetoxyscripenol (DAS), T-2 toxin and HT-2 toxin. DON contamination of corn and corn products in Canada, South Africa, Taiwan, the UK and the U.S. has been reported to be more than 1mg/kg in some lots of grain tested (Devegowda, *et al.*, 1998).

In Europe, the differences in climatic conditions among the northern, middle and southern parts, favor the development of different fungal species. Accordingly, different mycotoxins have gained considerable importance in respective European regions during the last two decades (Leibetseder, 1995). In the maize growing areas of southern and middle Europe (Sweden, Austria and Hungary) mainly fusariotoxins (DON, ZEA, T-2 toxin) cause illness and poor performance of livestock and poultry, whereas OTA is of greater importance in the northern part of Europe (Denmark and Poland).

Investigations in Germany demonstrated that 8.4% of 1,000 feed samples tested positive for trichothecenes. Fifteen-grain samples out of 966 contained ZEA (Gedek, 1988). A recent large-scale survey, where 1431 samples of wheat, barley, rye, oats and bran were analyzed for OTA in Denmark, showed that 40 % of the samples were contaminated with OTA. Among the commodities analysed, bran products showed a higher OTA contamination than cereal kernels. For example OTA was detected in wheat in 62 % of the bran samples and only 30 % of the samples of kernels (Hohler, 1999). These findings are typical for most of the mycotoxins, where cereals by products, especially bran, usually show higher mycotoxin levels than the whole cereal.

Aflatoxins, the most widespread of all the mycotoxins, are common in warm and humid climatic conditions like those existing in Latin American, Asian and African countries, southern regions of U.S. and certain parts of Australia. Aflatoxins occur in about 20% of the corn grain grown in the southern U.S. even in non-crisis years and in years with extreme weather conditions occurrence may be higher.

Extensive surveys conducted in India, Pakistan, Egypt and South Africa suggested that aflatoxins are often encountered in substantial levels in feeds and feed ingredients. The evidence comes from the fact that in southern parts of India, where hot and humid climatic conditions prevail during most parts of the year, certain feed ingredients and finished feeds were found to be positive for the presence of aflatoxin, OTA and T-2 toxin (Chandrasekaran, 1996). However, during the winter season in these countries high moisture conditions may result in other mycotoxins such as ZEA, DON, T-2 toxin, OTA, etc.

A survey of Chinese compound feeds and ingredients revealed that 88, 84, 77 and 60% of corn samples contained T-2 toxin, aflatoxin, fumonisin and OTA respectively. All corn samples contained ZEA and DON. The six major toxins were found in more than 90% of compound feeds (Wang, *et al.*, 2003).

In Latin American countries including Brazil, Peru, Mexico, Columbia, Venezuela and Argentina, reports exist on the presence of aflatoxins, OTA, T-2 toxin, DON, ZEA and other *Fusarium* toxins. In a recent Canadian survey for ergot alkaloids in various cereal products, individual alkaloids were found at low levels (<200 mcg/kg) (Devegowda, *et al.*, 1998). A maximum of 0.05% ergot alkaloid has been suggested in Canada as an acceptable level in wheat used for production of flour. Ergot poisoning is also seen in warm and humid regions of India, Ethiopia and the U.S.

Due to the increase in global trading of feedstuffs mycotoxins are no longer solely found in certain geographical regions but are now more widely distributed than before (Devegowda *et al.*, 1998a).

Significant mycotoxins in poultry

Some fungal strains are capable of producing more than one mycotoxin and also a single mycotoxin is produced by more than one fungus. The most important mycotoxins for poultry and the fungi producing them are given in the Table 1.

Table 1: Moulds and mycotoxins Important in intensive poultry production

Mycotoxins	**Moulds**
1. Aspergillus toxins	
Aflatoxins B_1, B_2, G_1 and G_2	*Aspergillus flavus and Aspergillus parasiticus*
Cyclopiazonic acid	*Aspergillus flavus*
Ochratoxins	*Aspergillus ochraceus*
Sterigmatocystin	*Aspergillus versicolor*
2. Pencillium Toxins	
Ochratoxins	*Penicillium viridicatum*
Citrinin	*Pencillium citrinum*
3. Fusarium Toxins	
T-2 Toxin, HT-2 Toxin, Diacetoxyscirpenol (DAS), Monoacetoxyscripenol (MAS) Deoxynivalenol (DON, vomitoxin)	*Fusarium tricinctum, Fusarium graminearum Fusarium solani*
Fumonisins B_1, B_2	*Fusarium moniliforme Fusarium proliferatum*
Moniliformin	*Fusarium moniliforme*
Zearalenone	*Fusarium graminearum, Fusarium roseum*

Effects of mycotoxins in Poultry

The effects of mycotoxins in poultry are discussed individually in the following sections. However, it should be noted that combinations of toxins, as found naturally in moldy feeds, cause greater adverse effects than feeds containing a single mycotoxin.

1. Aflatoxins

The most widespread and the most studied group of all the mycotoxins, aflatoxins are of concern in warm and humid climatic conditions as in Asian, Latin American, African countries, in the Southern region of U.S. and in certain parts of Australia. Though they are not considered to be a major problem in cold, temperate regions, caution needs to be exercised while feeding feedstuffs imported from warm and humid countries. Aflatoxins are primarily produced by fungi of the genus *Aspergillus* (*Aspergillus flavus* and *Aspergillus parasiticus*) and are found in poultry feeds and human food products. Major forms of aflatoxins include B_1, B_2, G_1 and G_2 with aflatoxin B_1 being the most common and biologically active toxin. Henceforth in this chapter, the term aflatoxin is used to refer to aflatoxin B_1 unless specified otherwise.

Impact on production performance: Economic losses associated with aflatoxin exposure include poor growth and feed conversion, increased mortality, decreased egg production, leg problems, and carcass condemnations in poultry. The frequent aflatoxin contamination of agricultural commodities and the chronic exposure of poultry to these toxins can mean the difference between profit and loss to the poultry industry (Hamilton, 1984; Devegowda *et al.*, 1998b).

Among poultry, ducks are most susceptible to aflatoxins followed by turkeys, broilers, laying hens and quails. Gooslings and pheasants are more sensitive than chicks and less sensitive than ducklings and turkey poults to aflatoxins. Clinically, the signs of aflatoxin toxicity include anorexia, decreased weight gain, decreased egg production, specific visceral hemorrhages, embryo toxicity, and increased susceptibility to environmental and microbial stressors. Histopathology reveals fatty liver, liver necrosis and bile duct hyperplasia as the most common findings in birds affected with aflatoxin.

Aflatoxin can have a wide range of effects on the metabolic system of poultry. Aflatoxin contamination of the diet decreases the activities of several digestive enzymes important in the digestion of starch, proteins, lipids and nucleic acids. On the other hand, the activities of a few metabolic enzymes like serum glutamate pyruvate transaminase (SGPT), serum glutamate oxalo-acetate transferase (SGOT) and gamma glutamyl transferase (GGT) are increased, primarily indicating hepatic damage. Also the reduction in the total proteins, total cholesterol and blood urea nitrogen are attributed to the toxic effects of aflatoxin in broiler chickens (Raju and Devegowda, 2000; Aravind *et al.*, 2003) (Table 2).

Table 2: Effect of feeding aflatoxin contaminated diet on serum biochemical parameters in broilers at five weeks of age

Aflatoxin 300ppb	Total proteins (g%)	Total cholesterol (mg %)	Blood urea nitrogen (mg %)
-	2.73^{bc}	114.8^{a}	2.22^{a}
+	1.45^{h}	57.3^{f}	1.01^{d}

Means with in each column bearing at least one common superscript do not differ significantly (P < 0.01)

(Raju and Devegowda, 2000)

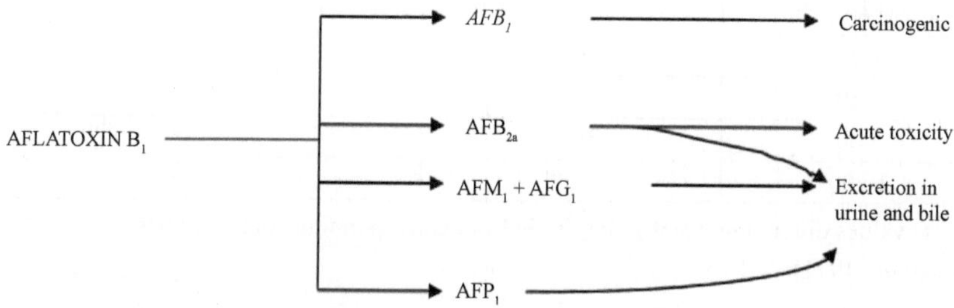

Aflatoxin is also known to interfere with the vitamin D metabolism contributing to reduced bone strength and leg weakness among the birds (Hamilton, 1987). Additionally, metabolism of several minerals including iron (causing hemolytic anemia), phosphorus (causing leg weakness) (Table 3) and copper are also affected by aflatoxin. Suppression of hepatic protein synthesis is the main factor resulting in growth suppression and reduced egg production seen in cases of aflatoxicosis. In aflatoxicosis, owing to reduced bile salt production, absorption of fat and carotenoid pigments is reduced. The resultant poor pigmentation of bird skin and egg yolk is generally referred to as "pale bird syndrome", which may sometimes be seen in ochratoxicosis too.

Table 3: Adverse effects of aflatoxin on 0-21 day old ducks.

Aflatoxin (mcg/ kg)	Weight Gain (g/100g of BW)	Leg Deformity Score	Liver Weight (g/100g BW)
60	602^{ef}	1.73^{b}	5.72^{b}
120	417^{g}	2.21^{a}	7.81^{a}
60	$642d^{e}$	1.23^{bc}	5.35^{bc}
120	597^{ef}	1.56^{b}	$5.32b^{c}$

$^{a-g}$ *Means within a column with different superscripts are significantly different.*

(Khajarern and Khajarern, 1999)

Bruising

Bruising is a significant cause of downgrading of broiler meat (Hess and Biligili, 1997), representing approximately 25 percent of the downgrades recorded. Mycotoxins, especially aflatoxins, are associated with bruising in chickens (Girish and Devegowda, 2004a). Aflatoxins have been shown to increase the fragility of capillaries, reducing the prothrombin levels thereby drastically increasing the incidence of bruising in carcasses (Tung *et al.*, 1971) (Table 4).

Table 4: Body weight and bruising during experimental aflatoxicosis

Aflatoxin (mg/g)	Body weight (g)	Bruising Energy (μ joules)
0	552	441
0.625	558	365*
1.25	547	314*
2.50	481*	229*
5.00	385*	212*
10.00	327*	206*

* These values differ significantly ($P < 0.05$) from corresponding control values.

(Tung *et al.*, 1971)

Broiler breeders

Feeding aflatoxin to broiler breeder hens has been reported to decrease egg production and hatchability (Afzali and Devegowda, 1999). Qureshi *et al.*, 1998, reported increase in the concentration of aflatoxin and its metabolites in the serum of hens and in eggs fed higher levels of aflatoxin. Further, drastic decreases in fertility and hatchability were observed within the first four days of feeding the contaminated feed (Table 5).

Table 5: Effect of aflatoxin on broiler breeder progeny performance

Aflatoxin[1] (mg/kg)	Fertile eggs (%)	Hatchability (%)	Phagocytic Macrophages[2] (%)
0	98.6[a]	82.8	35.8[a]
10	92.4[b]	35.3	9.7[b]

[ab] Means within a column with different superscripts are significantly different ($P < 0.05$)
[1] *In the diets of the hen.* [2] *To sheep red blood cells.* *(Qureshi, et al., 1998)*

Aflatoxin studies in other species of poultry

In a trial, gooslings and pheasants showed reduced weight gains as the level of aflatoxin was increased. All of the gooslings fed 4 mcg/g died by 2 weeks of age and 90% of the pheasants on the 4 mcg/g feed died by 3 weeks of age (Muller *et al.*, 1970). In another study involving poults, all the poults receiving the 1, 2 and 4 mcg/g diets were dead by the end of experiment (Muller *et al.*, 1970). As early as 1 week of age, high mortality and reduced weight gains were noted with higher levels of aflatoxin. Ducklings are most susceptible to aflatoxin injury of the species tested. One hundred percent mortality occurred at 2 weeks of age for the birds receiving the 2 and 4 mcg/g diets and at 3 weeks of age for the birds receiving the 1 mcg/g diet (Muller *et al.*, 1970).

Field study

Table 6 shows a study involving several poultry companies, where in the growers were grouped into three categories good, moderate, or poor, based on the performance (Jones *et al.*, 1982). A review of the records for the incidence of aflatoxin positive samples and the levels detected brought out a conclusive finding on the adverse effects of aflatoxin on growth of poultry, at all levels of occurrence. It is worthwhile to note here that, even at the low levels (6-14 mcg/kg), which may be considered 'practically safe' in some parts of the world, aflatoxin can cause considerable damage to the health and performance of the birds.

Table 6: Aflatoxin effects on production and processing characteristics

Parameters	Grower Classification		
	Good	Moderate	Poor
Number of growers	10	10	10
Number of birds	122,052	110,290	105,267
Average weight (lbs)	3.88	3.83	3.79
Average feed conversion	2.13	2.15	2.16
Livability (%)	95.98	95.61	92.78
Aflatoxin concentration (mcg/kg)	6.13	6.49	13.99
Aflatoxin Positive Samples (%)	18.04	22.08	31.25

(Jones *et al.*, 1982)

Immunosuppression

One of the major causes of worry is immunosuppression due to aflatoxin and the consequent increase in susceptibility to a wide variety of infectious diseases along with the accompanying vaccine failure and therapeutic drug failures. Immunosuppression caused by aflatoxins produces a cascading effect starting with depressed protein synthesis, lowered serum albumin and globulin levels, reduction in circulating antibody levels, impairment of the reticulo-endothelial system and reduced cell-mediated immunity, besides affecting the normal development of the thymus and bursa of Fabricius (Swamy and Devegowda, 1998) (Table 7). There is a large mass of evidence to suggest that aflatoxicosis (as also ochratoxicosis and T-2 toxicosis) can increase the susceptibility of the birds to salmonella infection, largely owing to lesser percentage of circulating leukocytes and their reduced ability to engulf the microorganisms. On the other hand, aflatoxicosis can even induce therapeutic failures. It has been found that aflatoxin can reduce the serum concentration of antibiotics (Miller and Wyatt, 1985), which may be attributed to the stepped-up efforts by the liver to maximize the systemic detoxification.

Table 7: Effect of aflatoxin B_1 on antibody titres against infectious bursal disease (IBD) and Newcastle disease (ND) at 6th week of age in broiler chickens

Aflatoxin ppb	IBD	ND
0	6180 ± 195^{e}	5800 ± 199^{g}
100	3800 ± 212^{c}	3025 ± 208^{cd}
200	3046 ± 220^{b}	2650 ± 214^{a}
400	2200 ± 225^{a}	1850 ± 217^{a}

Means bearing at least one common superscript in a column do not differ significantly ($P<0.05$)
(Swamy and Devegowda, 1998)

In poultry, the bursa of Fabricius, thymus and spleen and to a lesser extent the cecal tonsils and bone marrow constitute the organs contributing to humoral and cellular immunity. Various mycotoxins are known to adversely affect the immune system by depressing both the cell-mediated and humoral immune response.

Table 8: Mycotoxins that cause immunosuppression (In decreasing order of severity)

1.	Aflatoxin
2.	Vomitoxin, T-2 toxin, HT-2 toxin
3.	Ochratoxin
4.	Fumonisins

(Devegowda, 2001)

Aflatoxin has a direct adverse effect on both cellular and humoral immunity. While low levels of dietary aflatoxin may affect the cellular immunity, immunoglobulin production and antibody response are suppressed at higher levels (Afzali and Devegowda, 1999). Aflatoxin is considered to be a major contributor for immunosuppression with many disease outbreaks, vaccination failures and poor antibody titres being attributed to it (Raju and Devegowda, 2002).

Impact of aflatoxins on the immune system

- Reduction in size of bursa of Fabricius and thymus.
- Reduction in T-lymphocyte, B-lymphocyte and white blood cell counts.
- Reduction in total serum proteins and immunoglobulins.
- Reduction in antibody titers.
- Reduction in serum concentration of antibiotics.

Recent studies have implicated aflatoxin to cause immunosuppression at embryonic stage itself by instigating significant DNA damage to B and T-Lymphocytes at a stage when they are in rapid proliferation and differentiation (Qureshi *et al.,* 1998).

Residues

Aflatoxins are well absorbed and rapidly metabolized producing reactive epoxides, which are can further produce carcinogenic metabolites. The rate of aflatoxin residue excretion in poultry meat is much lower than that in ruminant milk. Level of residues in eggs is dose dependent with more residues concentrated in yolk than albumin (Table 9) (Jacobson and Wiseman, 1974). Due to lower rate of exposure to aflatoxins in Europe in line with the stringent regulations, the risk of undesirable residues in edible tissues is negligible.

Table 9: The relationship between the aflatoxin content of layer feed and the aflatoxin concentration in eggs.

Aflatoxin In feed (mcg/kg)	Aflatoxin In eggs (mcg/kg)
100	0.23
200	0.78
400	1.40

(Jacobson and Wiseman, 1974)

Permissible level in feeds

Many countries follow a maximum permissible level of 20 mcg/kg for aflatoxins in poultry feeds (CAST, 2003). Within effect from the year 2002, maximum permissible levels in the European Union for aflatoxins in agricultural commodities in general are 4 mcg/kg and maximum permissible levels for aflatoxin B_1 is 2 mcg/kg. In Japan, the regulation for aflatoxin is 10 mcg/kg for young and 20 mcg/kg for adult chickens. Most of the countries in the world have regulations for aflatoxins in poultry feeds.

2. Cyclopiazonic acid (CPA)

Cyclopiazonic acid (CPA) is primarily produced by *Aspergillus flavus* and is commonly found in combination with aflatoxin causing adverse effects on the performance of poultry. Urano and coworkers (1992) reported co-occurrence of CPA and aflatoxins in corn and peanuts in the U.S. In Indonesia, it was reported that CPA occurred in approximately 81% of samples analysed at poultry feed mill in Indonesia at levels up to 9 mg/kg (reference). The toxic effects of CPA have been summarized by Smith *et al.,* (1992). Recent toxicological studies have shown that the principal target organs of this mycotoxin are the liver, kidney and digestive system. Feeding trials with chickens have produced mucosal necrosis and inflammation in the crop, proventriculus and gizzard. In these chickens the kidneys often were swollen or distended (CAST, 2003). CPA is associated with hemorrhagic lesions seen on poultry thighs and is thought to be responsible for many hemorrhagic syndromes. CPA has been reported to markedly distribute to the skeletal tissue and having neurotoxic effects in poultry.

Turkeys

Cole (1986) has reappraised the etiology of the classical Turkey 'X' disease syndrome and has suggested that the arching of the neck and the head drawn back (opisthotonus), and the legs stretched (extended) fully backwards are effects produced by cyclopiazonic acid but not by aflatoxins. Thus, he concludes that this mycotoxin co-occurred with the aflatoxins in the Brazilian groundnut cake responsible for Turkey 'X' disease.

Laying hens

CPA chelates metal cations due to the presence of a tetramic acid moiety. The chelation of cations such as calcium, magnesium and iron is thought to be the main mechanism of CPA toxicity. Hens fed diets contaminated with CPA lay eggs with thin shells or visibly cracked shells due to impaired eggshell formation (Bryden 1991).

Residues

Dorner and coworkers (1994) reported that CPA was found in eggs after oral administration of CPA to laying hens. These findings indicate a potential source of human exposure via ingestion of eggs and meat containing residues of CPA.

3. Sterigmatocystin

This mycotoxin is produced by *Aspergillus versicolor*. It is also produced by toxigenic strains of *A. flavus* and *A. parasiticus*. Sterigmatocystin contains a xanthone nucleus and is considered to be a biosynthetic precursor of aflatoxin. Like aflatoxin, it contains the bis-dihydrofurofuran ring (the vinyl ether) and as would be expected is a carcinogen. The target organ for toxicity is the liver. Sterigmatocystin is found in commodities that are heavily contaminated with aflatoxin. Sterigmatocystin is also found in heavily molded grains, rice bran, sunflower meal, soybean meal, peanut meal etc.

4. Ochratoxin A (OTA)

Ochratoxin is one of the most toxic mycotoxins in poultry identified first by South African researchers in 1965. Several species of *Aspergillus* and *Pencillium* fungi produce ochratoxin. There are at least three types of ochratoxin with the most common being ochratoxin A and it is common contaminant found on a variety of feedstuffs in many countries. OTA is a highly carcinogenic toxin, and intoxications were reported already at concentration in feed of 0.05-0.1 mg/kg in chickens. The World Health Organisation (2001) proposed a general maximum limit of OTA of 5 mcg/kg in cereals and cereal products, which in the mean time has been established as official maximum limit in several countries for foods and feeds.

Ochratoxins are the most important storage toxins in temperate as well as in tropical areas. In tropical and subtropical countries ochratoxin A (the most prevalent derivative) is mainly produced by *Aspergillus* species, whereas in temperate countries, *penicillium* species (*Penicillium viridicatum)* is the major producer of ochratoxins (Devegowda *et al.,* 1998c).

Ochratoxin A is approximately three times more toxic to young broiler chicks than aflatoxin (Huff *et. al.,* 1974), and is implicated in significant field outbreaks of mycotoxicosis in poultry (Hamilton *et. al.,* 1982).

Impact on production performance

Ochratoxin A is primarily a nephrotoxin (Figure 8) that significantly suppresses feed intake, growth, feathering, egg production and feed conversion efficiency (Hamilton *et al.*, 1982). Feeding of the ochratoxin contaminated diet resulted in significant reduction in the body weight gain (17.6%), increased gamma glutamyl transferase (GGT) activity (38.5%), decrease in total proteins (16.4%) and in hematocrit values (11.3%) (Aravind and Devegowda, 2003) (Table 10). Though all the mycotoxins suppress body weight, ochratoxin produces the greatest body weight depression effect. Birds severely affected with ochratoxicosis show urate deposits in joints and abdominal cavity. Acute OTA toxicity results in acute renal failure leading to death. Polyurea leading to large volumes of wet feces, usually seen as 'loose droppings' or 'watery droppings' is another common observation with OTA.

Table 10: The effects of dietary ochratoxin on hematological and serum biochemical parameters

Ochratoxin 500 ppb	GGT (IU/L)	Proteins (g/100 ml)	Hematocrit (%)
-	8.3[a]	2.62[c]	36.0[b]
+	11.5[c]	2.19[a]	31.9[a]

Means with no common letters differ significantly (P < 0.05)

(Aravind and Devegowda, 2003)

Poor general resistance to disease and increased mortality are also observed among birds fed ochratoxin-contaminated diets. Young chicks in the initial few weeks of age are highly sensitive. Though older birds are less sensitive, laying hens show reduced egg production in a dose-related fashion with characteristic yellow staining of eggshells. Higher levels of ochratoxin A results in poor eggshell quality and higher incidence of eggs with blood and meat spots (Shirley and Tohala, 1983).

Decreased embryo viability, poor hatchability is observed in eggs from hens fed contaminated feed. The chicks from such eggs continue to perform below average in their post-hatch life. Delayed sexual maturity, susceptibility to even low-level exposures is commonly seen in chicks from hens exposed to OTA.

Since the main consumer of poultry product is the human species, it becomes relevant to view the problem of mycotoxin residues in poultry products from a point of human health as well (Table 11).

Table 11: Relevance of naturally occurring mycotoxins as residues in poultry products

Mycotoxin	Poultry Production	Carry over in Meat and Eggs
Aflatoxin B_1	+	Liver
Ochratoxin A	+	Hatching eggs
Cyclopiazonic acid	+	Meat and eggs
Deoxynivalenol	+	Hatching Eggs
Zearalenone	+	Eggs
T-2 toxin	-	-
Diacetoxyscripenol	-	-
Fusarochromanone (Fusarium toxin)	+	Hatching Eggs
Aurofusarin (pigment)	+	Eggs

Turkeys

Higher levels of OTA can have devastating effects on poultry. Table 12 shows the ochratoxicosis data from a turkey farm (Hamilton *et al.,* 1982). The farm lost over 50% of its flock in just 9 days. The level of ochratoxin in the feed was very high and it was reported that the wild birds foraging on the spilt feed on the ground, were dying before flying off the farm.

Table 12: Turkey mortality during an outbreak of ochratoxicosis

Age (Days)	Mortality (Number of Poults)
6	19
7	12
8	57
9	586
10	246
11	983
12	863
13	370
14	547
15	1033
16	826

(Hamilton et al., 1982).

Immune status

Ochratoxin is known to cause regression and cellular depletion (lymphocytes) of major lymphoid organs significantly affecting the cellular immunity in poultry. A lesser secondary suppression of humoral immunity with lower circulating immunoglobulins is observed in ochratoxicosis, as a result of depletion of immune system cells, especially the macrophages.

Significance of the problem

Ochratoxin has been detected in number of foods and feeds in various countries (Van Egmond and Spijers, 1994). A recent large-scale survey, where 1431 samples of wheat, barley, rye, oats and bran were analysed for OTA in Denmark (Hohler, 1999), showed that 40% of the samples were contaminated with OTA. Among the commodities analysed, bran products showed a higher OTA contamination than cereal kernels. For example OTA was detected in wheat in 62% of the bran samples and only 30% of the samples of kernels. These findings are typical for most of the mycotoxins, where cereal byproducts, especially bran, usually show higher mycotoxin levels than the whole cereal.

Residues

Ochratoxin A, cyclopiazonic acid and citrinin bind to plasma-proteins once absorbed, resulting in accumulation and a prolonged residence time in the animal body. Total body clearance varies considerably between species. Even though some E.U. member states specify regulations for ochratoxin levels in meat, it is generally accepted that the exposure of consumers towards OTA, CPA and citrinin originates predominantly from plant-derived foods and only to a relatively smaller percentage from animal derived foods (Veldman, 2003).

5. Citrinin

Citrinin is produced primarily by *Penicillium citrinum* and some species of *Aspergillus*. Citrinin is nephrotoxic and is often seen in combination with ochratoxin in cereals like maize, wheat, barely, oats, rice bran, sunflower and soybean meal. The major effects of citrinin toxicity are increased water consumption and watery diarrhoea (Table 13). Reduced body weight with post mortem lesions like mottled liver and enlarged kidney are the usual findings among the affected birds. Studies till date do not indicate any relation between citrinin and immunity in poultry.

Table 13: Individual and combined effects of ochratoxin and citrinin on water consumption of broiler chickens between 2 and 3 weeks of age.

Ochratoxin (mg/g)	Citrinin (mg/g)	Water Consumed (ml/bird)
0	0	631 ± 26[a]
0	400	2289 ± 53[b]
2.0	0	700 ± 18[a]
2.0	400	1181 ± 66[c]*

[a,b,c] Value within columns, values with different superscripts differ significantly (P < 0.5)

* Value that represent a significant (P < 0.5) interaction

(Manning et al., 1985)

Fusarium Mycotoxins

Fusarium mycotoxins are economically the most significant mycotoxins in foods and feeds on a global scale. Although more than 100 *Fusarium* mycotoxins are known, those mycotoxins of most concern based on their toxicity and occurrence, are trichothecenes (T-2 toxin, diacetoxyscripenol, monoacetoxyscripenol, HT-2 toxin, deoxynivalenol), zearalenone, fumonisins and moniliformin occurring on worldwide basis in cereal grains and poultry feeds (Hussein and Brasel, 2001). Furthermore, the trichothecenes mycotoxins themselves comprise a vast group of over 100 fungal compounds with the same basic structure. In many cases can be found in combination in contaminated feed with additive toxic effects (Raju and Devegowda, 2000 and Swamy *et al.*, 2002).

Trichothecenes [T-2 toxin, Diacetoxyscripenol (DAS), Monoacetoxyscripenol (MAS), HT-2 toxin and Deoxynivalenol (DON)]

Trichothecenes are proven tissue irritants with the major observation associated with their ingestion being oral lesions, dermatitis and intestinal irritation. The major physiological response to trichothecene mycotoxins is the loss of appetite thus earning them the name, “feed refusal toxins”. Swine is a more sensitive species to deoxynivalenol (DON) where as poultry is more sensitive to T-2 toxin and diacetoxyscripenol (DAS). Most trichothecenes cause necrosis and inflammation of the oral cavity (Smith *et al.*, 2001). Helicopter disease is a manifestation of altered feather structure, growth and appearance commonly observed with trichothecene-contaminated feeds in chicken.

Trichothecenes are the second most immunosuppressive mycotoxins next to aflatoxin. They affect primarily the cellular immune response by direct effects on bone marrow; spleen, lymphoid tissues, thymus and intestinal mucosa where actively dividing cells are damaged.

T-2 toxin

The T-2 toxin is a naturally occurring mycotoxin produced by several species of fungi in the genus *Fusarium* that are found in many cereals, cereal byproducts and feeds.

Indicators of T-2 toxicosis

Mouth lesions and associated productive losses caused by T-2 toxin are a major concern to the poultry industry (Wyatt *et al.*, 1975; Raju and Devegowda, 2000). As an indicator of T-2 toxicosis, oral lesions are about four folds more sensitive than growth inhibition. The lesions look like circumscribed proliferate yellow caseous plaques occurring at the margin of the beak, mucosa of the hard palate and the angle between the mouth and the tongue.

Even though the FDA is yet to establish advisory levels for T-2 toxin in poultry feeds, T–2 toxin at concentrations as low as 0.4 mg/kg causes oral lesions by affecting the epithelial cells of oral mucous membrane. T-2 toxin is highly irritant in nature and is known to cause gizzard erosion and necrosis of proventricular mucosa as reported by Brazilian workers (Santin and Fagundes, 2003). Recently it has been observed that T-2 toxin can also cause tibial dyschondroplasia in broiler chicken (Nascimento *et al.*, 2001).

Impact on production performance

The effects of T-2 toxicosis include decreased feed intake, body weight, egg production and poor shell quality, regression of ovaries and increased liver weight in laying hens (Manoj and Devegowda, 2000) (Table 14). Additionally, changes in plasma enzyme profile, loss of body weight and regression of ovary in laying birds are also observed (CAST, 2003). Further T-2 toxin is found to damage ovarian function in geese (Vanyi *et al.*, 1994) with resultant decrease egg production, reduced hatchability and high mortality of goslings and turkey poults (Fazekas *et al.*, 1993). T-2 toxin showed reduced body weight, changes in serum and plasma chemical values and hematological parameters in white Pekin duck broilers (Rafai *et al.*, 2000).

Table 14: Effect of T-2 toxin on laying hen performance.

T-2 toxin ppm	Egg prod.(%)	Egg wt.(gm)	Body wt.(gm)
0.0	96.29^{d}	52.45^{bc}	1331.8^{de}
0.5	93.81^{c}	51.77^{ab}	1312.5^{c}
1.0	91.75^{b}	51.35^{a}	1286.0^{a}
2.0	86.65^{a}	51.33^{a}	1284.9^{a}

$^{a-e}$ *means with differ superscripts are significantly different ($P < 0.05$)*
(Manoj and Devegowda, 2001)

A field case of T-2 toxicosis narrated here may be able to properly depict the adverse effects of T-2 toxins on productivity of poultry. In a flock of laying hens affected with T-2 toxins, the egg production went down by around 22% and the percentage of cracked eggs went up by 12%. The incidence of egg breakages during the transit was as high as 18% with eggs with blood spots moving up from 0 to 3%. Oral lesions were observable in more than 85% of the birds, in effect the farm had to be closed (Hamilton, 1987).

Muscovy ducklings are exceptionally sensitive to the dermatonecrotic effects of T-2 toxin. This extreme sensitivity renders them useful as bioassay animals to detect mycotoxins in contaminated grains. The findings of Shlosberg *et al.*, (1986) were reinforced by the studies made by Salyi and Glavits (1995) on Muscovy ducklings that were fed two levels of T-2 toxins in feed (0.75 and 1.5 mg/kg, respectively) between 4 and 26 days of age (Rafai *et al.*, 2000).

Inclusion of T-2 toxin in quail diet, significantly decreased the concentration of α-tocopherol, carotenoid level and ascorbic acid (Table 15) accumulation in the liver (Dvorska and Surai, 2001).

Table 15: Effect of T-2 toxin on antioxidants in the quail liver, mcg/g

Antioxidant	Control	T-2 toxin
α-tocopherol	18.4 ± 1.33^{a}	10.2 ± 0.96^{b}
Carotenoids	4.3 ± 0.13^{a}	2.7 ± 0.18^{b}
Ascorbic acid	166.4 ± 8.6^{a}	101.1 ± 5.1^{b}

Values within a row bearing superscripts are significantly different ($P < 0.05$).
(Dvorska and Surai, 2001)

Toxicity mechanism

The mechanisms of T-2 toxicity include effects on other metabolic functions of the body. For example, the chemical structure of T-2 toxin makes it fat soluble, which allows it to be incorporated in to cell membranes, potentially changing membrane structural and functional properties. Lipid peroxidation by T-2 toxin in the liver as also been identified as an important underling mechanism of T-2 toxin induced cell injury and DNA damage (Surai, 2002).

Impact of T-2 toxin on immunity

Decreased leucocyte count and regression of the bursa of Fabricius are common immunosuppressive effects associated with T-2 toxicosis. Increasing concentration of T-2 toxin derivatives reduces the macrophage viability (Kidd *et al.*, 1997). With aflatoxin as a co-contaminant, T-2 toxin can form the most immunosuppressive combination of mycotoxins for poultry (Raju and Devegowda, 2002).

Diacetoxyscripenol (DAS) and Monoacetoxyscripenol (MAS)

Diacetoxyscripenol (DAS) and monoacetoxyscripenol (MAS) are naturally occurring mycotoxins produced by several species of fungi in the genus *Fusarium* that are found in many cereals and feeds. Diacetoxyscripenol (DAS) and monoacetoxyscripenol (MAS) have been reported to cause mouth lesions, reduced feed intake and feed refusal in chickens and ducklings (Chi and Mirocha, 1978; Ademoyero and Hamilton, 1989). T-2 toxin and DAS are highly toxic for poultry. The LD_{50} values for DAS, T-2 toxin and HT-2 toxin in day old chicks are 2.0, 5.0 and 7.2 mg/kg, respectively.

Laying hens

Diaz *et al.,* (1994) reported a significant decrease in egg production and feed intake in commercial layers fed a diet containing 2 mg/kg DAS for 24 days. DAS has also been reported to reduce the hatchability of fertile eggs as well as the female related fertility in white leghorn hens (Allen *et al.*, 1982).

Deoxynivalenol (DON, vomitoxin)

Deoxynivalenol is produced by several *Fusarium* species of mold primarily *Fusarium graminearum* and may co-occur with other mycotoxins in contaminated commodities. In Austria maximum permissible level of DON is 1mg/kg in poultry feeds. Poultry birds are relatively more resistant to the effects of deoxynivalenol as compared to pigs and pet animals. However, in field situations the DON level is sometimes associated with reduced feed consumption in layers and broiler breeders. This means that DON may be an indicator that T-2 toxin or other unknown *Fusarium* mycotoxins are present.

Harvey *et al.* (1991) reported a decrease in serum antibody titer to Newcastle virus (NDV) after feeding a DON-contaminated diet (18mg/kg) to growing chickens for 18 weeks. Moreover, a dose-response related decrease in serum NDV-titers of broilers after feeding diets containing no DON, 7.5 mg and 15 mg DON/kg of diet was observed. Such changes in immune response might occur without interfering with performance, but should be viewed as an indication for adverse DON-effects on the health of the birds.

Residues in eggs

Deoxynivalenol is shown to appear in the body fat, muscles and the eggs laid with the egg concentration of deoxynivalenol being maximum between 24-96 hours of feeding on contaminated feed. Notably, only about 10% of the deoxynivalenol present in egg yolk can be detected thereby indicating a false low value of residues in eggs.

Fusaric acid

Fusaric acid is primarily produced by *Fusarium Moniliforme*. Despite its wide occurrence and possible interactions with trichothecenes, fusaric acid has not been analyzed in experimental diets involving contaminated grains or culture materials. The lack of information on the dietary fusaric acid content might explain the contradicting results observed in the earlier studies involving vomitoxin. Recent trials (Swamy *et al.,* 2002) have indicated that broiler chickens were susceptible when naturally contaminated grains were fed containing a combination of mycotoxins (DON and fusaric acid).

An increasing in redness of breast meat was observed in broiler chickens (Smith *et al.*, 2001) and in turkey poults fed *Fusarium* culture material (Wu *et al.,* 1994). The discoloration may be due to the effect of fusaric acid, which acts as a hypotensive agent. It was concluded that *Fusarium* mycotoxicosis could be observed in poultry with the feeding of naturally contaminated grains.

Fumonisins

The Fumonisins are relatively recently discovered group of mycotoxins, primarily produced by *Fusarium verticillioides* (*moniliforme*) and *Fusarium proliferatum.* The most toxic of this group is fumonisin B_1 (FB_1). Fumonisins are found in a wide range of commodities from millets to grains to banana fruits and are a major concern to food and feed producers since they directly affect both human and poultry health. Fumonisins are found worldwide, covering tropical, sub-tropical and temperate regions and also they have been found to co-occur in contaminated commodities with many other mycotoxins including aflatoxin, deoxynivalenol, zearalenone and ochratoxin. High incidence of human esophageal cancer observed in some countries (South Africa, China etc.) has been attributed to chronic exposure to high level of fumonisins (Smith *et al.,* 2001).

Increased liver sphinganine:sphingosine (SA:SO) ratios (Table 16), an early biomarker for fumonisin toxicosis, was observed in both broilers and turkeys fed diets that supplied 25 and 50 mg FB1/kg (Broomhead *et al .,* 1998).

Table 16: Effects of FB_1 on liver SA:SO ratio of broiler chicks and poultry poults

FB_1 (mg /Kg) diet	**SA:SO**	
	Broiler	**Turkey**
0	0.15^b	0.18^c
25	0.52^a	0.62^b
50	0.59^a	1.21^a

^{abc} values for variables within columns differ significantly.($P < 0.05$)
(Broomhead *et al.*, 1998)

Spiking mortality

"Spiking mortality or toxic feed syndrome" in poultry has been attributed to fumonisin toxicity. The symptoms of spiking mortality include paralysis, extended legs and neck, wobbly gait, gasping and poor growth.

Broilers and turkeys are relatively resistant to the acute toxic effects of FB1. In broiler chicks fed high levels of FB1, acute toxic effects included poor performance, increased organ weights, and multi focal hepatic necrosis. In turkey poults fed high levels of FB1, acute toxic effects include poor performance, increased organ weights, and hepatocellular hyperplasia (Weibking *et al.*, 1994).

Experiments with turkey poults using culture material with fumonisin B1 concentrations of 100 or 200 mg/kg gave results similar to those for broiler chicks. Turkey poults feed a diet with 200 mg/kg of fumonisin B1 were 25% less efficient than the controls (Ledoux *et al.*, 1992).

In field conditions fumonisin B1 at 20 mg/kg or more in diets is associated with elevated 10 and 30-day mortality, as well as feed refusal in commercial broiler flocks. In another experiment, birds fed the fumonisin toxin for four weeks responded much more poorly to an inactivated Newcastle vaccine. Investigation of the effects of fumonisin in poultry has been limited to the use of culture material contaminated with fumonisin, where the contaminated material was incorporated into the diet. Experiments with *F. moniliforme* (*verticillioides*) contaminated culture material can lead to confusing results and erroneous conclusions due to the high probability of other toxic metabolites being present in the contaminated material. Nevertheless, such recent experiments indicate that feed contaminated with fumonisin-producing fungi can cause some adverse responses in poultry (Ledoux *et al.*, 1992).

Residues

Due to poor absorption and rapid excretion following metabolism, fumonisin residues are of no major public health significance. Though well absorbed, trichothecenes are rapidly metabolized and excreted without considerable accumulation in animal tissues and thus a trichothecenes residue in animal origin foods is of no public health significance.

Moniliformin

Moniliformin is a mycotoxin produced by several *Fusarium* species including *Fusarium proliferatum*. Moniliformin is highly toxic to chicks with reported lethal dose of 4mg/kg body weight in day-old chicks. Exposure to moniliformin ranging from 144-575 mg/kg feed can lead to very high mortality rates of 80-100% in chicks, poults and ducklings (Engelhardt *et al.*, 1989). Cardiac injury and alterations in cardiac electrical conductance are shown to cause the mortality in affected birds (Nagaraj *et al.*, 1996). Even low levels of moniliformin can cause poor growth performance, increased serum pyruvate levels, enlarged hearts and cardiac lesions (Ledoux *et al.*, 1993), and poor immune response (Li *et al.*, 2000).

Fusarochromanone

Fusarochromanone, produced by *Fusarium equiseti,* is a mycotoxin associated with tibial dyschondroplasia of growing broiler chicks and turkeys. Auburn University (U.S.) publications indicate fusarochromanone to be the most likely cause of tibial dyschondroplacia. At 75mg/kg dietary level, fusarochromanones can cause tibial dyschodroplacia in 100% of the chicks exposed to contaminated feed. In breeder hens, fusarochromanone is transferred into eggs resulting in increased incidence of embryonic mortality with fertilized eggs.

Zearalenone

Zearalenone is produced primarily by *Fusarium graminearum* and *Fusarium roseum.* Zearalenone is responsible for reproductive disorders due to its estrogenic effect at high concentrations.Poultry are relatively more resistant to the effects of zearalenone as compared to pigs and cattle. At high dietary concentrations, however, vent enlargement and enhanced secondary sex characteristics are seen in turkeys and chickens.

Zearalenone, which often co-occurs with deoxynivalenol in naturally contaminated cereals, is even less toxic to laying hens than deoxynivalenol. Allen *et al.* (1981) did not find any detrimental effects of increasing dietary zearalenone-concentration up to 800 mg/kg of diet on laying performance or on productive performance, including growth of progeny. However, the feeding of zearalenone-contaminated feed to laying hens might cause residues of the toxin into egg yolk as indicated by an experiment by Dailey *et al.* (1980), who found radioactivity in egg yolks after an oral bolus of ^{14}C-labeled zearalenone. This could be important to human health because of the estrogenic and genotoxic properties of zearalenone. Moreover, a possible carryover of deoxynivalenol and zearalenone to eggs could adversely affect reproductive performance of hens as indicated by the investigations of Bergsj *et al.* (1993), who reported an increased incidence of chick developmental anomalies when hens were fed these mycotoxins.

Aurofusarin

Aurofusarin, a metabolite of *Fusarium graminearum* was first described in 1968, but only recently identified in feed ingredients in Ukraine, in particular in contaminated grains (Kotyk and Trufanova, 1998) to be characterized as a new crop contaminant. In particular this mycotoxin was shown to have a profound effect on egg quality with no clinical signs of toxicosis. On the other hand aurofusarin compromised the immune system of laying chickens (Sakhatsky, 1999) and quail and decreased fertility and hatchability of their eggs. On the biochemical level aurofusarin was responsible for significant changes in fatty acid and antioxidant profiles of quail eggs. Further more the antioxidant system of developing quail embryo was shown to be compromised as a result of aurofusarin inclusion in the maternal diet.

Aurofusarin pigment is transferred from feed to egg yolk, and due to its pH-dependent color change, can cause color change from yellow via red and pink to violet (Dvorska and Surai, 2003). Aurofusarin consumption is also associated with deterioration of chicken meat quality.

The LD_{50} values of some Mycotoxins for poultry

The LD_{50} values of some of the mycotoxins for poultry are presented in table 17. At much lower levels, and in combination, mycotoxins can cause significant damage to poultry in terms of health, productivity and economics.

Table 17: The LD_{50} values of some mycotoxins

Mycotoxins	LD_{50}[1] (μg/kg)
Aflatoxin	6.5
Ochratoxin	3.6
T-2 toxin	4.9 – 5.2
Moniliformin	5.4
DAS[2]	3.8 – 5.9
Citrinin	95
DON[3]	140
Fumonisin B_1	300*
CPA[4]	100

[1] LD_{50} = Dose in mg of aflatoxin per kg of body weight at which 50% of the test animals die.

[2] DAS = Diacetoxyscripenol, [3] DON = Deoxynivalenol, [4] CPA= Cyclopiazonic acid.

* Not LD_{50}. Fed this concentration had severe growth depression (Reduced body weight gain by 19% and increased liver weight by 30%)

Co-contamination of feeds by mycotoxins in poultry

More than single mycotoxins may simultaneously contaminate feed ingredient and finished feeds. The toxicity and clinical signs observed in poultry when more than one mycotoxin is present in feed are complex and diverse. Co-contamination of mycotoxins appears to exert greater negative impact on the health and productivity of poultry in comparison to their individual effect. Symptoms typical of mycotoxicosis are often seen in poultry despite analysis of the feed that indicates only very low concentration of mycotoxins. Toxicity may be due to toxicological interactions between different mycotoxins that exaggerate the toxicity.

The Brazilian workers Santin and Fagundes, 2003, demonstrated the symptoms and economical losses caused by combination of the mycotoxins to the professionals of different Brazilian poultry companies. They observed that the birds fed damaged corn, estimated to contain 15.3 of mcg/kg aflatoxin B_1, 11.6 mcg/kg of ochratoxin A, 1200 mcg/kg of zearalenone and 177 mcg/kg of T-2 toxin showed higher incidence of breast and thigh hemorrhage, liver steatosis and gizzard erosions in broilers.

In a survey on sunflower oil cake in India, 8% of the samples were found to contain T-2 toxin and ochratoxin simultaneously (Chandrasekaran, 1996). Similarly Ravindran *et al.*, 1996, reported co-occurrence of aflatoxin, fumonisin and zearalenone in Australian maize.Over several years considerable amount of research has been conducted into the co-occurrence of mycotoxin in feeds. Mycotoxin co-contamination can occur in many combinations, some of which are listed below. Co-contamination is a natural phenomenon, persistent in most cases than we can imagine, since the fungi that produce mycotoxins do not exist in nature as pure cultures.

Co-contamination of mycotoxins in Poultry

- Aflatoxins and Ochratoxin
- Aflatoxins and T-2 toxin
- T-2 toxin and Diacetoxyscripenol
- Ochratoxin and Citrinin
- Vomitoxin and Fusaric acid

(Devegowda et al., 2003)

The microenvironment of feed is very complex and consists of many types of fungi, all competing for the available nutrients. A feed sample positive for a particular mycotoxin not only confirms the presence of that mycotoxin, but also signifies the fact that, at a point of time, that crop or that harvest lot was under conditions favoring the growth of fungi and toxin production by them. At such an interval, it becomes pertinent to check that sample for the presence of other mycotoxins as well, recent findings strongly support of this line of thought. The mycotoxin interactions scientifically examined are presented in Table 18.

Table 18: Impact of co-contamination by mycotoxins in poultry

Mycotoxins	Species tested	Production effects	References
Aflatoxin & Ochratoxin	Broiler chicks	Synergism	Huff et al., 1992
Aflatoxin & Diacetoxy-scripenol	Broiler chicks	Synergism	Kubena et al., 1993
Aflatoxin & Deoxyniva-lenol	Broiler chicks	Additive	Huff et al., 1986
Aflatoxin & T-2 toxin	Broiler chicks	Synergism	Aravind et al., 2003, Girish & Devegowda, 2004b
Aflatoxin & Ochratoxin	Broiler chicks	Synergism	Kubena et al., 1989, Raju & Devegowda, 2000
Ochratoxin & T-2 toxin	Broiler chicks	Synergism	Raju & Devegowda, 2000
Deoxynivalenol & Monili-formin	Turkey Poults	Moniliformin effect only	Morris et al., 1999
Deoxynivalenol & Fusaric acid	Broiler chicks	Synergism	Smith et al., 2000, Swamy et al., 2002
Fumonisin B_1 & Monili-formin	Turkey Poults	Moniliformin effect only	Li et al., 2000
Fumonisin B_1 & T-2 toxin	Turkey Poults	Additive	Kubena et al., 1995
Fumonisin B_1 & Diacetox-yscripenol	Turkey Poults	Additive	Kubena et al., 1997
Ochratoxin & Citrinin	Broiler chicks	Antagonism	Manning et al., 1985

Aflatoxins vs. Ochratoxin

Both aflatoxin and ochratoxin are extremely toxic to poultry and they interact synergistically (Campbell *et al.*, 1983 and Raju and Devegowda, 2000). The toxicity resulting from dual exposure to aflatoxin and ochratoxin is much greater than the sum of the individual toxicities of these mycotoxins (Table 19). This may be one reason why very low levels of aflatoxin in the field sometimes produce significant effects in poultry compared to laboratory studies where only aflatoxin is evaluated. The symptoms of this co-mycotoxicosis in poultry are totally different than those observed with only aflatoxin. Ochratoxin, when in combination with aflatoxin, suppresses the symptomatic manifestation of aflatoxin mediated liver damage, fatty, yellow, enlarged, and friable liver making the diagnosis of aflatoxicosis difficult (Huff and Doerr, 1981) (Table 20). The target organ of the interaction between aflatoxin and ochratoxin in poultry appears to be the kidney.

Table 19: Effect of dietary aflatoxin and ochratoxin A on body weight of three week old broiler chickens

Aflatoxin (µg toxin/g diet)	Ochratoxin (µg toxin/g diet)	Body weight (g)
0	0	625.8 ± 9.7[1]
0	2.0	549.1 ± 11.7[2]
2.5	0	551.1 ± 10.7[2]
2.5	2.0	380.4 ± 5.5[3*]

[1-2-3] within columns, values without a common superscripts number differ ($P < 0.05$).

*Values that represent a significant ($P < 0.05$) interaction between aflatoxin and ochratoxin A.

(Huff and Doerr, 1981)

Table 20: The individual and combined effects of dietary aflatoxin and ochratoxin A on liver lipid of broiler chickens.

Aflatoxin (µg toxin/g diet)	Ochratoxin (µg toxin/g diet)	Liver lipid (% dry wt)
0	0	16.49 ± .51[1]
0	2.0	14.59 ± .20[1]
2.5	0	24.48 ± 1.58[2]
2.5	2.0	17.25 ± .53[1*]

[1-2] Within columns, values without a common superscripts number differ ($P < 0.05$).

Values represent the mean + SEM of six groups of 10 birds.

* Values that represent a significant ($P < 0.05$) interaction between aflatoxin and ochratoxin A.

(Huff and Doerr, 1981)

Aflatoxins vs. T-2 toxin

Both aflatoxins and T-2 toxin are important to the poultry industry because of their toxicity and co-occurrence in feeds. These two mycotoxins have been found to co-contaminate grain samples and causing significant synergistic interaction on body weight, relative organ weights and antibody titers in broiler chickens (Huff *et al.*, 1988; Raju and Devegowda, 2002; Girish and Devegowda 2004b).

T-2 toxin and Diacetoxyscripenol

The co-occurrence of T-2 and DAS was reported in mixed diet and grains with concentrations ranging from 0.2 to 5.8 mg/kg for T-2 toxin and 0.5 to 2.1 mg/kg for DAS. A survey in Canada showed concentration of 0.11 –2.27 mg/kg DAS occurring in less than 10% of grains samples analysed, while T-2 toxin concentration ranged from 0.16 to 0.31 mg/kg in the same samples (Stratton *et al.*, 1993). T-2 and DAS are more toxic than aflatoxin and comparable in toxicity to ochratoxin in chickens (Huff *et al.*, 1974). Additive lethal toxicity has been reported in chickens given DAS and T-2 toxin in combination (Hoerr *et al.,* 1981). The effects of T-2 and DAS were additive in laying hens for feed intake, oral lesions, mild changes in plasma enzyme activities and reduced egg production (Diaz *et al.,* 1994) and in broilers for body weight gain and feed intake (Hoerr *et al.,* 1981).

Ochratoxin vs. Citrinin

Citrinin is a nephrotoxin similar to ochratoxin and some of the fungi that produce ochratoxin also produce citrinin. This is an important mycotoxin interaction to understand since it is very likely that when one is present the other mycotoxin will, in all probability, be present. The interaction between these two mycotoxins can be characterized as antagonistic. The toxicity that results when these two mycotoxins are present in feeds is much less than the sum of the toxicity of these two individual mycotoxins. It is essential at this point to note that even though the interaction is antagonistic, the birds have much lower performance in the presence of the two toxins as compared to the exposure to a single toxin. One of the symptoms of citrinin toxicity in poultry is a dramatic increase in the amount of water consumed and excreted by these birds, which is of a significant diagnostic value in identifying the condition. However, ochratoxin prevents this very important diagnostic index of citrinin, making the diagnosis in case of co-contamination difficult.

Deoxynivalenol and Fusaric acid

The feeding of the contaminated grains (DON and fusaric acid mainly) synergistically depressed broiler growth rate and feed intake. There was significant increase in the breast meat colour. In laying hens the feeding of the contaminated grains resulted in significant reduction in feed consumption, egg production and alleviated blood uric concentration (Smith *et al.,* 2003).

Safe/permissible level of mycotoxins in poultry feeds

What is a safe level? What level do you recommend? If I cannot feed it to poultry, can I feed it to cattle? Can I blend it with good quality feed? How much loss will be there by feeding such type of feed? These are some of the questions commonly asked by all those people involved in poultry and livestock farming (Hamilton, North Carolina State University).Strictly speaking there is no *safe level.* With reference to mycotoxins the risk directly depends on the level of the major mycotoxins and also on the presence and levels of other mycotoxins in feeds. A mycotoxin level considered safe in one farm may not be safe in another farm because of differences in management and disease prevalence. Additionally, factors like interaction of mycotoxins with pathogens, genetic variability, environmental conditions (high temperature, humidity, ammonia etc.) sex difference and nutritional status etc., influence the severity of the manifestation of mycotoxicosis.

In order to reduce the toxic and economical impact of mycotoxins, several countries regulate the levels of some mycotoxins in foods and feeds. Worldwide food and feed legislation safeguards the health of consumers and the economic interests of animal producers and traders. Virtually all countries with fully developed market economies have regulations with the exception of some African countries.

Control of the adverse effects of mycotoxins

Mycotoxins are produced at only certain stages of mold growth. Mycotoxin molecules are generally quite resistant to chemical or thermal treatments capable of destroying mold spores. The presence or absence of visible mold spores, therefore, does not always serve as a reliable guide to presence or otherwise of toxins and their levels.

Practical mycotoxin control involves two main stages: prevention of fungal growth and toxin production in feedstuffs, and decontamination of existing mycotoxins in feeds. Several strategies, to be adopted in a coordinated manner, have been proposed to reduce the impact of mycotoxins, which include: plant breeding for mold resistance, efficient harvesting and storage practices to minimize contamination and decontamination process for the contaminated commodities (Devegowda and Aravind, 2002)

The most effective method of neutralizing mycotoxins that are already present in feed is by binding them to an inert compound before they can be absorbed from the intestine. The question that feed manufacturers, livestock and poultry producers are asking is: "which mycotoxin binder is most effective?" The "ideal" features of good mycotoxin binder are:

- Ability to bind a wide range of mycotoxins
- Low effective inclusion rate in feed
- Rapid and uniform dispersion in the feed during mixing
- Heat stability during pelleting, extrusion, and during storage
- No affinity for vitamins, minerals or other nutrients
- High stability over a wide pH range and
- Bio-degradability after excretion

1. Nutritional modifications

Nutritional approaches for protection against mycotoxins include methionine, selenium and vitamin supplementation of affected diets and some plant and herbal compounds including chlorophyll derivatives, aspartame etc. Mycotoxins, upon being absorbed, get detoxified in liver-utilizing glutathione (selenium containing compound), which is composed of cystine (derivative of methionine). Hence the metabolic level of methionine is depleted, leading to poor growth and feed efficiency. Higher levels of methionine, selenium and vitamins supplementation in feed, therefore, have been found to be beneficial.

2. Herbal mold inhibitors

Certain herbs and herbal extracts exert inhibitory effect on mold growth and toxin production. Aqueous extracts of garlic, onion, turmeric, neem etc., are shown to exert anti fungal activity and/or inhibit aflatoxin production. Though beneficial to some extent, standardization and practical implementation of this method is not easy and a lot of research work is required in this direction.

3. Chemical detoxification

Among the chemicals tested for their ability to detoxify/inactivate mycotoxins ammonia, sodium bisulfite, peroxide acids, bases and gases are most effective. However, most of the chemical methods are impractical and do not generally comply with the requirements of the ideal detoxifying agent, especially the safety of reaction products and the palatability of the feed.

4. Application of mineral clays

Many clays have been tested for counteracting mycotoxins, and among the successful, very few are used commercially. These include bentonites, zeolites and aluminosilicates. Several studies have demonstrated that sodium aluminosilicate, sodium calcium aluminosilicate, and sodium bentonites can adsorb aflatoxins (Phillips *et al.*, 1988 Doerr, 1989; Kubena *et al.*, 1990; Araba and Wyatt, 1991; Schiedeler, 1993; Santurio *et al.*, 1994 and Mahesh and Devegowda, 1996). The chemisorption of aflatoxin to HSCAS involves the formation of complex by the Beta-keto-lactone or bilactone system of aflatoxin with uncoordinated metal ions in HSCAS (Phillips *et al.*, 1990). The degree of adsorption depends on chemical structure of the clay material with the adsorption capacities varying between 0% to 87% with various mineral clay materials (Schiedeler, 1993; Santurio *et al.*, 1994).

The high inclusion rates and narrow range of binding efficacy are the main disadvantages of the mineral clays. They are mainly effective against aflatoxins

(Kubena *et al.,* 1990; Huff *et al.,* 1992; Ledoux *et al.*, 1999 and Girish and Devegowda 2004a) and appear to have little or no beneficial effect against:

- Zearalenone (Volkl and Karlovsky, 1998)
- T-2 Toxin (Dvorska and Surai 2001, Girish and Devegowda 2004a)
- Ochratoxin (Santin *et al.*, 2002)
- Diacetoxyscirpenol-DAS (Kubena *et al.*, 1993)
- Fescue Toxin (Chestnut *et al.,* 1992).

Despite being shown that the clays do not adsorb several mycotoxins *in vitro* or *in vivo*, the poultry industry has used aluminosilicates to control mycotoxicosis for quite long time because of an impression that the altered chemical structure of some aluminosilicates might be able to adsorb other mycotoxins than aflatoxin. Further, it is demonstrated that the mineral clays reduce the utilization of minerals like Manganese, Zinc and Magnesium (Chestnut *et al.*, 1992), Chloride (Schiedeler, 1993), Copper and Sodium (Kramer, 1993), which suggests that the use of mineral clays may not be wise at all.

5. Natural and organic binder

In the early 1990s, commercially yeast culture preparation of *Saccharomyces cerevisiae*[1026], which was earlier noted as a nutritional aid and a growth promoter, was found to improve hatchability (McDaniel, 1991) and broiler body weights (Stanley *et al.*, 1993). Further investigations lead to the establishment of yeast culture preparation's ability to bind aflatoxins in poultry feeds (Devegowda *et al.*, 1994 & 1995).

This work was a landmark that signaled the beginning of a set of new strategies that use yeast-derived products to overcome problems associated with mycotoxin-contaminated feeds. Several researchers confirmatively proved that the modified glucomannan, a derivative of the yeast cell wall, is able to bind higher levels of several important mycotoxins at a lower inclusion rates as compared to the limited narrow range binding abilities of inorganic binders (Mahesh and Devegowda, 1996; Volkl and Karlovsky, 1998; Trenholm *et al.*, 1996; Dawson *et al.*, 2001). Some interesting recent research findings are listed below:

Modified glucomannan supplementation is beneficial in reducing the individual and combined adverse effects of aflatoxin, ochratoxin and T-2 toxin in broilers Apart from improving the body weights and antibody titres suppressed by combined dietary mycotoxins, modified glucomannan also improves serum biochemical and hematological parameters (Raju and Devegowda, 2000).

In broiler chicken fed feeds naturally contaminated with different mycotoxins supplementation of modified glucomannan improves the performance (Smith *et al.*, 2001; Swamy *et al.*, 2002; Aravind *et al.*, 2003).

Feed containing wheat and barley contaminated with T-2 and DON reduced the body weight gains by 5.8%. The addition of modified glucomannan completely protected the broilers from the performance depressing effects of the mycotoxins (Smith *et al.*, 2001).

Modified glucomannan can effectively counteract dietary diacetoxyscirpenol (DAS) in broiler chickens Addition of modified glucomannan reverses the toxic effects of DAS on body weight gain of broilers (Pavicic *et.al.*, 2001) (Table 21).

Table 21: Modified glucomannan and diacetoxyscripenol (DAS) in broiler chicken

Diacetoxyscripenol (mg/kg)	Modified glucomannan (%)	Body weight (gm)
0	0	1681
1	0	1374
0	0.1	1794
1	0.1	1678

(Pavicic et al., 2001)

Modified glucomannan is also proven to be beneficial against the sorghum ergot alkaloid (SEA) on poultry performance and has shown to improve the body weights suppressed by dietary SEA (Deo *et al.*, 1999).

Murthy and Devegowda (2004) demonstrated the rapid absorption of aflatoxin and T-2 toxin (Reddy and Devegowda, 2004) by modified glucomannan in a biological system at different time intervals after ingestion of feed in broiler chickens. They clearly showed the ability of modified glucomannan to rapidly adsorb mycotoxins within 30 minutes of feeding.

Feeding broilers with diets containing aflatoxin (2 mg/kg) and T-2 toxin (1 mg/kg), significantly reduced feed intake, weight gain and feed efficiency, weights of thymus and bursa of Fabricius, antibody titers against Newcastle disease and infectious bursal disease. Modified glucomannan (1kg/ton feed) significantly improved body weight, feed intake, antibody titers, weights of thymus and bursa of Fabricius suggesting action against both aflatoxin and T-2 toxin. Hydrated sodium calcium aluminosilicate (10 kg/ton of feed) showed improvement against AF without much protection against T-2 toxin (Girish and Devegowda 2004b). With dietary treatments of four concentrations of T-2 toxin (0, 0.5, 1.0, and 2.0 mg/kg) and two concentrations (0 and 0.1%) of modified glucomannan.

Manoj and Devegowda (2001) observed that modified glucomannan reversed the suppression of egg production by T-2 toxin on egg production. Even at the highest concentration of T-2 toxin (2 mg/kg) wherein egg production was reduced to less than 90% of the control, modified glucomannan-restored production to more than 95% of the control.

Ducklings are the most susceptible species to aflatoxins with very high mortality rate and suppression of serum total protein, serum albumin and relative bursal weights. Biological trials with supplementation of modified glucomannan to aflatoxin containing diets can very effectively reduce the aflatoxin induced mortality as well as significantly improve other parameters comparable to that of normal ducklings (Devegowda *et al.*, 1994) (Table 22).

Table 22: Effect of Yea-Sacc[1026] on weight of bursa of Fabricius, total serum protein and albumin in ducklings fed diets containing aflatoxin. *

Parameters	**Control**	**100 µg/kg aflatoxin**		**200 µg/kg aflatoxin**	
		Yea-Sacc[1026] %			
		0	**0.1**	**0**	**0.1**
Bursal weight, g / 100g BW	0.25[c]	0.19[b]	0.24[c]	0.11[a]	0.23[c]
Total protein, g / dl	1.94[d]	1.11[b]	1.92[d]	0.81[a]	1.81[c]
Albumin, g / dl	0.49[c]	0.37[b]	0.51[d]	0.29[a]	0.47[c]

[ab] ($P < 0.05$)

(Devegowda et al., 1994)

In ducklings, modified glucomannan supplementation can reverse the growth suppression induced by dietary aflatoxin modified glucomannan inclusion can also improve feather score, incidence of leg deformity, and web toe hemorrhage scores which are adversely affected by higher levels of dietary aflatoxin (Khajarern and Khajarern, 1999).

T-2 toxin is known to decrease the levels of innate anti-oxidants in birds and increase the lipid peroxidation in liver. Recent studies have revealed that modified glucomannan supplementation helps maintain the levels of systemic antioxidants and prevents hepatic lipid peroxidation in growing quails while zeolite supplementation may not be beneficial (Dvorska and Surai, 2001).

Conclusions

Under practical conditions, no poultry feed is virtually free from mycotoxins. Additionally, no feed can be expected to contain only one mycotoxin. The adverse effects of mycotoxins on poultry are manifold indicating a clear and persistent danger.

A strong recommendation is made hereby to view the problem in its natural way i.e., co-contamination of feeds and feedstuffs by mycotoxins, rather than a narrow approach of dealing with one mycotoxin at a time. It is therefore essential to take all the necessary precautions:

- Prevention of fungal growth on crops in the field, at harvest of crop, during storage of feedstuffs and processing of feed.
- Time to act is not after the birds are affected, but before the contaminated feed is consumed.
- Application of appropriate mycotoxin binder (which is safe to the birds, to the environment and to the consumers) in order to achieve good productivity and economy.

References

Ademoyero, A. A. and Hamilton, P. B. 1989. Research note: Influence of degree of acetylation of scirpenol mycotoxins on feed refusal by chickens. Poultry Science, 68: 854-856.

Afzali, N. and Devegowda, G. 1999. Ability of modified mannanoligosaccharide to counteract aflatoxicosis in broiler breeder hens. Poultry Science, 78 (Suppl. 1): 228. (Abstr.)

Allen, N. K., Jevne, R. L., Mirocha, C. J. and Lee, Y. W. 1982. The effect of Fusarium roseum culture and diacetoxyscripenol on reproduction of white leghorn females. Poultry Science, 61: 2172-2175.

Allen, N. K., Mirocha, C. J., Aakhus-Allen, S., Bitgood, J. J., Weaver, G. and Bates, F. 1981. Effect of dietary zearalenone on reproduction of chickens. Poultry Science, 60: 1165-1174.

Araba, M. and Wyatt, T. D. 1991. Effects of sodium bentonite, hydrated sodium calcium aluminosilicate (Novasil) and ethical on aflatoxicosis in broiler chickens. Poultry Science, 70: S6. (Abstr.)

Aravind, K. L., Patil, V. S., Devegowda, G., Umakantha, B. and Ganpule, S. P. 2003. Efficacy of modified glucomannan to counteract mycotoxicosis in naturally contaminated feed on performance, serum biochemical and hematological parameters in broilers. Poultry Science, 82: 570-576.

Aravind. K. L. and Devegowda, G. 2003. Use of glucomannan to reduce the effects of ochratoxin A in broilers. In: Proc. of Second World Mycotoxin Forum, The Netherlands. pp : 122.

Bauer, J. 1998. Krankheit and Leistungsdeppression in der schweine haltung durch Mycotoxine. Tierarstliche Praxis Suppl. 3: 40-47

Bergsj, B., Herstad, O. and Nafstad, I. 1993. Effects of feeding deoxynivalenol-contaminated oats on reproduction performance in white leghorn hens. British Poultry Science, 34: 147 – 159.

Broomhead, J. N., Ledoux, D. R., Bermudez, A. J. and Rottinghaus, G. E. 1998. Effects of Fumonisin B_1 in broilers and turkeys fed dietary treatments to market age. UMC Animal Sciences Departmental Report. 107 – 110.

Bryden, W. L. 1991. Occurrence and biological effects of cyclopiazonic acid. In K. Mixe and J. L. Richard (Eds.). Emerging Problem Resulting from Microbial Contamination. National Institute of Hygienic Science, Tokyo, Pp. 127–147.

Campbell, M. L., May, J. D., Huff, W.E. and Doerr, J. A. 1983. Evaluation of immunity of young broiler chickens during simultaneous aflatoxicosis and ochratoxicosis. Poultry Science, 62: 2138-2144.

Chandrasekaran, D. 1996. Survey on the presence of T-2 toxin and ochratoxin in feed/ingredients in Namakkal area. In: Proc. 20th World's Poultry Congress, New Delhi, India 4:268.

Chestnut, A.B., Anderson, P. D., Cochran, M. A., Fribourg, H. A. and Twinn, K. D. 1992. Effects of hydrated sodium calcium aluminosilicate on fescue toxicosis and mineral absorption. Journal of Animal Science, 70: 2838-2846

Chi, M. S. and Mirocha, C. J. 1978. Necrotic oral lesions in chickens fed diacetoxyscripenol, T-2 toxin and crocotin. Poultry Science, 57: 807 – 808.

Cole, R. J. 1986. Etiology of turkey "X" disease in retrospect: A case for the involvement of cyclopiazonic acid. Mycotoxin Research, 2: 3 – 7.

Council for Agricultural Science and Technology (CAST). 2003. Mycotoxins: Risks in Plant, Animal, and Human Systems. Ames, Iowa, USA.

Dailey, R. E., Reese, R. E. and Brouwer, E. A. 1980. Metabolism of ^{14}C zearalenone in laying hens. Journal of Agriculture and Food Chemistry, 28: 286-291.

Dawson, K. A., Evans, J.and Manoj, K. 2001. Understanding the absorption characteristics of yeast cell wall preparations associated with mycotoxin binding. In: Biotechnology in the Feed Industry: Proceedings of Alltech's 17th Annual Symposium (T. P. Lyons and K.A. Jacques, eds). Nottingham University Press, Nottingham. pp. 169-181.

Deo. P., Blaney, B. J. and Dingle, J. G. 1999. Effects of mineral and organic adsorbents in meat chicken diets contaminated with sorghum ergot alkaloid. In: Proceedings of Queensland Poultry Science Symposium, 8.

Devegowda, G. 2001. Mycotoxins: Economic risks and their control. In: Handbook of Poultry Nutrition. (Eds. V. Ramasubba Reddy and Dinesh T. Bhosale) Published by American Soybean Association, pp. 246-260.

Devegowda, G. 2002. Mycotoxins: A worldwide threat. Feeding times .Vol 7: pp. 2-3.

Devegowda, G. and Aravind, K. L. 2002. Global mycotoxins problem: Biological solutions. In: proc.150th year celebration, Institute Superior de Agronomia., Lisbon, Portugal. pp. 30-45.

Devegowda, G., Aravind, B. I. R., Morton, M.G. and Rajendra, K. 1995. A biotechnological approach to counteract aflatoxicosis in broiler chickens and ducklings by the use of Saccharomyces cerevisiae. In: Proc. Feed Ingredients Asia '95, Singapore. pp, 161-171.

Devegowda, G., Aravind, K. L., Murthy, T. N. K. and Reddy, B. N. 2003. Mycotoxins: Economic risk and control-The biological solutions. In: 3rd International poultry show and seminar, World's Poultry Science Association, Bangladesh. pp. 94-98.

Devegowda, G., Arvind, B. I. R., Rajendra, K., Morton, M. G., Baburathna, A. and Sudarshan, C. 1994. A biological approach to counteract aflatoxicosis in broiler chickens and ducklings by the use of Saccharomyces cerevisiae cultures added to feed. In: Biotechnology in the Feed Industry: Proceedings of Alltech's 10th Annual Symposium (T. P. Lyons and K.A. Jacques, eds). Nottingham University Press, Nottingham. pp. 235-245.

Devegowda, G., Raju, M. V. L., Afzali, N.and Swamy, H. V. L. N. 1998a. Mycotoxin picture worldwide: Novel solutions for their counteraction. Feed Compounder, 18 (6): 22-27.

Devegowda, G., Raju, M.V.L.N. and Swamy, H.V.L.N. 1998c. Mycotoxins: Novel solutions for their counteraction. Feedstuffs, 70 (50): 12-17.

Devegowda, G., Raju, M.V.L.N., Afzali, N. and Swamy, H.V.L.N. 1998b. Mycotoxin picture worldwide: Novel solutions for their counteraction. In: Biotechnology in the Feed Industry: Proceedings of Alltech's 14th Annual Symposium (T. P. Lyons and K.A. Jacques, eds). Nottingham University Press, Nottingham, pp 241-255.

Diaz, G. J., Squires, E. J., Julian, R. J. and Boermans, H. J. 1994. Individual and combined effects of T-2 toxin and DAS in laying hens. British Poultry Science, 35: 393-405.

Doerr, J. A. 1989. Effect of an aluminosilicate on broiler chickens during aflatoxicosis, Poultry Science, 68: S 45. (Abstr.)

Dorner, J. W., Cole, R. J., Erlington, D. J., Susksupath, S., McDowell, G. H. and Bryden, W. L. 1994. Cyclopiazonic acid residues in milk and eggs. Journal of Agriculture and Food Chemistry, 42: 1516 – 1518.

Dvorska, J. E. and Surai, P. F. 2003. Aurofusarin, a Fusarium graminearum pigment: oxidative stress and protective effect of modified glucomannan. In: Biotechnology in the Feed Industry: Proceedings of Alltech's 19th Annual Symposium (T. P. Lyons and K.A. Jacques, eds). Nottingham University Press, Nottingham. pp. 27-32.

Dvorska, J.E. and Surai, P. F. 2001. Effect of T-2 toxin, zeolite and mycosorb on antioxidant systems of growing quail. Asian – Australian Journal of Animal Science, 14: 1752-1757.

Engelhardt, J. A., Carton, W. W. and Tuite, J. f. 1989. Toxicity of Fusarium moniliforme var. subglutinans for chicks, ducklings and turkey poults. Avian Diseases, 33: 357-360.

Fazekas, B., Tanyi, J., Salyi, G., Bistyak, A. and Kerekes, L. 1993. Effect of T-2 toxin on the hatching ability of turkey eggs and viability of day old turkey poults. Magy. Allatorv, Lapja. 48: 221 – 225.

Gedek, B. 1998. Pilzifte lauern in Futtergetxeide. Tierzuchter. 40: 26-28

Girish C. K. and Devegowda, G. 2004b. Efficacy of modified glucomannan (Mycosorb) and clay (HSCAS) to alleviate the individual and combined toxicity of aflatoxin and T-2 toxin in broilers. In: 22nd World's Poultry Congress, Istanbul, Turkey, pp 591

Girish C. K., and Devegowda, G. 2004a. Evaluation of modified glucomannan (Mycosorb) and hydrated sodium calcium aluminosilicate to ameliorate the individual and combined toxicity of aflatoxin and T-2 toxin in broiler chickens. Australian Poultry Science Symposium, Sydney, Vol (16): pp 126-129.

Hamilton, P. B. 1987. Why the animal industry worries about mycotoxins. Presented at a Symposium on "Recent Developments in the study of Mycotoxins". Kaiser Chemicals, Illinois.

Hamilton, P. B., Huff, W. E., Harris, J. R. and Wyatt, R. D. 1982. Natural occurrences of ochratoxicosis in poultry. Poultry Science, 61: 1832-1841.

Hamilton, P. B.1984. Determining safe levels of mycotoxins. Journal of Food Protection, 47: 570 –575.

Harvey, R. B., Kubena, L. F., Huff, W. E., Elissalde, M. H. and Phillips, T. D. 1991. Hematologic and immunologic toxicity of deoxynivalenol (DON)-contaminated diets to growing chickens. Bulletin of Environmental Contamination and Toxicology, 46: 410 – 416.

Hess. J. B. and Biligili, S. F. 1997. Mycotoxins: Hidden culprit in bruising. Broiler Industry. 60(11): 20 – 21.

Hoerr, F. J., Carlton, W. W. and Yagen, B. 1981. Mycotoxicosis caused by a single dose of T-2 toxin or diacetoxscirpenol in broiler chickens. Veterinary Pathology, 18: 652- 664.

Hohler, D. 1999. A brief survey on important mycotoxins and possible detoxification methods. World poultry Misset, 15 (11): 13-15

Huff, W. E. and Doerr, J. A. 1981. Synergism between aflatoxin and ochratoxin A in broiler chickens. Poultry Science, 60: 550.

Huff, W. E., Harvey, R. B., Kubena, L. F. and Rottinghaus, G. E. 1988. Toxic synergism between aflatoxin and T-2 toxin in broiler chickens. Poultry Science, 67:1418–1423.

Huff, W. E., Kubena, L. F., Harvey, R. B. and Phillips, T. D. 1992. Efficacy of hydrated sodium calcium aluminosilicate to reduce the individual and combined toxicity of aflatoxin and ochratoxin A. Poultry Science, 71: 64-69.

Huff, W. E., Kubena, L. F., Harvey, R. B., Hagler Jr, W. M., Swanson, S. P., Phillips, T. D. and Creger, C. R. 1986. Individual and combined effects of aflatoxin and deoxynivalenol (DON, vomitoxin) in broiler chickens. Poultry Science, 64: 1291-1298.

Huff, W. E., Wyatt, R. D., Tucker, T. L. and Hamilton, P. B. 1974. Ochratoxicosis in broiler chickens. Poultry Science, 53: 1585.

Hussein, H. S., and Brase, J.M. 2001. Toxicity, metabolism, and impact of mycotoxins on humans and animals. Toxicology, 167: 101-134.

Jacobson, W. C. and Wiseman, H. G. 1974. Transmission of aflatoxin B_1 into eggs. Poultry Science, 53: 1743

Jelinek, C. F., Pohland, A. E. and Wood, G. E. 1989. Worldwide occurrence of mycotoxins in foods and feeds-an update. Journal - Association of Official Analytical Chemists, 72: 223–230.

Jones, F T., Hagler, W. M. and Hamilton, P. B. 1982. Association of low levels of aflatoxins in feed with productivity losses in commercial broiler operations. Poultry Science, 61: 861-868.

Khajarern. J. and Khajarern, S. 1999. Protective effects of Mycosorb against aflatoxicosis in ducklings and broilers. In: Poster presentation of Alltech's 15th Annual Symposium on Biotechnology in the Feed Industry, Lexington, KY.

Kidd, M.T., Qureshi, M.A., Hagler Jr, W.M. and Ali, R. 1997. T-2 tetraol is cytotoxic to a chicken macrophage cell line. Poultry science, 76(2): 311-313.

Kotyk, A. N. and Trufanova, V. A. 1998. Detection of naphthoquinone fusariotoxin aurofusarin in wheat. Mycology and Phytopathology, 32: 58-61.

Kramer, K., Anke, M., Glei, M. and Muller, M. 1993. Effects of oral bentonite offer on macro and trace element incorporation of different parts of the body and the milk. Trace Elements in Man and Animals. Germany: Verlag Medica Touristik, Gersdorf, pp.466-469.

Kubena, L. F., Edrington, T. S., Kamps-Holtzapple, C., Harvey, R. B., Elissalde, M. H. and Rottinghaus, G. E. 1995. Effects of feeding fumonisin B_1 present in Fusarium moniliforme culture material and aflatoxin singly and in combination to turkey poults. Poultry Science, 74: 1295-1303.

Kubena, L. F., Harvey, R. B., Buckley, S. A., Edrington, T. S. and Rottinghaus, G. E. 1997. Individual and combined effects of moniliformin present in Fusariumfujikuroi culture material and aflatoxin in broiler chicks. Poultry Science, 76: 265–270.

Kubena, L. F., Harvey, R. B., Huff, W. E., Corrier, D. E., Phillips, T. D. and Rottinghaus, G. E. 1989. Influence of ochratoxin A and T-2 toxin singly and in combination on broiler chickens. Poultry Science, 68: 867–872.

Kubena, L. F., Harvey, R. B., Huff, W. E., Corrier, D. E., Phillips, T. D. and Rottinghaus, G. E. 1990. Efficacy of a hydrated sodium calcium aluminosilicate to reduce the toxicity of aflatoxin and T toxin. Poultry Science, 69: 1078 - 1086.

Kubena, L. F., Harvey, R. B., Huff, W. E., Yersin, A. G., Elissalde, M. H. and Witzel, D. A. 1993. Efficacy of a hydrated sodium calcium aluminosilicate to reduce the toxicity of aflatoxin and diacetoxyscirpenol. Poultry Science, 72(1): 51–59.

Ledoux, D. R., Bermudez, A. J. and Rottinghaus, G. E. 1993. Effects of Fusarium fujikuroi culture material containing known levels of moniliformin on turkey poults. Poultry Science, 72 (Suppl. 1): 68. (Abstr.)

Ledoux, D. R., Rottinghaus, G. E., Bermudez, A. J. and Alonso Debolt, M. 1999. Efficacy of a hydrated sodium calcium aluminosilicate to ameliorate the toxic effects of aflatoxin in broiler chicks. Poultry Science, 78: 204-210.

Ledoux, D. R., Weibking, T. S. and Rottinghaus, G. E. 1992. Effects of Fusarium moniliforme culture material containing known levels of fumonisin B_1 on turkey pouts. Poultry Science, 71(Suppl.1): 162.

Leibetseder, J. 1995. The European perspective on mycotoxins. In: Biotechnology in the Feed Industry: Proceedings of Alltech's 11th Annual Symposium (T. P. Lyons and K.A. Jacques, eds). Nottingham University Press, Nottingham. pp. 65-74.

Li, Y. C., Ledoux, D. R., Bermudez, A. J., Fritsche, K. L. and Rottinghaus, G. E. 2000. The individual and combined effects of fumonisin B1 and moniliformin on performance and selected immune parameters in turkey poults. Poultry Science,79: 871–878. 16:253–260.

Mahesh, B. K. and Devegowda, G. 1996. Ability of aflatoxin binders to bind aflatoxin in contaminated poultry feeds-an in vitro study. In: Proceedings XX World's Poultry Congress, New Delhi, India, 4: 296.

Manning, R. O., Brown, T. P., Wyatt, R. D. and Fletcher, O. J. 1985. The individual and combined effects of citrinin and ochratoxin A in broiler chicks. Avian Diseases, 29: 986–997.

Manoj, K. B. and Devegowda, G. 2001. Use of esterified glucomannan to reduce the effects of T-2 toxin in laying hens. In:Proc. of The World Mycotoxin Forum, The Netherlands. pp. 71.

Manoj, K.B. and Devegowda, G., 2000. Efficacy of esterified glucomannan to ameliorate the toxic effects of T-2 toxin in layer hens. Poultry Science, 79(Suppl 1), p.270.

McDaniel, G. 1991. Effect of Yea-Sacc[1026] on reproductive performance of broiler breeder males and females. In: Proc. Alltech's 7th Annual Symposium on Biotechnology in the Feed Industry. Alltech Technical Publications, Nicholasville, Kentucky, USA.

Miller, B. L. and Wyatt, R. D. 1985. Effect of dietary aflatoxin on the uptake and elimination of chlortetracycline in broiler chicks. Poultry Science, 64: 1637-1643.

Morris, C. M., Li, Y. C., Ledoux, D. R., Bermudez, A. J. and Rottinghaus, G. E. 1999. The individual and combined effects of feeding moniliformin, supplied by Fusarium fujikuroi culture material, and deoxynivalenol in young turkey poults. Poultry Science, 78: 1110–1115.

Muller, R. D., Carlson, C. W., Semeniuk, G. and Harshfield, G. S. 1970. The response of Chicks, Ducklings, Goslings, Pheasants and Poults to graded levels of aflatoxins. Poultry Science, 49: 1346 – 1350.

Murthy, T. N. K. and Devegowda, G. 2004. Efficacy of modified glucomannan (Mycosorb) to adsorb aflatoxin B_1 in gut conditions of broiler chickens. In: 22nd World's Poultry Congress, Istanbul, Turkey: pp 471

Nagaraj, R. Y., Wu, W., Will, J. A. and Vesonder, R. F. 1996. Acute cardio toxicity of moniliformin in broiler chickens as measured by electrocardiography. Avian Diseases, 40: 223 – 227.

Nascimento, J.A.F.B., Nunes, V.A., Guedes, R.M.C. and Rachid, M.A. 2001. T-2 toxin and disturbed endochondral bone growth in broiler chicken. Arquivo Brasileiro de Medicina Veterinária e Zootecnia, 53: 332-341.

Pavicic, P., Spring, P., Fuchs, N. and Nemanic, A. 2001. In: 13th European Symposium Poultry Nutrition, World's Poultry Science Association, Blankenberge, Belgium.

Phillips, T. D., Kubena, L. F., Harvery, R. B., Taylor, D. R. and Heidelbaugh, N. D. 1988. Hydrated sodium calcium aluminosilicate: A high affinity sorbent for aflatoxin. Poultry Science, 67: 243 – 247.

Phillips, T. D., Sarr, A. B., Clement, B. A., Kubena, L. F. and Harvery, R. B. 1990. Prevention of aflatoxicosis in farm animals via selective chemisorption of aflatoxin. In: G. A. Bray and D. H. Ryan, ed. Penningto Center Nutrition Series Volume 1, Mycotoxins, Cancer, and Health, Louisiana State Univ. Press, Baton Rouge, LA. pp. 223-237.

Qureshi, M. A., Brake, J., Hamilton, P. B., Hagler, W. M. and Nesheim, S. 1998. Dietary exposure of broiler breeders to aflatoxin results in immune dysfunction in progeny chicks. Poultry Science, 77: 812-819.

Rafai, P., Pettersson, H., Bata, A., Papa, Z., Glavits, R., Tubolys, S., Vanyi, A. and Sooss, P. 2000. Effect of dietary T-2 fusariotoxin concentrations on the health and production of white pekin duck broilers. Poultry Science, 79: 1548-1556.

Raju, M. V. L. N. and Devegowda, G. 2000. Influence of modified glucomannan on performance and organ morphology, serum biochemistry and hematology in broilers exposed to individual and combined mycotoxicosis (Aflatoxin, Ochratoxin and T-2 toxin). British Poultry Science, 41: 640-650.

Raju, M. V. L. N. and Devegowda, G. 2002. Esterified glucomannan in broiler chicken diets contaminated with aflatoxin, ochratoxin and T-2 toxin: evaluation of its binding ability (invitro) and efficacy as immunomodulatory. Asian – Australian Journal Animal Science, 15(7): 1051-1056.

Ravindran, P., Gill, R. J. and Bryden, W. L. 1996. Aflatoxin, fumonisin and zearalenone contamination of Australian maize. Proceedings 20th World's Poultry Congress. New Delhi, India, 4: 273.

Reddy, N. B. and Devegowda, G. 2004. Ability of modified glucomannan (Mycosorb) to sequestrate T-2 toxin in the gastrointestinal tract of chicken. Asian-Australian Journal Animal Science, 17(1).

Sakhatsky, I.M. 1999. Effect of Fusarium graminearum mycotoxins on reproduction and immunity of laying hens. Veterinary Medicine Ukraine, 9: 34-35.

Sályi, G. and Glávits, R., 1995. A barbari kacsa kísérletesen elõidézett T-2 toxikózisa. Magy. Állatorv. Lapja, 50: 202-208.

Santin, E. and Fagundes, F. 2003. Practical demonstration of the effects of mycotoxins in poultry: Mycotoxin Workshops.

Santin, E., Maiorka, A., Krabbe, E.L., Paulillo, A.C. and Alessi, A.C., 2002. Effect of hydrated sodium calcium aluminosilicate on the prevention of the toxic effects of ochratoxin. Journal of Applied Poultry Research, 11(1): 22-28.

Santurio, J.M., Mallmann, C.A., Baldissera, M.A., Ewald, C. and Heer, A. 1994. Níveis de adsorção de Aflatoxina B1 in vitro de aluminosilicatos e bentonitas comercializados no Brasil. In I Congresso Latino-Americano de Micotoxicologia (pp. 10-11).

Schiedeler, S. E. 1993. Effects of various types of aluminosilicates and aflatoxin B_1 on aflatoxin toxicity, chick performance, and mineral status. Poultry Science, 72: 282 – 288.

Shirley, H. V. and Tohala, S. H. 1983. Ochratoxicosis in laying hens.1982. Annual science progress report 83-08. University of Tennessee Agriculture Experiment Station.

Shlosberg, A. S., Klinger, Y.and Malkinson, M. H. 1986. Muscovy ducklings, a particular sensitive avian bioassay for T-2 toxin and diacetosxyscirpenol. Avian Diseases, 30: 820 – 824.

Smith, E. E., Kubena, L. F., Braithwaite, C. E., Harvey, R. B., Philips, T. D. and Reine, A. H. 1992. Toxicological evaluation of aflatoxin and cyclopiazonic acid in broiler chickens. Poultry Science, 71: 1136 – 1144.

Smith, T. K., Mac Donald, E. J. and Haladi, S. 2001. Esterified glucomannan: Growth and neurological response of pigs given fusariotoxin contaminated diets. In: Science and Technology in Feed Industry. Eds: Lyons, T. P and Jacques. K. A, Nottingham University Press, Loughborough, Leics, UK.

Smith, T. K., Modirsanei, M.and Macdonald, E. J. 2000. The use of binding agents and amino acid supplements for dietary treatment of Fusarium mycotoxicosis. In: Biotechnology in the Feed Industry. Eds: Lyons, T. P. and Jacques, K. A., Nottingham University Press, Loughborough, Leics, UK, pp. 383-390.

Smith, T. K., Swamy, H. V. L. N., Chowdhary, S. R. and Raymond, S. L. 2003. In vivo demonstrations of the efficacy of Mycosorb^{TM} in prevention of Fusariummycotoxicoses. The Second World Mycotoxin Forum, 17-18 February. pp. 63-64.

Stanley, V.G., Ojo, R., Woldesenbet, S. and Hutchinson, D.H. 1993. The use of Saccharomyces cerevisiae to suppress the effects of aflatoxicosis in broiler chicks. Poultry Science, 72: 1867-1872.

Stratton, G. W., Robinson, A. R., Smith, H. C., Kittilsen, L., and Barbour, M. 1993. Levels of five mycotoxins in grains harvested in Atlantic Canada as measured by high performance liquid performance liquid chromatography. Archives of Environmental Contamination and Toxicology, 24: 399 – 409.

Surai, P. F. 2002. Natural Antioxidants in Avian Nutrition and Reproduction. Nottingham University Press, Nottingham.

Swamy H. V. L. N., Smith, T. K., Cotter, P. F., Boermans, H. J. and Seftons, A. E. 2002. Effects of feeding blends of grains naturally contaminated with Fusarium mycotoxins on production and metabolism in Broilers. Poultry Science, 81: 966-975.

Swamy, H.V.L.N. and Devegowda, G. 1998, Ability of mycosorb to counteract aflatoxicosis in commercial broilers. Indian J. Poultry Science, 33: 273-278.

Trenholm, H. L., Charmley, L. L. and Prelusky, D. B. 1996. Mycotoxin binding agents: An update on what we know. In: Biotechnology in the Feed Industry Eds: Lyons. T. P and Jacques. K. A, Nottingham University Press, Loughborough, Leics, UK.

Tung, H. T., Smith, J. W. and Hamilton, P.B. 1971. Aflatoxicosis and bruising in chickens. Poultry Science, 50: 795-800.

Urano, T., Trucksess, M.W., Beaver, R.W., Wilson, D.M., Dorner, J.W. and Dowell, F.E., 1992. Co-occurrence of cyclopiazonic acid and aflatoxins in corn and peanuts. Journal of AOAC International, 75(5): 838-841.

Van Egmond, H. P. and Spijers, G. J. A. 1994. Survey of data on the incidence and levels of ochratoxin A in food and animal feed. World wide: Journal of Natural Toxin 3:125-144.

Vanyi, A., Glavits, R., Bata, A. and Kovacs, F., 1994. Pathomorphological changes caused by T-2 trichothecene fusariotoxin in geese. Acta Veterinaria Hungarica, 42(4): 447-457.

Veldman, B. 2003. Effects of dietary mycotoxins on the quality of animal products and on human health. In: proceedings of the Second World Mycotoxin Forum, The Netherlands. pp: 52-54.

Volkl, A. and Karlovsky, P. 1998. Biological detoxification of fungal toxins and its use in plant breeding, feed and food production. Natural Toxins 7: 1-23.

Volkl, A. and Karlovsky, P. 1998. Zearalenone and feed additives: adsorption and desorption as a function of PH. University of Hohenheim, Struttgart, Germany. Personnel communication.

Wang, R., Miao, C., Chong, R., Sawatwiroj, N., Dawson, K., Fu, S. and Feng, D. 2003. Feed and feed ingredient mycotoxin contamination in China: A survey. In: Proceedings of Alltech's 17th annual Asia pacific lecture tour.

Weibking, T. S., Ledoux, D. R., Bermudez, A. J. and Rottinghaus, G. E. 1994. Individual and combined effects of feeding Fusarium moniliforme culture material containing known levels of fumonisin B_1 and aflatoxin B_1 in the young turkey poult. Poultry Science, 73:1517–1525.

World Health Organisation (WHO). 2001. Safety evaluation of certain mycotoxins in food. Geneva, Switzerland.

Wu, W., Jerome, D. and Nagaraj, R.1994. Increased redness in turkey breast muscle induced by Fusarial culture materials. Poultry Science, 73: 331 – 335.

Wyatt, R. D., Hamilton, P. B. and Burmeister, H. R. 1975. Altered feathering of chicks caused by T-2 toxin. Poultry Science, 54:1172 (Abstr.)

14

Application of in-ovo Technology in Poultry

Vignesh G., Gajendiran K. and Srinivasan G.

Department of Poultry Management, Suguna Institute of Poultry Management Post Box No.44,23/A, 24, Chinnapappanoothu Village, Vilamarathupatti (PO) Anaimalai Road, Udumalpet Taluk, Tirupur (Di), Tamil Nadu-642 207

Introduction

Poultry industry is one of the quickest developing sectors in India. Poultry involves a remarkable position in the livestock economy of India by coexistence of intense technology, capital, and scale with integrated production, marketing and the others based on the traditional knowledge and practices. The annual growth rate is more than 11% and 8 % in broiler production and egg production respectively. The general development rate of poultry industry is around 7-8% for every annum, most outstanding among all sectors of agriculture. In poultry industry, poultry meat accounts for two third of the value of output and one third by eggs. Poultry industry generates direct employment for more than 3.5 million people and indirect employment for another 3.5 million people in different facets of allied activities. India is the third most noteworthy egg producer and fifth biggest poultry meat producer. This makes poultry part as the quickest developing segment among all livestock sectors. The broilers in India are reared for 35-40 days to a market weight of 1.8 to 2.2 kg. The feed conversion ratio for modern broilers has been improved considerably through continuous selection programme, precision nutrition by adopting biosecurity measures from 2.2 to 1.6.

In-ovo feeding of nutrients has gained more attention recently. *In-ovo* feeding of nutrients would be a more effective option, and this is the approach that has been developed by Uni and Ferket (2003). The first administration of *in ovo* delivery of exogenous material was reported in the 1980s for vaccination against Marek's disease (Sharma and Burmester, 1982). At early stages of development, day zero or on or before day seven of incubation, the preferable site of injection is the air cell or albumen part of the egg, which may be termed '*in ovo* administration'. Pre-hatch birds naturally consume the amniotic fluids on 18th day of incubation. Therefore addition of a nutrient solution to the embryonic amniotic fluid would deliver essential nutrients into the embryo's intestine. These early advancements have prompted expanded research on *in ovo* methods in poultry to enhance starting weights, better feed utilization, faster growth rate and higher final weight.

Some of the challenges faced by broilers chicks include weakness, reduced feed intake, impaired growth, susceptibility to disease, and mortality. These symptoms may be due to limitations in some nutrients and energy and to immature digestive system unable to reload depleted energy reserves from consumed feed. Supplementing the amnion fluid with appropriate nutrients (by in-ovo feeding) is a novel way to feed critical dietary components to embryos a 'jump-start' development of the chick. In-ovo feeding technology has established a new science of perinatal nutrition that will open opportunities for greater production efficiency and animal welfare.

Necessity for in ovo feeding

In any commercial production system, the first few weeks are most critical period in a chicks life, which has a significant varying on the survivability and growth of the bird, newly hatched chicks are often subjected to undue stress that makes them more susceptible to pathogens.The potential period, the last four days before hatch and the first four days after hatch is most critical period for development and survival of commercial birds. It's the period during which the nutritional conditioning and perinatal programming can occur. The perinatal chick makes the metabolic and physiological transition from the nutrition supplied in the egg to feed, and it's functionally programmed to adopt its environment. The chick's first meal occurs when it consumes the amnion fluid before internal piping at about 18 days of incubation.

In commercial hatcheries, hatchlings are commonly held for 36 to 72 hours from the time of actual hatch to placement this is due to the wide hatching "hatching window" hatchlings are not removed, until maximum number of eggs has been hatched. This causes most hatchlings to be fasted for 48hours or more before they access to first feed and water. This makes hatchlings become more susceptible to pathogens, have decreased body weight and have restricted development of the intestine. In-ovo feeding of nutrients especially carbohydrates replenishes the glycogen stores depleted during the prenatal period and also increase body weight.

Principle

Epigenetic programming refers to the influence produced by the exposure to specific conditions during critical periods of early life that modify the developmental pathways of the organism, leading to stable and long-lasting alterations that have effects when the individual reaches adulthood.

In poultry, epigenetic programming, which allows an animal to metabolically or physiologically adapt to specific dietary or environmental conditions, can occur during two critical periods: when embryo consumes the amniotic fluid prior to hatch, and when the chicks absorb residual yolk and feed during the first few days after hatch.

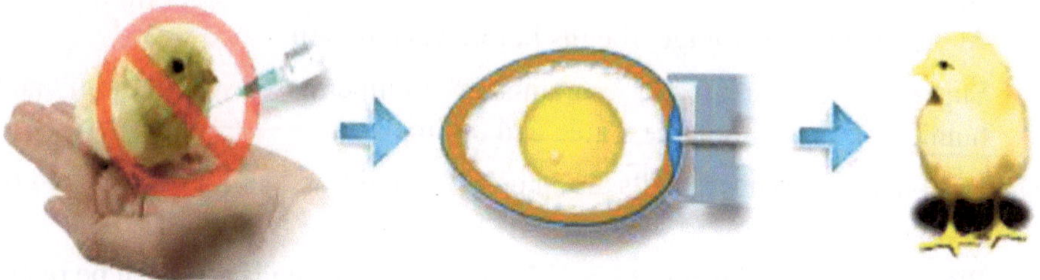

Nutrients that have been applied for in-ovo injection

1. Amino acids
2. Carbohydrates
3. Vitamins
4. Trace mineral
5. Fatty acids
6. feed additives

Various potential nutrient supplements can be included in the *in-ovo* feeding solution. Carbohydrates can be used as a source for glucose, which is crucial for the hatching process and hatchling development. Na^+ and Cl^- ions play a major role in the activity of apical and basolateral transporters and in the absorption of glucose and amino acids. β-hydroxy-β-methylbutyrate (HMB), a leucine metabolite which affect muscle satellite cells and increases carcass yield, is a good candidate for the *in-ovo* feeding solution, as are minerals and vitamins which support the development of skeletal, immune and digestive systems in chickens. Many nutrients were evaluated for their contribution to poultry hatchability, chick quality and production performance.

Indeed, any selected nutrients can be applied for *in-ovo* feeding and that includes all amino acids, carbohydrates, vitamins, fatty acids, and other modulators. A large variety of nutrients or supplements can potentially be included in the *in-ovo* feeding solution. Limitations are volume, timing, osmolality and viscosity of *in-ovo* feeding formulation.

Important Points should be considered before applying in ovo injection

- The stage of development of the embryos.
- Site of injection
- Dose of injection and knowing the stage of development of the embryos is essential to determine the correct time to achieve the best hatchability.
- Avoid prolonged storage of eggs before vaccination.
- Supervise the incubator parameters (temperature, ventilation, and humidity): they should be stable and optimal.
- Use only eggs whose shells are in perfect condition, do not use cracked or broken eggs.
- Place the eggs in the correct position (upright); the eggs will then be ready for injection.
- Use sterile techniques and follow the vaccine manufacturer's instructions to prepare the nutrients.
- Have personnel qualified in aseptic techniques for this operation.

Sites of Injection

- Air cell
- Amniotic sac (recommended)
- Yolk sac
- Embryo itself

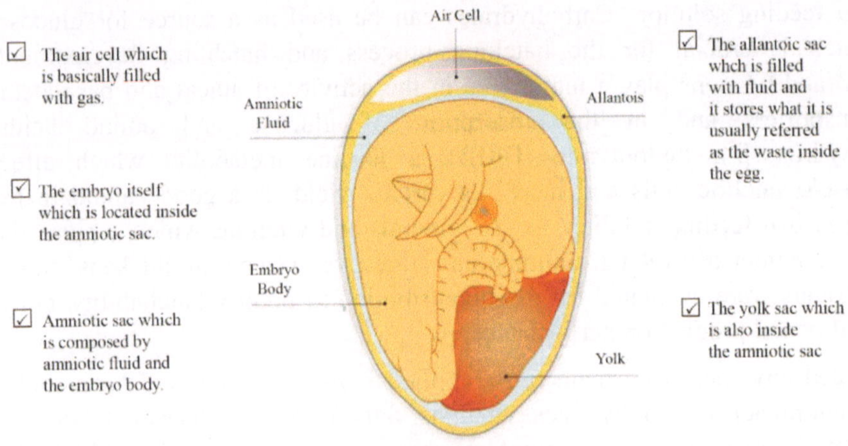

Sites of injection

The ideal site for in-ovo injection

At early stages of development, from 0-7 days of incubation, the preferable site of injection is the air cell or albumin part of the egg. At 18th day amniotic sac is preferable.

The ideal time for in-ovo injection

Vaccines or nutrients is recommended to be at 18 days of incubation, Pre-hatch embryos consume the amniotic fluids till hatch, In-ovo nutrient injection will help the embryos absorb the nutrients before hatch

Procedure

- Clean the eggs and wipe with 70% ethanol
- The amnion in the in egg was identified by candling
- Inject, with In-ovo feeding solution using a 21-gauge needle after making a pin head size (0.30 mm diameter) hole
- After the eggs were injected, the injection holes were sealed with cellophane tape or with parafilm wax.

Note: (0.1 ml and up to 0.2 ml volumes have been used to avoid embryonic death or failure)

(21 gauge needle for performing in ovo)

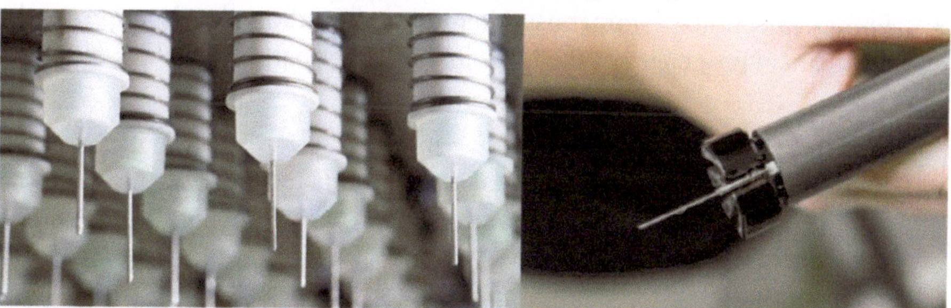

Research studies carried out

Nutrient injected	**Stage of incubation**	**Location of injection**	**Result**	**Reference**
Threonine	18th day	yolk	Improves post-hatching growth and humoral responses of broiler chicks.	Kadam et al., 2008.
Arginine	18th day	Amniotic sac	Improves hatch weight, chick/egg weight ratio & placement weight and provides enough nutrition	Nayak et al., 2016.

Probiotic, prebiotic and synbiotics	18th day	Amniotic sac	Improves the gut health	Survase Swapnil Harishchandra,2018 M.V.Sc thesis, TANUVAS
Nano dicalcium phosphate and Vitamin D3	18th day	Amniotic sac	Better bone development and overall economic index	Yadav Sunil Machendra, 2019 M.V.Sc thesis, TANUVAS

Benefits of *In-ovo* feeding

- It may lead to improved digestive capacity, increased growth rate and feed efficiency, reduced post hatch mortality and morbidity, improved immune responses to enteric antigens, reduced incidence of developmental skeletal disorders, increased muscle development and breast meat yield, increase liver glycogen status, higher glycogen reserves, body weight, pectoral muscle weight and body weight gain.
- *In-ovo* fed bird's exhibit increased length of villus, thereby increase absorption of nutrients thereby increase the overall performance of the birds.
- *In-ovo* injection of amino acids, trace elements or fatty acids and vitamins modulate the cell mediated immune response.
- *In-ovo* injection of minerals, vitamins and carbohydrates improve the mechanical properties of the bone in the earlier part of the chicks life.

Limitation

- Requirement of skilled persons to carry out this technology
- Time consuming process
- Commercial interventions are not up to the expected level
- Lack of automation
- Lack of Facilities, equipment availability and cost

Future Potential

Further research is required to adapt *in-ovo* feeding technique for application at commercial scale in farm conditions, to understand the embryonic development and nutrient metabolism process more precisely, and understand how early nutrition affects specific genes responsible for performance, intestinal health, and overall health-related traits in poultry.

Conclusion

The degree of response to *In-ovo* feeding may depend upon genetics, breeder hen age, and egg size and incubation conditions.The *In-ovo* injection of important nutrients or substances into the amnion is a novel way to feed critical dietary components to embryos. Indeed, *In-ovo* feeding may "jump-start" development, improving the nutritional status of the perinatal chick. The *In-ovo* feeding technique has several advantages, including improvements of total digestive tract capacity; increased body weight, growth rate, and feed efficiency; reduction of post-hatch mortality and morbidity; improvements in the immune system and the response to enteric antigens; reduction in incidence of developmental skeletal disorders; and increase in muscle development and breast meat yield. The next step in the early nutrition could be to imprint genes of a bird at a very early age and turn it into a more efficient animal later.

15

Nutritional Factors Affecting Fertility and Hatchability of Eggs

Manzoor A. Wani, S. Adil, M.T. Banday and I.U. Sheikh

Division of Livestock Production Management
Faculty of Veterinary Science and Animal Husbandry, Shuhama, Alusteng, Srinagar, Sher-e-Kashmir University of Agricultural Sciences and Technology of Kashmir

Introduction

Poultry production is practiced at levels ranging from subsistence to large scale commercial operations. Commercial operations depend on hatcheries for the supply of day-old chicks while the subsistence farmers hatch their chicks by natural incubation. The hatchery plays a central role in the poultry production chain. Optimization of hatchery and breeder farm management can lead to improvement of the result throughout the production chain (Heier and Jarp, 2001). Generally, the success of hatchery management is monitored by the percentage of eggs set that are hatched (hatchability) and the number of chicks that are placed for grow-out (saleable chicks). Fertility and hatchability are two major parameters that influence the supply of day old chicks. Hatchability is influenced by many factors, some of these are the responsibility of the breeding farm and others are the responsibility of the hatchery. Reasons for low hatchability could be improper management of the breeder flock, an incorrect incubation procedure, or a failure within any step between the breeder flock and the final hatch. Breeder factors that affect hatchability include strain, health, nutrition and age of the flock, egg size, weight and quality, egg storage duration and conditions, egg sanitation, and season of the year (Kirk *et al.*, 1980; Wilson, 1991, 1997; Elibol *et al.*, 2002; Tona *et al.*, 2005, 2007).

The growth and development of normal embryo depends on a complete supply of all required nutrients within the egg. This supply of nutrients originates in the maternal diet and metabolism, which is further determined by the effectiveness of their deposition into the egg. Genetic variation in absorption-metabolism-deposition has long been recognized as a factor in nutrient effects on embryo viability (Lillie *et al.*, 1951). Maw, 1954 has found genetic basis for inadequate deposition of riboflavin in the egg of chicken. The transfer of adequate and balanced supply of nutrients to the egg required for normal development of the embryo requires the parent birds must be on a balanced diet. Marginal deficiencies may affect the embryos of only the most susceptible hens as well as result in predominantly late incubation deaths or other late occurring effects. However, mortality during 8 to 14 days of incubation is a sensitive indicator of breeder diet deficiencies as mortality is normally very low during this period (Leeson *et al.*, 1979b). Not only the deficiencies, but excesses of certain nutrients or egg constituents may cause serious problems and as either nutritional deficiencies or excesses get progressively more severe, the effects on the embryo also become more severe and occur at earlier stages of development. In this chapter, the nutritional factors affecting fertility and hatchability of poultry eggs will be discussed in detail;

1. Energy and protein

Nutrition can play a major role in fertility and hatchability of eggs. The energy and protein form the two major components of the diet, comprising more than 90% of the total diet of poultry. The composition of hen diet has an effective factor on egg production (Khajali *et al.*, 2008; Perez-Bonilla *et al.*, 2012), egg weight (Whitehead *et al.*, 1991, Zimmerman 1997; Shim *et al.*, 2013) and hatching characters (Danicke *et al.*, 2000) in poultry. The amount of energy and protein varies according to the growth and production of the bird. As per BIS 2007, broiler breeder female and male requires 2800 and 2750 kcal/kg Metabolizable energy (ME) and 16 and 15% crude protein (CP) respectively, whereas layer breeder female and male requires 2600 Kcal/kg ME and 17 and 16% CP respectively. Breeders fed a low energy-high protein diet tend to produce eggs with lower hatchability (Pearson and Herron, 1982; Leeson and Summers, 1991). This decrease appeared to result from increased embryonic mortality in mid-incubation and unhatched pips. But, energy and protein levels of the breeder diet did not affect the incidence of malpositions or malformations. Li *et al.,* (2013) reported ranges of estimated optimum ME and CP intake were 2591 to 2683 kcal/kg and 15.58% to 16.64% CP for optimizing egg production of lohmann Brown laying hens. Diets containing high protein and low energy were found to have a negative effect on egg weight and egg production (Li *et al.*, 2013; Steenhuisen and Gous, 2016). It was reported that there is a positive relationship between egg weight and hatching weight (Ozcan *et al.*, 2001; Tona *et al.*, 2004). So, the relationship between egg weight and protein levels of hen diet should be taken into consideration for hatching chick weight. Spratt & Leeson (1987) reported a reduction in egg weight and consequently in chick weight when dietary protein content was reduced from 16.70% to 12.70% for broiler breeder hens. It was also reported by Leeson & Caston (1996) that the egg weight decreased when dietary protein content was reduced from 16.80%

to 14.40% in iso-energetic hen diets. The levels of protein in a breeder diet form an important factor for hatching characters and embryonic mortality. A study on chukar partridge reported the general tendency increase infertility with high protein levels (CP 17%), and in contrary hatchability decreased under the same condition (Cufadar *et al.,* 2010). However, Mohiti-Asli *et al.,* (2012) found that fertility, hatchability of total and fertile eggs, and embryonic mortality of hen diet with high protein (CP 17.40%) were higher than those of hen diet with low protein (CP 14.50%). Also, a number of authors reported negative effects of a high compared to a low daily dietary crude protein (CP) intake (27 vs. 23, 26 vs. 21, and 25 vs. 16 g/day) during the laying period on fertility and hatchability of eggs (Pearson and Herron (1982), Whitehead *et al*., 1985 and Lopez and Leeson (1995a). Also, a high compared to a low daily protein intake (27 vs. 23 g/day) during the laying period, resulted in an increased mortality and malformation of embryos (Pearson and Herron, 1982). Ekmay *et al.* (2013) showed in a dose-response study that higher levels of dietary lysine and isoleucine at peak production resulted in a reduction in fertility.

Van Emous *et al.,* 2015, found that broiler breeder pullets fed rearing diets with a decrease of dietary protein levels show a decreased fertility of early hatching eggs. Walsh and Brake (1997) also found that a low dietary crude protein level (11 or 14 versus 17%) during the rearing period decreased fertility of hatching eggs during the entire laying period. Contrary to this, Hocking *et al*., (2002) did not find an effect of different dietary protein levels (13 versus 15.5% weighted average) during the rearing period on fertility. Van Emous *et al.,* 2015, also observed that broiler breeders fed the medium protein diet (14%) had a reduced hatchability of fertile eggs, which was caused by an increased embryonic mortality between 18 and 21 day of incubation. An increased embryonic mortality during that stage of the incubation period could be due to respiratory failure, poor resorption of the yolk sac, embryo malposition or abnormalities.

Body weight at the end of the rearing period is also mentioned as a potential factor that might affect fertility and hatchability of hatching eggs. Renema *et al*. (2001a) demonstrated that a higher body weight (BW) during the rearing and laying period increased fertility and hatchability and decreased embryonic mortality, although these effects were not observed in other studies (Fattori *et al.,* 1991; Hocking *et al*., 2002; De Beer and Coon, 2007; Zuidhof *et al*., 2007; Ekmay *et al*., 2012).

Table 1: Nutritional requirements for Breeder chicken (BIS, 2007)

Characteristics	Broiler Breeder feed				Layer Breeder feed			
	Chick	Grower	layer	Male	Chick	Grower	layer	Male
ME (kcal/kg)	2800	2750	2800	2750	2800	2600	2600	2600
CP (%)	20	16	16	15	20	16	17	16
Calcium (%)	1.0	1.0	3.5	1.0	1.0	1.0	3.5	1.0
Available Phosphorous (%)	0.45	0.45	0.40	0.40	0.45	0.40	0.40	0.40
Lysine (%)	1.0	0.8	0.85	0.80	0.95	0.70	0.70	0.80
Methionine (%)	0.45	0.40	0.45	0.40	0.40	0.40	0.40	0.40

2. Fat and Fatty Acids

The fatty acid composition of the diet has been shown to affect the fatty acid composition of the yolk, which in turn can affect embryonic development and hatchability (Vilchez *et al.*, 1990a,b). Palmitic acid appears to increase yolk oleic acid levels, to affect transport across the yolk sac membrane, and to spare linoleic acid for embryonic growth and hatchability. Adding corn oil, palmitic acid, oleic acid, or linoleic acid to a basal diet increased hatchability and decreased late embryonic mortality. Subsequent studies have indicated that palmitic acid facilitates increased yolk mobilization by the embryo (Vilchez *et al.*, 1992). Low hatchability in young broiler breeders has been associated with reduced mobilization of yolk lipids by the embryo as well as an altered fatty acid composition of the yolk (Noble and Yafei, 1988; Tullett, 1990). Increasing egg cholesterol by 70% did not significantly affect hatchability (Jiang *et al.,* 1990). Field problems have been observed with diets containing cottonseed or kapok seed meal as ingredients or contaminants (Tullett, 1990). These materials contain cyclopropenoid fatty acids and cause yolks with putty-like consistency as well as the release of iron from the yolk producing pink albumen. The ratio of stearic to oleic acid changed from about 7:43 to 20:30. The embryonic effects were hatchability reduced almost to zero, very high mortality in 2nd week and to a lesser extent in 1st week, and very poor blood and circulatory system formation. Besides, it is also suggested by some researchers that a certain proportion of body fat in broiler breeders at the onset of lay is necessary for an adequate reproductive performance (Sun and Coon, 2005; De Beer, 2009).

3. Vitamins and Minerals

Vitamins and minerals are crucial nutrients for metabolic and physiological processes and thereby for animal productive and reproductive performance (Tufarelli and Laudadio, 2016). Suboptimal levels of these nutrients in commercial diets are known to result in negative responses to both parent and offspring performance. They account for about 4% of the cost of a breeder feed, so economising on their inclusion rates is rarely an option. Vitamins improve the immune status in birds and defend against diseases and stress. Fat soluble-vitamins like A and E positively influence egg production (i.e., number, weight or egg quality) and hatchability. Vitamin A is responsible for maintaining the integrity of epithelia of male and female reproductive tract (khan *et al.*, 2012). Insufficient levels of vitamin A results in increased atresia, ovulation of degenerated eggs and also with an abnormal development of the embryo. Whereas, excess of vitamin A intake leads to a decrease in egg production and an increase of congenital abnormalities in embryos. The main role of Vitamin E is protecting the cells against oxidative damage and therefore it is essential for male and female fertility. Deficiency of vitamin E supplementation results in decrease of fertile eggs and egg hatchability. Vitamin E has been found to be transferred to the egg yolk (Surai *et al.,* 1997; Vieira, 2007) so, its supplementation in broiler breeder diets would increase its content in the yolk, and sbsequently in chicks (Surai *et al.,* 1999, 2001; Surai, 2000). This would protect the developing chicks against oxidative stress and improves immune response (Gore and Qureshi, 1997). Also, interaction between vitamin E and selenium increase the production of the Glutathione peroxidase (GPx), which is part of the antioxidant protection system (Surai, 2000; Skrivan *et al.,* 2008). Vitamin D, which is involved in absorption of calcium from intestine, its deposition onto bones, as well as resorption from bone tissues when plasma calcium levels are low. Vitamin D_3 level in the hens diet has been found to be positively correlated with vitamin D_3 and 25-OH vitamin D_3 contents within the egg yolk. The enzyme 25-hydroxyvitamin D-1α-hydroxylase, which is responsible for the hydroxylation of 25-OH vitamin D_3 to 1, 25$(OH)_2$ D_3 is present as early as 12 days of incubation and increases in specific activity during further embryonic development. This signifies the importance of this nutrient to the developing embryo. However, even with diets sufficient in vitamin D activity (2,200 IU), the addition of 1,100 IU of 25-OH vitamin D_3 to the diet of turkey breeders increased egg hatchability as compared with dietary vitamin D_3 alone. This may be related to the fact that 25-OH vitamin D_3 is more efficiently absorbed by the bird than vitamin D_3, which may also be the case for the chick embryo. Providing the broiler breeder hen with dietary 25-OH vitamin D_3, may increase the absorption efficiency of Ca from the gut, leading to increased eggshell quality and less reliance on bone Ca as the bird ages. In addition, maternal supplementation of 25-OH vitamin D_3, increases deposition of 25-OH vitamin D_3 into the egg and may result in increased egg hatchability and chick quality, which could in turn result in increased growth and efficiency of the broiler chick. The recommended levels of vitamins in the diets of breeders are given in table 2 and effects of vitamins deficient in the diet on hatchability has been presented in Table 3.

Table 2: Suggested levels of vitamins in the diets breeder chicken

Ingredient	Broiler Breeder				Layer Breeder			
	Chick	Grower	Layer	Male	Chick	Grower	Layer	Male
Vitamins (I.U./Kg)								
Vitamin A	12000	12000	15000	12000	12000	12000	15000	12000
Vitamin D_3	2500	2500	3000	2500	2500	2500	3000	2500
Vitamin E	20.00	20.00	50.00	20.00	20.00	20.00	50.00	25.00
Vitamins (mg/Kg)								
Vitamin K	2.00	2.00	3.00	2.00	2.00	2.00	3.00	2.00
Thiamine B_1	2.00	2.00	2.00	2.00	2.00	2.00	3.00	2.00
Riboflavin B_2	4.00	4.00	4.00	4.00	5.00	5.00	6.00	5.00
Nicotinic Acid	40.00	40.00	50.00	40.00	40.00	40.00	50.00	40.00
Pantothenic Acid	15.00	15.00	25.00	15.00	15.00	15.00	25.00	15.00
Pyridoxine B_6	2.00	2.00	2.00	2.00	5.00	5.00	6.00	5.00
Biotin	0.10	0.10	0.10	0.10	0.20	0.20	0.20	0.20
Folic Acid	0.50	0.50	0.50	0.50	3.00	3.00	4.00	3.00
Choline	1200	1000	1200	1000	800	800	600	800
Vitamin B_{12} μg/Kg	15.00	15.00	15.00	15.00	20.00	20.00	30.00	20.00

Table 3: Effects of some important vitamins deficient in the diet of breeders on Hatchability of eggs

Vitamins	Effects on Hatchability
Vitamin A	• Increased incidence of malposition's in embryos. • Abnormal circulatory system development. • Death of embryos within 2-3 days.
Vitamin D	• Beak deformities and inadequate skeletal formations, shortened upper mandible. • Late embryonic mortality, mostly on 18th and 19th day of hatch.
Vitamin E	• Cloudy spots in the eyes, blindness. • Abnormal vascular system (Exudative diathesis). • Embryonic mortality 2 to 5 days.
Vitamin K	• Haemorrhage's in the embryo. • Increased blood clotting time (Lavelle *et al.*, 1994)
Riboflavin	• Embryos may show oedema, increased mortality, clubbed down, haemorrhages, dwarfing, micromelia, and anaemia

Thiamine	• Polyneuritis and embryonic mortality at early and late at ≥19 days
Pantothenic acid	• Embryonic mortality peaks have been reported to occur after 18th day (Gillis *et al.,* 1947). • Subcutaneous haemorrhages, oedema, hydrocephalus, poor feathering, twisted legs, decreased hatchability, and chicks with muscular incoordination, swollen hocks.
Niacin	• Hypoplasia of skeletal muscles, nervous and vascular abnormality. • Abnormal embryonic development & hatchability (Briggs *et al.,* 1946) • Excesses of Nicotinamide have also caused embryonic mortality and loss of hatchability (Romanoff and Romanoff, 1972). • Mortality during 8-14days.
Biotin	• Mortality of embryos is increased during the 1st and 3rd week of incubation (Leeson *et al*., 1979b). • Chondro-dystrophy or micromelia condition, shortened bones and "parrot beak".
Folic acid	• Embryonic abnormalities include shortened bones, beak defects. • Most embryos appeared normal but died after pipping the air cell. • Mortality after 17thday of hatch.
Vitamin B12	• Embryonic mortality occurred in the 1st week of incubation. • Abnormalities include oedema around the eyes, poor leg muscle development, haemorrhages, dwarfing and shortened beak.

The supply of trace minerals (TM) such as Zinc, Manganese, and Copper, in poultry diets is essential for maintenance of bird health, immune stimulation, expression of production potential (Smith and Akinbamijo, 2000), as well as better eggshell quality (Yenice *et al.,* 2015). Trace minerals are typically included in poultry diets as inorganic salts, such as carbonates, sulphates and oxides (Sirri *et al.,* 2016). Broiler breeder diets with insufficient TM levels have reduced egg production, increased embryonic mortality, impaired eggshell quality and production of unviable chicks. Also, Trace minerals in broiler breeders feed are deposited in the egg yolk (Kidd, 2003; Dibner *et al*., 2007), and are utilized by embryos for their development. These trace minerals are constituents of several proteins involved in intermediary metabolism, hormone secretion, and the immune system (Savage, 1968) and are required in small amounts in the diet. In conventional feedstuffs, mineral concentration can fluctuate widely because of the trace mineral composition in soils, geographic area, climate and crop yield (Hodgson *et al.,* 1962). Thus, in practical poultry formulations, nutritionists usually include a wide margin of safety for trace minerals to ensure appropriate bird growth and maximize performance (Dale and Strong Jr., 1998). In breeder hens, Zn is important as a component of carbonic anhydrase, which is involved in the supply of carbonate ions during eggshell formation (Nys *et al.,* 1999). Other important

Zn metalloenzymes include carboxypeptidases and DNA polymerases, which are important in immune responses, skin and wound healing, and hormone production. Breeder diets that are deficient in Zn can lead to a decrease in egg production and eggshell quality, as well as in hatchability (Kienholz *et al.*, 1961). Manganese plays a significant role in the formation of chondroitin sulphate, which is essential for formation of bone cartilage. Manganese-deficient avian embryos exhibit shortening of the long bones, parrot beak, and wiry down (Caskey *et al.*,1939). The involvement of Cu in the synthesis of hemoglobin, erythrocuprein, and other plasma proteins is well known (Leeson, 2009). Moreover, Cu is closely associated with iron metabolism because it is a part of ceruloplasmin. Copper also plays an important role in eggshell membrane formation, which in turn influences eggshell structure, texture, and shape (Baumgartner *et al.*, 1978). The recommended levels of minerals in the diets of breeders are given in table 4 and effects of some minerals deficient in diet on hatchability has been presented in Table 5.

Table 4: Suggested levels of minerals in diets of breeder chicken

Substance	Broiler Breeder				Layer Breeder			
	Chick	**Grower**	**Layer**	**Male**	**Chick**	**Grower**	**Layer**	**Male**
Minerals (%)								
Phosphorus, Total	0.70	0.70	0.70	0.70	0.65	0.60	0.60	0.60
Sodium Chloride	0.50	0.50	0.50	0.50	0.50	0.50	0.50	0.50
Potassium	0.20	0.20	0.20	0.20	0.20	0.20	0.20	0.20
Magnesium	0.05	0.05	0.05	0.05	0.05	0.05	0.05	0.05
Micro-minerals (mg/Kg)								
Copper	12.00	12.00	12.00	12.00	12.00	12.00	12.00	12.00
Iodine	1.50	1.50	1.50	1.50	1.50	1.50	1.50	1.50
Iron	80.00	80.00	80.00	80.00	80.00	80.00	80.00	80.00
Manganese	100.00	100.00	100.00	100.00	100.00	100.00	100.00	100.00
Zinc	80.00	80.00	80.00	80.00	80.00	80.00	80.00	80.00
Selenium	0.15	0.15	0.20	0.15	0.15	0.15	0.20	0.15

Table 5: Effects of some macro and micro-minerals deficient in the diet of breeders on hatchability of eggs

Minerals	Effects on Hatchability
Calcium (Ca)	• The level of Calcium in breeder diet affects embryonic development primarily through eggshell quality (Landauer, 1967; Romanoff and Romanoff, 1972). • Poor egg shells results in excessive egg weight loss accompanied by increased mortality during 1st week. • Embryos with stunted growth, poor bone development and increased mortality at the end of incubation (McDaniel *et al.*, 1979; Wilson, 1993). • Increasing the dietary calcium level from 0.99 to 1.77% resulted in improved hatchability in turkey eggs (Potter *et al.*, 1974). • Normal hatchability was obtained with Quail birds fed 2.5 to 3.0% calcium with 0.8% phosphorus (Nelson *et al.*, 1964) and in broiler breeders on litter floor fed 2.25 to 6.00% calcium (Wilson *et al.*, 1980).
Phosphorus (P)	• It is necessary for support of normal embryonic bone development and hatchability (Waldroup *et al.*, 1967). • Caged laying hens had depressed hatchability when fed a diet containing 0.19% phosphorus (O'Rourke *et al.*, 1954) and supplementing the diet to provide 0.18% inorganic and 0.30% total phosphorus improved hatchability. • Singsen *et al.* (1962) suggested that caged layers require 0.4% phosphorus for normal hatchability, whereas Wilson *et al.* (1980) found that broiler breeders on litter floor had normal hatchability with 0.31% phosphorus. • Breeders on litter floors appear to recycle considerable amounts of phosphorus by coprophagy (Wilson et al., 1980). • Phytic acid phosphorus does not support normal hatchability but does prevent embryonic rickets (Waldroup *et al.*, 1967). • Inorganic phosphorus has been reported to be required for maximum hatchability in turkey eggs (Sewell *et al.*, 1972; Ferguson *et al.*, 1974) and 0.19% inorganic dietary phosphorus has been suggested for maximum hatchability of caged laying hens (Waldroup *et al.*, 1967). • Excess phosphorus intake through a combination of dietary and coprophagic sources may reduce shell quality and indirectly decrease hatchability (Wilson *et al.*, 1980). • Mortality during 14-16 days of incubation.
Manganese (Mn)	• Reduced hatchability and embryonic abnormalities almost identical to those of biotin deficiencies. • Ataxia in the form of a tetanic spasm of the opisthotonic type has been described in manganese-deficient embryos (Caskey *et al.*, 1944). • Chondrodystrophy, parrot beak resulting from a disproportionate shortening of the lower mandible is also seen

Iodine (I)	• Excess dietary iodine will also cause hatchability problems, resulting in embryonic mortality, unhatched pips, and extended incubation periods (Arrington *et al.*, 1967).
Selenium (Se)	• Deficiency causes decrease in hatchability, chicks hatched were weak and had gizzard muscle myopathy and legs extended backward and curved upward. • Abnormalities due to excess of selenium include dwarfing, short or missing lower beak, and shortened bones of the legs and wings. • Supplementation of Organic Se in diets of laying hen increase hatchability of fertile eggs (Hanafy *et al.*, 2009). • Organic selenium in layer diets improved the environment of the sperm storage tubule in hens oviduct allowing the sperm to live for longer time which increases the fertility (Agate *et al.* 2009). • In breeder nutrition, vitamin E, carotenoids and selenium received most of attention as a way of improving stress resistance of poultry.
Boron	• Feeding high levels of boron in the form of boric acid or borax to broiler breeder hens decreased hatchability, but did not affect egg production (Rossi *et al.*,1993). • Males fed high levels of boron had an increased incidence of abnormal spermatozoa.

Conclusion

Nutrition of breeder stock has a crucial role in subsequent development and hatching of embryos. Over and undersupply of nutrients into and through lay can have a very significant impact on breeder production and quality of progeny. Hence, greater attention must be given on the nutrition of the breeder stock providing the balanced diet without neglecting the vitamins and minerals and to provide appropriate feed allocation in lay. Therefore, it should be a standard practice to sample all batches of breeder feed for routine analysis and as an aid in troubleshooting hatchability and production problems. Diseases, parasitic infections, chemical and biological toxins, poisons, malabsorption syndromes, or drugs may also cause nutritional or pseudo nutritional problems in hatchability or chick quality. In addition to above factors environmental factors, genotypes, and interactions among the numerous factors are also common

References

Agate, D.D., O'dea, E.E. and Rustad, M.E. 2000. Effects of dietary selenium on laying hen fertility as assessed by the periviteline sperm hole assay. In Proceedings of the poultry research and production symposium, Alberta poultry research centre (pp. 1-4).

Arrington, L.R., Santa Cruz, R.A., Harms, R.H. and Wilson, H.R. 1967. Effects of excess dietary iodine upon pullets and laying hens. The Journal of Nutrition, 92(3), pp.325-330.

Caskey, C.D., Norris, L.C. and Heuser, G.F. 1944. A chronic congenital ataxia in chicks due to manganese deficiency in the maternal diet. Poultry Science, 23(6), pp.516-520.

Danicke, S., Jeroch, H., Bottcher, W. and Simon, O. 2000. Interactions between dietary fat type and enzyme supplementation in broiler diets with high pentosan contents: effects on precaecal and total tract digestibility of gross energy, digesta viscosity and weights of small intestine. Animal Feed Science and Technology, 84: 879-294.

De Beer, M. and Coon, C.N. 2007. The effect of different feed restriction programs on reproductive performance, efficiency, frame size, and uniformity in broiler breeder hens. Poultry Science, 86(9): 1927-1939.

De Beer, M. and Coon, C.N. 2009. The effect of feed restriction programs and growth curves on reproductive performance, in vitro lipogenesis and heterophil to lymphocyte ratios in broiler breeder hens. International Journal of Poultry Science, 8: 373-388.

Ekmay, R.D., De Beer, M., Mei, S.J., Manangi, M. and Coon, C.N. 2013. Amino acid requirements of broiler breeders at peak production for egg mass, body weight, and fertility. Poultry Science, 92(4): 992-1006.

Ferguson, T.M., Sewell Jr, C.E. and Atkinson, R.L. 1974. Phosphorus levels in the turkey breeder diet. Poultry Science, 53(4): 1627-1629.

Gillis, M. B., Heuser, G. F. and Norris, L. C. 1947. The pantothenic acid requirement of hens for reproduction. Poultry Science, 26:540. (Abstr.)

Hanafy, M. M., El-Sheik, A. M. H. and Abdalla, E. A. 2009. The effect of organic selenium supplementation on productive and physiological performance in local strain of chicken. Egyptian Poultry Science, 29:1061–1084

Heier, B.T. and Jarp, J. 2001. An epidemiological study of the hatchability in broiler breeder flocks. Poultry Science, 80(8): 1132-1138.

Hocking, P.M., Bernard, R. and Robertson, G.W. 2002. Effects of low dietary protein and different allocations of food during rearing and restricted feeding after peak rate of lay on egg production, fertility and hatchability in female broiler breeders. British Poultry Science, 43(1): 94-103.

Jiang, Z., Cherian, G., Robinson, F. E. and Sim, J. S. 1990. Effect of feeding cholesterol to laying hens and chicks on cholesterol metabolism in pre- and posthatch chicks. Poultry Science, 69:1694–1701

Khajali, F., Khoshouie, E.A., Dehkordi, S.K. and Hematian, M. 2008. Production performance and egg quality of Hy-line W36 laying hens fed reduced-protein diets at a constant total sulfur amino acid: lysine ratio. Journal of Applied Poultry Research, 17(3): 390-397.

Khan, R.U., Rahman, Z.U., Javed, I. and Muhammad, F. 2012. Effect of vitamins, probiotics and protein on semen traits in post-molt male broiler breeders. Animal Reproduction Science, 135(1-4): 85-90.

Kienholz, E. W., Turk, D. E., Sunde, M. L. and Hoekstra, W. G. 1961. Effects of zinc deficiency in the diets of hens. Journal of Nutrition, 75: 211–221

Kirk, S., Emmans, G.C., McDonald, R. and Arnot, D. 1980. Factors affecting the hatchability of eggs from broiler breeders. British Poultry Science, 21(1): 37-53.

Landauer, W. 1967. The hatchability of chicken eggs as influenced by environment and heredity. Monograph 1 (Revised). Storrs Agricultural Experiment Station, Storrs, CT.

Lavelle, P.A., Lloyd, Q.P., Gay, C.V. and Leach Jr, R.M. 1994. Vitamin K deficiency does not functionally impair skeletal metabolism of laying hens and their progeny. The Journal of nutrition, 124(3): 371-377.

Leeson, S. 2009. Copper metabolism and dietary needs. World's Poultry Science Journal, 65(3): 353-366.

Leeson, S. and Summers, J. D. 1991. Commercial Poultry Nutrition. University Books, Guelph, ON, Canada

Leeson, S., Reinhart, B. S. and Summers, J. D. 1979b. Response of White Leghorn and Rhode Island Red breeder hens to dietary deficiencies of synthetic vitamins. 2. Embryo mortality and abnormalities. Canadian Journal of Animal Science, 59: 569-575.

Lillie, R. J., Olsen, M. W. and Bird, H. R. 1951. Variation in reproductive response of hens to dietary deficiency. Poultry Science, 30: 92–97.

Lopez, G. and Leeson, S.1995. Response of broiler breeders to low-protein diets. 1. Adult breeder performance. Poultry Science, 74: 685–695.

McDaniel, G.R., Roland Sr, D.A. and Coleman, M.A. 1979. The effect of egg shell quality on hatchability and embryonic mortality. Poultry Science, 58(1): 10-13.

Noble, R. C. and Yafei, N. 1988. An association between low embryo hatchability in eggs from young broiler birds and aspects of lipid metabolism. Pages 640–641 in: Proceedings 18th World's Poultry Congress. Nagoya, Japan.

O'Rourke, W. F., Bird, H. R., Phillips, P. H. and Cravens, W. W. 1954. The effect of low phosphorus rations on egg production and hatchability. Poultry Science, 33: 1117–1122

Pearson, R. A. and Herron, K. M. 1982. Effects of maternal energy and protein intakes on the incidence of malformations and malpositions of the embryo and time of death during incubation. British Poultry Science, 23: 71–77

Pérez-Bonilla, A., Novoa, S., García, J., Mohiti-Asli, M., Frikha, M. and Mateos, G.G. 2012. Effects of energy concentration of the diet on productive performance and egg quality of brown egg-laying hens differing in initial body weight. Poultry Science, 91(12): 3156-3166.

Potter, L.M., Leighton Jr, A.T. and Chu, A.B. 1974. Calcium, phosphorus and Nopgro as variables in diets of breeder turkeys. Poultry Science, 53(1): 15-22.

Renema, R.A., Robinson, F.E., Goerzen, P.R. and Zuidhof, M.J. 2001. Effects of altering growth curve and age at photostimulation in female broiler breeders. 2. Egg production parameters. Canadian journal of animal science, 81(4): 477-486.

Romanoff, A. L., and Romanoff, A. J. 1972. Pathogenesis of the Avian Embryo. Wiley Interscience, New York, NY

Rossi, A.F., Miles, R.D., Bootwalla, S.M., Wilson, H.R. and Eldred, A.R. 1993. The effect of feeding two sources of boron on broiler breeder performance. Poultry science, 72(10): 1931-1934.

Sewell Jr, C.E., Atkinson, R.L., Couch, J.R. and Ferguson, T.M. 1972. The effect of supplemental phosphorus on the reproductive performance of turkey hens and the subsequent effect upon the poults. Poultry science, 51(3): 792-796.

Shim, M.Y., Song, E., Billard, L., Aggrey, S.E., Pesti, G.M. and Sodsee, P. 2013. Effects of balanced dietary protein levels on egg production and egg quality parameters of individual commercial layers. Poultry science, 92(10): 2687-2696.

Singsen, E.P., Spandorf, A.H., Matterson, L.D., Serafin, J.A. and Tlustohowicz, J.J. 1962. Phosphorus in the nutrition of the adult hen: 1. Minimum phosphorus requirements. Poultry science, 41(5): 1401-1414.

Sirri, F., Maiorano, G., Tavaniello, S., Chen, J., Petracci, M. and Meluzzi, A. 2016. Effect of different levels of dietary zinc, manganese, and copper from organic or inorganic sources on performance, bacterial chondronecrosis, intramuscular collagen characteristics, and occurrence of meat quality defects of broiler chickens. Poultry Science, 95(8): 1813-1824.

Skøivan, M., Marounek, M., Dlouhá, G. and Ševèíková, S. 2008. Dietary selenium increases vitamin E contents of egg yolk and chicken meat. British Poultry Science, 49(4): 482-486.

Sun, J. and Coon, C.N. 2005. The effects of body weight, dietary fat, and feed withdrawal rate on the performance of broiler breeders. Journal of Applied Poultry Research, 14(4): 728-739.

Surai, P.F. 2000. Effect of selenium and vitamin E content of the maternal diet on the antioxidant system of the yolk and the developing chick. British poultry science, 41(2): 235-243.

Surai, P.F. and Sparks, N.H.C. 2001. Comparative evaluation of the effect of two maternal diets on fatty acids, vitamin E and carotenoids in the chick embryo. British Poultry Science, 42(2): 252-259.

Surai, P.F., Noble, R.C. and Speake, B.K. 1999. Relationship between vitamin E content and susceptibility to lipid peroxidation in tissues of the newly hatched chick. British Poultry Science, 40(3): 406-410.

Tona, K., Onagbesan, O., Bruggeman, V., Mertens, K. and Decuypere, E. 2005. Effects of turning duration during incubation on embryo growth, utilization of albumen, and stress regulation. Poultry Science, 84(2): 315-320.

Tufarelli, V. and Laudadio, V. 2016. Antioxidant activity of vitamin E and its role in avian reproduction. Journal of Experimental Biology and Agricultural Sciences, 4(3): 266-272.

Tullett, S. G. 1990. Science and the art of incubation. Poultry Science, 69:1–15

Van Emous, R.A., Kwakkel, R.P., Van Krimpen, M.M., Van den Brand, H. and Hendriks, W.H. 2015. Effects of growth patterns and dietary protein levels during rearing of broiler breeders on fertility, hatchability, embryonic mortality, and offspring performance. Poultry Science, 94(4): 681-691.

Vilchez, C., Touchburn, S.P., Chavez, E.R. and Chan, C.W. 1990. The influence of supplemental corn oil and free fatty acids on the reproductive performance of Japanese quail (Coturnix coturnix japonica). Poultry Science, 69(9): 1533-1538.

Vilchez, C., Touchburn, S.P., Chavez, E.R. and Chan, C.W. 1992. Effect of feeding palmitic, oleic, and linoleic acids to Japanese quail hens (Coturnix coturnix japonica). 2. Maternal diets and stage of incubation on the lipid metabolism of quail embryos. Poultry Science, 71:1032–1042

Vilchez, C., Touchburn, S.P., Chavez, E.R. and Chan, C.W.1990b. Dietary palmitic and linoleic acids and reproduction of Japanese quail (Coturnix coturnix japonica). Poultry Science, 69: 1922–1930

Waldroup, P.W., Simpson, C.F., Damron, B.L. and Harms, R.H. 1967. The effectiveness of plant and inorganic phosphorus in supporting egg production in hens and hatchability and bone development in chick embryos. Poultry Science, 46(3): 659-664.

Whitehead, C.C., Bowman, A.S. and Griffin, H.D. 1993. Regulation of plasma oestrogen by dietary fats in the laying hen: relationships with egg weight. British Poultry Science, 34(5): 999-1010.

Whitehead, C.C., Maxwell, M.H., Pearson, R.A. and Herron, K.M. 1985. Influence of egg storage on hatchability, embryonic development and vitamin status in hatching broiler chicks. British Poultry Science, 26(2): 221-228.

Wilson, H.R. 1991. Interrelationships of egg size, chick size, posthatching growth and hatchability. World's Poultry Science Journal, 47(1): 5-20.

Wilson, H.R. 1993. Hatchability problem analysis. University of Florida, Institute of Food and Agricultural Sciences, Florida Cooperative Extension Service.

Wilson, H.R. 1997. Effects of maternal nutrition on hatchability. Poultry Science, 76(1): 134-143.

Wilson, H.R., Miller, E.R., Harms, R.H. and Damron, B.L. 1980. Hatchability of chicken eggs as affected by dietary phosphorus and calcium. Poultry Science, 59(6): 1284-1289.

Yenice, E., Mizrak, C., Ceylan, N., Yildiz, T., Gültekin, M. and Atik, Z. 2015. Effects of dietary sodium bentonite and mannan oligosaccharide supplementation on performance, egg quality, blood and digestion characteristics of laying hens fed aflatoxin contaminated diet. Kafkas Univ Vet Fak Derg, 2: 211-218.

16

Feed Technological Interventions for Augmenting Poultry Productivity

Y.A. Beigh, A.M. Ganai, S. Adil, M.T. Banday and Z. Haq

Faculty of Veterinary Science and Animal Husbandry, Sher-e-Kashmir University of Agricultural Sciences and Technology of Kashmir, Shuhama, Alusteng Srinagar-190 006, Jammu and Kashmir, India

Introduction

The Indian poultry industry has emerged as the most dynamic and fastest expanding segment in animal husbandry sector with an annual growth rate of 23% in broiler chickens and 5% in egg production. The production performance of birds in terms of meat and egg has also improved significantly; however, the sector has crippled many times due to various reasons among which the important ones were rising feed cost, non-availability og feed ingredients, fluctuating market price of produce (eggs and broilers) and emergence of new or re-emerging of existing diseases. In future, poultry industry may face more such challenges.

The cost of feed accounts for 65-70% of broiler and 75-80% of layer production cost and is a major means of manipulating the production cost. The feeding cost alone being the major constraint in poultry enterprise, every effort is directed to maintain feed quality, contain feed cost and utilize every bit of the feed to convert into food for the mankind. The cost, easy availability and nutritional quality of feed coupled with genetically potent feed efficient stocks to produce safe food from poultry are the need of time. The ways to curtail feeding cost for maximizing profitability and reduce wastage of nutrients for lowering soil/ water pollution due to loss of the nutrients through excretion are establishment of optimal nutrient requirements to keep up with genetic improvements, and efficient utilization of nutrients/feed through feed technological interventions. The interest in the application of feed technology has increased, as the industry continues to search for ways of optimizing feed utilization and improving production efficiency. Various technological innovations in the area of poultry nutrition include:

1. Feed processing interventions in poultry feeding

i. *Particle size reduction*: This process is known to influence a number of aspects of poultry production, including bird performance, digestive tract development, gut health and functionality. In commercial feed industries this is done with hammer mill. The particle size and efficiency of the hammer mill is influenced by a number of factors, including grain type, grain moisture content, screen size and area, hammer peripheral speed, hammer length, number of hammers, hammer tip to screen clearance, feed rate, power of the motor and speed of air flow through the mill (Martin, 1985). Size is defined as the average diameter of individual particles of feed or "fineness of grind" of the feed. ASAE (1983) has developed method to describe particle sizes wherein the particle size is expressed as geometric mean diameter (GMD), in mm or microns (μm) and the variation as geometric standard deviation (GSD), with a larger GSD representing lower uniformity. GMD and GSD are accurate measures only when particle size distribution is expressed as log data, and when the distribution is normal. Feed particle size is typically determined by dry sieving of a 100-gram representative sample (Baker and Herrman, 2002) using sieves of different pore size. The suggested GMD of cereal grains for broiler chickens for age 1 to 7 d, 7 to 21 and 21 plus days is 900-1100, 1100 -1300 and 1300-1500 microns respectively. Particle size is more critical in mash feeds than for pelleted / crumbled feed. In today broilers production industry, the use of mash feed has nearly replaced with crumble or pellet feed. However, nutrition research in broilers is carried out using mash feed, wherein the particle size will be very useful.

ii. *Pelleting/crumbling*: Broilers fed pelleted diets have greater feed intake, better FCR and greater weight gain (Corzo et al., 2011) due to improved nutrients digestibility (Zalenka, 2003), reduced feed wastage and energy spent for eating. The better performance can only be achieved, if the pellets maintain their integrity till ingested by the birds. Pellet quality is measured as "Pellet durability index" (PDI) using "Holmen pellet tester" which measures the percentage of intact pellets or fines subjected to mechanical forces. Poor-quality pellets disintegrate, resulting in a feed consisting of a few pellets and fines. The geometric mean diameter (GMD) of fine particles is equal or lower than that of mash diets (Mckinney and Teeter, 2004). Several factors affect pellet quality, such as dietary nutritional composition, feedstuff particle size, conditioning time and temperature, feed moisture content, compression rate of pellet die, gap between the pellet press roll and die (Colovic, 2010) or interactions among these factors etc. The extend of contributor (in %) to pellet quality is Formulation-40,

Particle size-20, Mixing-5, Die specification-10, Conditioning-20 and cooling-5.

Particle size reduction influences pellet quality, however the influence of size does not influences the performance. Reducing particle size increases particle surface area thereby increasing the number of contact sites among particle and increases penetration of heat and moisture to the centre of the feed particle. Dozier, (2001) suggested that for broiler diets based on corn and soybean meal, the optimal GMD for pellet durability should be between 650 μm and 700 μm, Reece et al. (1986) reported ideal GMD between 680 and 1024 μm. The upper range of particle size is preferred as they increased gizzard development and improves gizzard motility. Very fine reduction of particle size of feedstuffs may not be beneficial to pellet quality.

With respect to feed formulation on pellet quality, it should be noted that starch is a natural adhesive when heat and moisture are applied, protein can be positive and significant effect, although it seems to be dependent on the source (zein protein in corn and gluten protein in wheat) and the other ingredients in the diet. Need for fat Inclusion: High fat in the formulation results in less pellet durability. Fat reduces the contact of the meal with die-hole walls, facilitating quick passage of feed through the die and thereby reducing feed compaction inside the die holes (Fahrenholz, 2012). The addition of fat before conditioning causes partial encapsulation of feed particles and hinders the penetration of steam, thus reduces starch gelatinization and weakens capillary adhesion forces (Fahrenholz, 2012). The amount of added fat should be limited to 0.5-1 % of feed to produce good quality pellet (Leaver, 2008). Fairfield 2003 observed adding more than 2 % fat in the mixer previous to pelleting decreases the PDI of diets based on corn and soybean meal. The post pellet liquid fat application (PPLA) of supplemental fat is an alternative to maintain the integrity of the pellets.

iii. *Crumbling:* The cooled pellet, if it has to be reduced in size for feeding of young chicken, they need to be crumbled. Before the pellet is send to the crumbler, the fines of the pellet are sieved. A crumbler is a roller mill with rolls specially designed for breaking up pellets into smaller particles. Usually the crumbler consists of two corrugated rolls situated below the cooler/drier exit. The pellets can then be diverted into the crumbler, if crumbles or granules are desired, or they can by-pass it. The principle of Feed Pellet Crumbler is it has quick and slow roller, transmission mechanism, roll gap adjusting mechanism and tightening devices. The cooled feed pellets travels through the feeding roller to the open valve and between the two rollers. The rollers runs in differential speed making the pellet materials to be squeezed, cut and tore between the two rollers, resulting in crushing effect. The size of the pellet can be reduced to meet the different requirement, the size achieved here can be 0.6-1.5 mm (fine type) or 1-2.5 mm (normal type).

2. Incorporation of feed additives in poultry diets

Excessive and extensive use of antimicrobials and heightened interest in public security has given rise to concern about the development of antimicrobial-resistant human pathogenic bacteria. As a result, the use of in-feed antimicrobials in poultry diets as feed additives to enhance growth was banned in the EU in 2006. This was followed by a worldwide drive to use antimicrobials purely as therapeutic agents to treat bacterial infections. An effective alternative to antimicrobials should be safe for both the animal and consumer, have a significant and sustainable beneficial impact on poultry production and be easy to apply and store. Cost is obviously a major criterion, due to the low profit margins of poultry. Alternatives to antimicrobials promote gastrointestinal health by mechanisms such as altering pH, selecting for beneficial organisms and against pathogens and improving nutrient uptake and immune responses. Feed additives that can reduce gastrointestinal pH in the bird, such as organic acids and polyunsaturated acids, are advantageous because pathogenic bacteria cannot flourish at low pH.

There are also a number of feed additives that have a direct impact on microbiota balance in the bird like essential oils for example cavacrol from oregano, can suppress pathogenic bacteria and help maintain the structure of the gut. Phytogenic feed additives (often also called phytobiotics or botanicals) are plant-derived compounds incorporated into diets to improve the livestock productivity through amelioration of feed properties, promotion of the animals' production performance, enhancement of immunity and improving the quality of food derived from those animals. For the reason, various phytogenic compounds as feed additives have been used in poultry diets in terms of claimed antioxidative and antimicrobial actions, beneficial effects on palatability and gut functions, and growth-promoting efficacy (Windisch *et al.*, 2008).

The use of pro- and pre-biotics in poultry nutrition is a hot topic. Probiotics are cultures of living organisms that can enhance stability of the beneficial microbiota and reduce growth of pathogens and promote gut health and immunity. Prebiotics provide energy for the favorable bacteria which helps to eliminate the pathogens; the most common prebiotics are small chain sugars called oligosaccharides. Yeasts are promising alternatives to antimicrobials because they show diverse biological activities against pathogens, such as reducing pH, preventing them binding to the gut and releasing compounds that directly attack them, as well as being rich in β-glucans which enhance immunity. There are conflicting results with the application of these different feed additives, and a great deal more research needs to be conducted in this field. It must also be noted that nutritional strategies alone cannot overcome the issues caused by removing antimicrobials, good management practices are also required.

Exogenous enzymes are almost ubiquitous in poultry diets, as the birds are not able to produce sufficient endogenous enzymes themselves, or produce them in the correct locations, to facilitate absorption of all components in normal feed or reduce the anti-nutritional factors in feed that limit digestion. The use of enzymes such as xylanases, phytases and β-glucanases can reduce variability and enhance digestibility by releasing encapsulated nutrients, namely starch and protein, and reduce viscosity in the gastrointestinal tract. Exogenous enzyme supplementation to cereal-based diets can significantly improve chick performance by increasing the rate of gain, efficiency of feed utilization, the apparent metabolizable energy and digestibilities of dry matter, fat and protein, with excellent improvements being obtained with diets containing rye, oats and barley. Less dramatic results are often obtained with wheat. In addition, enzyme treatment decreases the moisture content of excreta, which, together with improved dry matter digestibility, reduces the total amount of excreta produced and therefore reduces management and environmental problems. Enzyme supplementation also improves the nutritional value of lupins, and reduces the length and size of various sections of the gastrointestinal tract and the size of the pancreas of chickens (Marquardt *et al.*, 1996).

3. Use of wastes as alternate feeds in poultry rations

In both developed and developing countries, continued growth of the by-product industry is anticipated. This means that large quantities of various waste-products of animal and vegetable/fruit origin will be available. These wastes are generated particularly by the agricultural and industrial segments. For reason of better utilization of these by-products/wastes to curtail the increasing costs and increased consciousness of environmental protection, the use of waste in practical livestock and poultry diets should be increased thereby decreasing the competition for food between humans and poultry.

Wastes can be utilized either directly (as a diet ingredient, such as citrus pulp or feather meal) or indirectly (upgrading by micro-organisms such as algae, larvae house-fly, earthworm, solid state fermentation etc.) for livestock and poultry feeding. Since many by-products or wastes have a substantial potential value as a diet ingredient in livestock diets this kind of utilization may be economically worthwhile especially in developing countries where traditional and often expensive feedstuffs can be replaced to reduce animal/poultry feeding costs and lower prices for animal products. It also contributes to self-sufficiency in nutrients from locally present wastes. Therefore, the system of feed from waste makes possible a vertical, mutually complemented integration of animal production among individual species which can in turn solve some problems of local waste disposal and thus some problems of pollution (Muller, 1980).

In different animal studies, most of the tested fruit wastes either as fresh or dried served as excellent alternate feed resources for livestock and poultry (Wadhwa and Makkar, 2013). Edwards *et al.* (1986) reported that cooked potatoes could be used up to 40 percent in poultry rations. Dried citrus pulp could replace 5-10 percent concentrate in poultry diets (Mourao *et al.*, 2008).

4. *In-ovo* feeding interventions

One of the earliest recommendations for providing feed at hatch was to provide it in the hatching trays (Sklan *et al.*, 2000). This practice is fraught with problems owing to the tight regulation of environmental factors in the hatchery. High-quality diets containing many supplements have also been developed for provision to the chicks once they reach the farm. Generally, feeding immediately post-hatch has been shown to be more beneficial than feeding high-quality diets after a delay in feeding. *In ovo* feeding of nutrients is more effective option, and this is the approach that has been developed by Uni and Ferket, (2003). The nutrients are supplemented to the developing embryo through the amniotic sac at a later stage of development (day 18 of incubation) to provide a continuous supply of critical nutrients during the first few days (3–4 days) of the post-hatch period, thereby facilitating enteric development and metabolism. This is distinct from other methods of *in ovo* nutrient administration. *In ovo* nutrient administration appears to have a significant effect on hatching weights, but the responses in terms of final weights and feed conversion efficiency are not consistent. This failure to obtain tangible benefits may be due to a lack of suitable nutritional products for administration, but there are also fears of a reduction in hatchability as a result of *in ovo* feeding of some nutrients.

The genetic potential of the bird is dictated by early nutrition. Carcass traits from a bird are judged at 42 days of age when the bird spends 33% of its life in the egg. Nutritional intakes of the hen dictates the ability of the bird to meet its' genetic potential. Feeding hens a diet varying in a myriad of nutrients impacts early chick development and carcass development (Kidd, 2003). It has been claimed that this technique has much potential to yield several advantages, among them reduced post-hatch mortality and morbidity; greater efficiency of feed nutrient utilization at an early age; improved immune response to enteric antigens; reduced incidence of developmental skeletal disorders; and increased muscle development and breast meat yield (Noy and Uni, 2010). Many potential nutrients have been tested in this direction, and new findings are being reported. Although response at the neonatal stage is typically observed, whether such advantage is lost at a later stage is not well established. The use of *in ovo* feeding for poultry may also gain from identification of more suitable and effective nutrients. There are still some inconsistencies in the benefits of different nutrients that have been assessed. This may be due to the impact of the treatment on osmotic pressure or other physical effects on the developing embryo. Chicks may also benefit more from a combination of *in ovo* nutrient administration and early post-hatch feeding (Shariatmadari, 2012). It is likely that future research will increasingly focus on the ways in which genes are affected by nutrients that are introduced into the egg.

5. Nutrigenomics in poultry production

Nutrition has always been known to induce metabolic changes in muscle which are reflected in tissue remodelling, increased protein turnover, and muscle atrophy. From a production point of view, these changes influence efficiency of production and meat quality. As a result, they are of tremendous economic importance. It is often difficult to rapidly diagnose nutritional limitations associated with particular dietary components and management strategies. The concept of nutritional genomics or specifically the term nutrigenomics developed at the turn of the 21st century to describe the trend in human nutrition research towards individualized dietary formulation. Nutrigenomics refers to study of the effects of nutrients/bioactive food on gene expression of an individual. The study of how genes and gene products interact with dietary chemicals to alter phenotype and conversely, how genes and their products metabolize nutrients is called nutritional genomics or nutrigenomics. In nutrigenomics, nutrients are signals to specific cells in the body, when interpreting the information of such a nutrient, the cell reacts by sending biochemical information from DNA or genes (the science of genomics) to RNA (the science of transcriptomics) which is in turn translated into specific proteins (science of proteomics) and ultimately determines the metabolic pathways.

Dietary fats have profound effects on gene expression. Effect of specific fatty acid to regulate transcription factors have been identified in bacteria, amphibians and mammals. In mammals, these factors include peroxisome proliferator-activated receptors (PPAR α, -β/δ, and -γ), oestrogen receptors

(ERs) and sterol regulatory element binding proteins (SREBPs). At the cellular level, the physiological response to fatty acids will depend on the quantity, chemistry and duration of the fat ingested. Protein-rich diets cause a shortage of mRNA necessary for expression of the fatty acid synthase gene in the adipocytes, resulting in the moderation of total body fat. Such an effect cannot be observed in the liver tissue (Clarke, 1993). Hepatic fat synthesis, in turn, can be inhibited by providing unsaturated fatty acids in the diet. Likewise, bivalent metals strongly influence gene expression. For instance, either parenteral and oral zinc or cadmium application enhances the transcription rate of the metallothionein (MT) gene in intestinal tissue (Ouellette *et al.*, 1982). Cadmium acts also in prolonging the half-life of MT mRNA in hepatocytes. This effect on the half-life prolongation of MT mRNA is metal and tissue specific: the influence of cadmium is stronger than that of zinc.

6. Use of synthetic amino-acids in poultry feeding

Protein is a costly nutrient in poultry feeds. Broiler diets are usually formulated using linear least cost software frequently setting a minimum concentration of crude protein (CP) in a strategy to have minimum levels of indispensable and dispensable amino-acids intakes so that performance is not limited. The increasing cost of feed ingredients and the competition with the bio-fuel industry indicates a scenario of increased costs for plant based ingredients in the future. Additionally, the composition of amino-acids in the diets is variable according to ingredient inclusion; different protein sources (plant or animal), and inclusion of synthetic and crystalline amino-acids. Formulating diets with a reduced CP level is possible with the use of supplemental amino-acids if commercially available at competitive prices. Using the ideal protein concept also allows for a greater precision in formulation and ensures that a balanced amino-acids profile is formulated to optimise growth performance and breast meat yields. This formulating approach has been increasing among nutritionists and targets the reduction in imbalances between the limiting amino-acids and other dietary amino-acids (Vieira and Angel, 2012).

The main commercially available supplemental amino-acids sources used in poultry diets are L-Lysine (L-Lys), DL-Methionine (DL-Met) or Methionine analogues (Met-ana), and L-Threonine (L-Thr). These are usually included in diets as digestible amino-acids maintaining ratios to digistible lysine (Lys) to satisfy the ideal protein concept (Baker and Han, 1994). Nutritionists also have to consider the opportunities for commercial use of crystalline valine (L-Val) and isoleucine (L-Ile), which can further reduce minimum dietary CP, as these are fourth- and fifth-limiting amino-acids added to maize-soy diets (Berres *et al.*, 2010).

7. Use of chelated minerals in poultry rations

Organic minerals are considered the most significant event regarding commercial forms of minerals targeting animal supplementation in the last decades. Minerals, especially metals, are usually supplemented in poultry feeds using cheap saline sources and have never required a lot of attention in terms of quality. On the other hand, definitions of organic minerals are very broad and frequently lead to confusion when decision-making becomes necessary. Organic minerals include any mineral bound to organic compounds, regardless of the type of existing bond between mineral and organic molecules. Proteins and carbohydrates are the most frequent candidates in organic mineral combinations. Organic fraction size and bond type are not limitations in organic mineral definition; however, essential metals (Cu, Fe, Zn, and Mn) can form coordinated bonds, which are stable in intestinal lumen. Metals bound to organic ligands by coordinated bonds can dissociate within animal metabolism whereas real covalent bonds cannot. Chelated minerals are molecules that have a metal bound to an organic ligand through coordinated bonds; but many organic minerals are not chelates or are not even bound through coordinated bonds. Utilization of organic minerals is largely dependent on the ligand; therefore, amino acids and other small molecules with facilitated access to the enterocyte are supposed to be better utilized by animals. Organic minerals with ligands presenting long chains may require digestion prior to absorption. After absorption, organic minerals may present physiological effects, which improve specific metabolic responses, such as the immune response.

Results demonstrate a clear trend for a better utilization and higher bioavailability for chelated mineral supplements. Differences between traditional trace mineral sources are due to the salt source and, at least for zinc and copper, oxides have minimal contribution for poultry (Han and Baker, 1993). Zinc-methionine supplemented to corn-soybean meal diets presented 206% bioavailability, but only 117% when included in a purified diet without phytate (Wedekind *et al.*, 1992). Zinc-methionine usually has higher bioavailability than inorganic sources, and can be absorbed in its intact form, therefore potentially altering zinc balance in metabolism. Independently of the involved mechanisms, improvements were shown in some cell functions related to disease resistance when zinc-methionine was supplemented in broiler or breeder feeds (Kidd, 1996). Mineral chelates are currently more expensive than the traditional mineral supplements. However, there are indications that, at least in some situations, chelated minerals can achieve biological objectives better than inorganic sources (Patton, 1997).

8. Biotechnological application in poultry nutrition

Applications of biotechnology in the poultry industry is useful in improving productivity through increased growth, carcass quality and reproduction, improved nutrition and feed utilization, improved quality and safety of food, improved health and welfare of animals, and reduced waste through more efficient utilization of resources. Besides, biotechnology also play role in development of new and improved feedstuffs, as well as in microbiology as related to food and bioremediation. In poultry nutrition, biotechnology is more useful in the following areas of:

a) *Feed additives:* The use of biotechnological products is relatively well established in the feed industry and shows considerable potential for further growth. A wide range of applications, both current and potential includes silage inoculants, supplementation of amino acids, diagnostics for food safety (i.e. mycotoxins), removal of anti-nutritional factors and toxins through enzymes, enzymes for increased digestibility of nutrients (monogastric and ruminant), enzymes for increased digestibility of non-starch polysaccharides, supplementation of endogenous enzymes for improved digestion, supplementation of immune products such as disease-specific antibodies, supplementation of hormones and prebiotics to promote gut growth and health, supplementation of probiotics and supplementation of enzymes to reduce nutrient content in waste.

b) *Nutrients:* Grain based feeds for poultry are deficient in several amino acids including methionine and tryptophan. The deficiency of nutrients in the feed and growing intensification of the poultry production systems has required an extensive use of several nutrients in the developing world. For instance, the amino acid market present in India alone is worth a total of 5 million US dollars. Many of these essential amino acids are being produced from *Escherichia coli* through recombinant DNA technology (http://www.fao.org/biotech/c16doc.html). Non-traditional applications of amino acids may involve the use of arginine and aspartic acid (Kuhara et al., 1991) as potent stimulants of pituitary somatotropin release and enhance growth and carcass quality.

c) *Enzymes:* By the aid of biotechnology, more effective exogenous enzyme preparations can now be produced in large amount and relatively inexpensively. Therefore, supplementation of these enzymes as a means of improving nutritive value is becoming commonplace. Their major purpose is to improve the nutritive value of available diets, especially when poor-quality like, roughage and usually less expensive, ingredients is incorporated. Amino acid digestibility is improved with phytase enzyme supplementation. Cellulase enzymes can be used to break down cellulose, which is not degraded by endogenous mammalian enzymes. Enzymes are essential for the breakdown of cell-wall carbohydrates to release the sugars necessary for the growth of the lactic acid bacteria. Supplementation of a wheat byproduct diet with cellulase increased the digestibility of non-starch polysaccharides from 0.192 to 0.359 and crude protein from 0.65 to 0.71 (Mc Donald *et al.*, 2010).

d) *Transgenic feeds:* Many developed and developing countries adopted the cultivation of the transgenic crops for human and animal nutrition. In 2007, a total of 23 countries cultivated transgenic plants on around 114 million hectares which represented about 5% of arable land worldwide. These areas were concentrated very strongly on five countries in the North and South America in where 88% of the acreage was located (USA: 57.7 million hectares; Argentina: 19.1 million hectares; Brazil 15.0 million hectares; Canada: 7.0 million hectare; Paraguay: 2.6 million hectares), India (6.2 million hectares), China (3.8 million hectares) and South Africa (1.5 million hectares). Even after 12 years of cultivation only two genetic traits, i.e. herbicide tolerance (HR) and insect resistance to *Bacillus thuringiensis* (Bt), either alone or in combination, account for 99.9% of cultivated genetically modified plants, in only four crop varieties (51.3% soybean, 30.8% maize, 13.1% cotton, and 4.8% rapeseed/canola) (http://www.tab.fzk.de/en/ projekt/zusammenfassung/ab128.htm) Many animal studies were conductedto assess the nutritive values of the first generation (feed plants with changed tolerance or resistance and with minor changes in the content of valuable and desirable ingredients) genetically modified plants (GMP) such as Bt-maize, Bt-potatoes, Pat-maize, Patsugar beet and roundup ready Soybeans, and the second generation plants. From the results it was concluded that there was no significant difference in the nutritive value between isogenic and first generation transgenic feeds (Flachowsky *et al.*, 2007). Very few companies in developing countries are supplying transgenic soybean protein as an animal feed (e.g., Shandong Rongfeng Biotechnology Development Co., Ltd. China). Further research and extension is required to reduce the cost and to adapt the transgenic crops technology in the field conditions.

e) *Immune product supplements:* Immune products may be included in feeds to alter microbial flora and to reduce the effect of pathogens. One of these products is spray dried plasma protein containing antibodies that provide protection, sometimes variable, against common pathogens. Spray dried plasma protein consistently improves feed intake and growth in animals weaned early. This product is derived from blood collected at slaughter plants, and therefore the protection provided depends on the exposure to pathogens prior to slaughter. Laying hens can be vaccinated against specific viral and bacterial pathogens commonly responsible for high morbidity and mortality in weaning pigs (Yokoyama *et al.*, 1992). The egg yolk, rich in disease-specific antibodies, is spray dried and fed to weaning pigs with the added advantage that a highly nutritious product is provided.

9. Biological processing of poultry feeds

Generally, the by-products from plant origin are rich in nutrients. There are many reports on the utilization of these agro-byproducts as poultry feed and nutrient enrichment can be performed by solid state fermentation and bio-processing technologies. Most of the reports show that nutritional and nutraceutical properties of the agro-byproducts as solid substrates were improved by fermentation. Thus, scope exists for microbial upgradation of low-quality agro-wastes and development of healthy poultry feed supplements. The production of poultry feed from agro-residues represents one of the economically beneficial methods due to the continuous and huge demand for feeds. The production of animal feed from agro-residues will be one of the most sustainable technologies for better economic resources of local agro-communities and also for the better management of environmental pollution.

Potato pulp is the industrial waste produced during starch extraction from potatoes and its discharge has become an environmental-pollution problem and is a decisive cost factor due to stricter environmental legislation and associated expenses in the potato-starch industry. Recently, a model was developed to assess potato pulp for use as a new poultry feed, which will help starch factories to decrease waste discharge (Wang *et al.*, 2010). Animal feed produced by solid state fermentation of wastes from potato pulp has been assessed for its toxicity, nutritional quality and its effect on growth performance of poultry farming.

Apple pomace, a by-product from the apple-processing industry, is not a suitable feed since it is deficient in digestible protein. Growth of yeast on the apple pomace increases protein and vitamin contents. However, the low level of fermentable sugars limits protein enrichment of the pomace by yeasts. It was reported that co-culture of *Candida utilis* and *A. niger* on dried and pectin-extracted apple pomace increased the protein content to 20% and 17%, respectively (Bhalla and Joshi, 1994).

10. Nutritional manipulations for quality poultry products (Designer foods)

In the recent years people have become more conscious of the relation between food and their health. In this regard, they started to show more interest in the foodstuffs they consume, and so also in the quality of poultry meat and eggs. Primarily, the main concern of consumers is that the food they consume is safe and healthy, i.e. free of substances which could directly affect their health (microorganisms, mycotoxins, pesticides, antibiotics, etc.). Secondly, consumers have shown special interest in poultry products which have reduced content of substances which can pose risk to human health which in turn developed production of poultry meat and eggs with reduced fat and cholesterol content. In the third phase, consumers expect to derive additional benefit by enriching with substances beneficial for their health and poultry meat and eggs have huge potential in this aspect. In case of poultry, there are two types of value addition of products:

- Pre-slaughter value addition i.e. value addition before the product is produced. Products like, designer / organic / functional eggs and meat fall under this category.
- Post-slaughter value addition i.e. value addition after the product is produced.

These types of value addition can be done mostly by combination of managemental and nutritional manipulations. Dietary manipulation is the major step in producing the pre-slaughter value added poultry products through: Omega-3 fatty acids enrichment, lowering cholesterol content, enrichment with carotenoids and enrichment with immunomodulators etc.

The development of nutrient enriched value added poultry eggs and meat greatly increased the context of functional foods for human health. By manipulating the diet of chicken with nutritional interventions like supplementation of chromium, copper, herbs, probiotics, n-3 fatty acids, antioxidants etc. value added and health promoting chicken egg, meat and their products can be made available to the consumers. The designing must take into consideration the production facilities, available materials, technical know-how, economic resources of the producers and environmental impacts with welfare issue.

11. Poultry feed formulation softwares

Feed formulation is one of the important aspects of animal feed industry. Balancing the feedstuffs is big challenge faced by the industries when the costumers and requirement increases. Development of animal feed industry depends upon the quality of feed and quality of feed is based upon the raw material used to formulate feed (ration). The first ever computer used for feed formulation was made in 1951 when F.V. Waugh published a paper titled "The Minimum-Cost Dairy Feed". Dent and Casey (1967) authored the first published book on computer-based formulation entitled as "Linear

Programming and Animal Nutrition." In 1970, feed industries started using computers for practical feed formulation. In 1980s, computerized linear program was developed for least cost feed formulation. In the present age, feed formulation without the use of computers is very rare.

Presently, a number of software and mathematical models are developed for finding least cost and maximizing the profit. Many software (WinFeed2.8, FeedMU2, Eco-MIX, AFSO, Feed-Mixer etc) are not free and only trial versions are available but they have student offers, where "Feed Formulation" and "Feed Assist" are free and easily downloaded by giving minimum information.WinFeed 2.8 is the only software which uses Stochastic method in feed formulation and gives the 99% assurance of meeting the nutrient requirement. Software which uses linear programming is FeedMU2, Eco-MIX, AFSO, Feed-Mixer, and WinFeed. Win Feed is the only software which formulates the feed by both the methods. Many feed formulation software have some specific requirement of hardware and platform without which, the user cannot run them. The introduction of cloud computing has increased the use of feed formulation where the user buy a service and can connect through internet and access the database stored in the cloud and perform formulation. Feed formulation software is easy to use, saves time and minimizes the human error of calculation.

Conclusion

Feed technological interventions in the poultry industry has improved productivity through increased growth, carcass quality and reproduction, improved nutrition and feed utilization, improved quality and safety of food, improved health and welfare of animals, and reduced waste through more efficient utilization of resources. Use of feed formulation softwares for balanced diet formulation is easy to use, saves time and increases accuracy.

References

Baker, D.H. and Han, Y. 1994. Ideal amino acid profile for chicks during the first three weeks posthatching. Poultry Science, 73: 1441-1447.

Berres, J., Vieira, S.L., Kidd, M.T., Taschetto, D., Freitas, D.M., Barros, R. and Nogueira, E.T. 2010. Supplementing l-valine and l-isoleucine in low-protein cornsoybean meal all-vegetable diets for broilers. Journal of Applied Poultry Research, 19: 373-379.

Bhalla, T.C. and Joshi, M. 1994. Protein enrichment of apple pomace by co-culture of cellulolytic moulds and yeasts. World Journal of Microbiology and Biotechnology, 10: 116-117.

Edwards, S.A., Fairbairn, C.B. and Capper, A.L. 1986. Liquid potato feed for finishing pigs: feeding value, inclusion rate and storage properties. Animal Feed Science and Technology, 15: 129-139.

Flachowsk, Y.G., Aulrich, K., Bohmea, H. and Hall E, I. 2007. Studies on feeds from genetically modified plants (GMP) – Contributions to nutritional and safety assessment. Animal Feed Science and Technology, 133, 2-30.

Hahn, M. and Baker, D.H. 1993. Growth and plasma zinc response of young pigs fed pharmacologic levels of zinc. Journal of Animal Science, 68: 3020-3024.

Kidd, M.T. 2003.A treatise on chicken dam nutrition that impacts progeny. World´s Poultry Science Journal, 59: 475-494.

Kidd, M.T., Ferket, P.R. and Qureshi, M.A. 1996. Zinc metabolism with especial reference to its role in immunity. World´s Poultry Science Journal, 52: 309-324.

Marquardt, R.R., Brenes, A., Zhang, Z. and Boros, D. 1996. Use of enzymes to improve nutrient availability in poultry feedstuffs. Animal Feed Science and Technology, 60: 321-330.

Mc Donald, P., Edwards, R.A., Greenhalgh, J.F.D., Morgan, C.A. and Sinclair, L.A. 2010 Animal Nutrition. Pearson Books.

Mourao, J.L., Pinheiro, V.M., Prates, J.A.M., Bessa, R.J.B., Ferreira, L.M.A., Fontes, C.M.G.A. and Ponte, P.I.P. 2008. Effect of dietary dehydrated pasture and citrus pulp on the performance and meat quality of broiler chickens. Poultry Science, 87: 733-743.

Muller, Z.O. 1980. Feed from animal wastes: state of knowledge. FAO Animal Production and Health Paper, Rome, Italy, p. 195.

Noy, Y. and Uni, Z. 2010. Early nutritional strategies. World´s Poultry Science Journal, 66:639–646.

Ouellette, A.J., Aviles, L., Burnweit, C.A., Frederick, D. and Malt, R.A. 1982. Metallothionein mRNA induction in mouse small bowel by oral cadmium and zinc. American Journal of Physiology, 243: 396403.

Patton, R. 1997. Efficacy of chelated minerals: review of literature. Proceedings of the 2nd Conference of the Nutrition Advisory Group of the American Zoo and Aquarium Association on Zoo and Wildlife Nutrition, 16-19 out; Ft. Worth, Texas. EUA- 1979. pp.14-31.

Shariatmadari, F. 2012. Plans of feeding broiler chickens. World´s Poultry Science Journal, 68: 21–30.

Sklan, D., Noy, Y., Hoyzman, A. and Rozenboim, I. 2000.Decreasing weight loss in the hatchery by feeding chicks and poults in hatching trays. Journal of Applied Poultry Research, 9: 142-148.

Uni, Z. and Ferket, P.R. 2003. Enhancement of development of oviparous species by in ovo feeding. US Regular Patent US 6:B2

Vieira, S.L. and Angel, C.R., 2012. Optimizing broiler performance using different amino acid density diets: what are the limits. Journal of Applied Poultry Research, 21: 149-155.

Wadhwa, M. and Makkar, M.P.S. 2013. Utilization of fruit and vegetable wastes as livestock feed and as substrates for generation of other value-added products. FAO publication, RAP Publication 2013/04, E-ISBN 978-92-5-107632-3.

Wang, T.Y., Wu, Y.H., Jiang, C.Y. and Liu, Y. 2010. Solid state fermented potato pulp can be used as poultry feed. British Poultry Science, 51: 229-234.

Wedekind, K.J., Hortin, A.E. and Baker, D.H. 1992. Methodology for assessing zinc bioavailability: efficacy estimates for zinc-methionine, zinc sulfate, and zinc oxide. Journal of Animal Science, 70: 178-187.

Windisch, W., Schedle, K., Plitzner, C. and Kroismayr, A. 2008. Use of phytogenic products as feed additives for swine and poultry. Journal of Animal Science, 86 (E. Suppl.): E 140–E148.

Yokoyama, H., Peralta, R.C., Diaz, R., Sendo, S., Ikemori, Y. and Kodama, Y. 1992. Passive protective effect of chicken egg yolk immunoglobulins against experimental enterotoxigenic Escherichia coli infection in neonatal piglets. Infection and Immunity 60: 998-1007.

[illegible] 2012. [illegible] ... temperature ... [illegible].

[illegible] ... National Research Council ... [illegible].

[illegible] ... [illegible].

[illegible] ... [illegible].

17

Solid State Fementation of Feed for Poultry

Ramesh Sharma

Professor and Head, Division of Animal Nutrition, FVSc & AH, SKUAST-Jammu Jammu and Kashmir, India

Introduction

The huge nutritious potential of agricultural based byproducts has generated an interest of nutritionist for utilizing them in efficient ways in order to improve the production of animals. In this concern, solid state fermentation (SSF) is a promising and novel technique. The lignocellulosic structural characters of plant residues provide them a solid support and act as substrates for the microbial fermentation to produce certain value added products through SSF. The scope of SSF in the field of animal nutrition is wide, in terms for the production of enzymes, bioactive components, organic acids, vitamins, and feed additives, bio-transforming products, biological degradation and detoxification of agricultural residues/wastes. The inclusion of SSF biomass has a huge impact on nutritive composition of feed, performance, hemobiochemical status, gut morphology, gut microbiota, carcass attributes and rumen fermentation along with the reduction in enteric methane emission of animals and poultry birds.

Types of Fermentation

There are two type of fermentation process namely solid state fermentation (SSF) and Liquid or submerged state fermentation (SmF). Solid state fermentation (SSF) is a process that takes place in a solid matrix (inert support or substrate) without or with smaller quantity of free water. Moisture is needed to support the growth and metabolic activity of microorganisms on solid substrate. However, in liquid-state fermentation (LSF) the substrate is solubilized or suspended as free particles in a large volume of water. The differentiating feature between SSF and SmF has been described in Table 1.

Table 1: Differentiating points between SSF and SmF

Features	SSF	SmF
Medium	Not free- flowing	Free flowing
Deepness	Shallow	Greater
Nutrients	Solid substrate	Employed
Water	Medium absorbed	Medium is dissolved
Temp, ph.	Not uniform	Uniform
Contamination	less	Higher
System	3 phase	2 phase
Intra particle resistances	Present	No such resistances
Culture distribution	Adhere to solid and grow	Uniformly distributed
Bioreactors	Small	Large
Measurement of biomass	Lots of difficulties	Online sensors are available
Product	Highly concentrated	Low concentration
Liquid waste	Not produced	High quality

Source: Prabakar *et al.*, 2005; Koyani and Rajput, 2015

Solid State Fermentation

Solid state fermentation (SSF) is the fermentation process, where microorganisms are grown in an environment in absence of free water, or with very low content of free water on solid substrate and complex material is converted into simpler forms. The solid substratum itself acts as carbon/energy source. Egyptians were reported to make bread using this notable technique of SSF and has been used in Asian continent from the ancient times. In natural condition with little moisture or in near absence of water, the microorganisms obtain carbon, nitrogen and other nutrients for growth and show degradative activity. In recent years, SSF has shown much development in bio processing in food, pharmaceutical, textile, biochemical and bioenergy. Solid state fermentation is processed through fungi, bacteria or yeast. With increase in the expansion of agro-industrial activity, accumulates of bulk quantity of residues are left behind. This agricultural based biomass is highly lignified as per the composition and are lignocellulosic in nature, thus causing an elimination issue with ultimate environmental pollution.

Table 2: Some lingocellulosic wastes with their percentage compositions.

Lignocellulosic waste	**Cellulose (wt%)**	**Hemicellulose (wt%)**	**Lignin (wt%)**
Barley straw	33.8	21.9	13.8
Corn cobs	33.7	31.7	6.1
Corn stalks	35.0	16.8	7.0
Cotton stalks	58.5	14.4	21.5
Oat straw	36.2	27.1	17.5
Rice straw	36.2	19.0	9.9
Rye straw	37.6	30.5	19.0
Soya straw	34.5	24.8	19.8
Sugarcane straw	40.0	27.0	10.0
Sunflower straw	42.1	29.7	13.4
Wheat straw	32.9	24.0	8.9

(Nigam *et al.*, 2009)

There is a worldwide bid of animal based products augmenting on a blooming rate thus emphasizing the inevitability of applying strategies to improvise animal productivity. The major constraints in growth of livestock sector is the lack of availability of feed resources, poor quality of available feed sources, and high feed cost particularly in tropical countries. The worsening animal health and their sustainability have necessitated the use of certain substitutes such as agricultural by products, crop residues and grasses as a feed source for livestock. These agro industrial residues used for animal feeds have highly lignified fiber, low nitrogen content and minerals reduced digestibility and contain anti nutritional factors. Owing to this these, are not utilized judiciously and therefore they are receiving more consideration for quality control. Due to their high nutritional perspective these residues are not described as a waste but known to be as raw materials for further product formation and developments. With an advance, in a field of animal nutrition, animal nutritionist has developed various physical, chemical and biological methods to overcome the problems associated with animal feed stuffs. SSF biomass is one such technique which revealed to enhance the nutritive value by relaxing the fiber matrix with increase nitrogen content of residues. On supplementation in animal feeds it improves nutrient utilization, health status of animal, gut health and productive performance along with the reduction in methane emission. Feed fermentation has been divided into two phases by Canibe and Jensen (2003). The first phase, which is characterized by low levels of lactic acid bacteria and yeasts, high pH and a blooming of enterobacteria while the second phase of the fermentation process is characterized by high levels of lactic acid bacteria and yeasts, low pH and low counts of enterobacteria.

Table 3: Application of SSF in Animal nutrition

Economic Sector	Application	Examples
Industrial Fermentation	Enzyme production	Amylases, amyloglucodidase, cullulases, proteases, pectinases, xylaneses, glucoamylases
	Bioactive products	Mycotoxins, gibberlins, alkaloids, antibiotics, harmones
	Organic acid production	Citric acid, fumaric acid, itaconic acid, lactic acid
	Biofuel	Ethnol production
	Miscellaneous compounds	Pigments, biosurfactants, vitamins, xantham
Agro-Food Industry	Biotransformation of crop residues	Traditional food fermented (koji, sake, ragi, tempeh), protein enrichment and single cell protein production, mushroom production.
	Food additives	Aroma compounds, dye stuffs, essential fat and organic acids.
Environmental control	Bioremediation & biodegradation of hazardous compounds	Caffeinated residues, pestiscides, polychlorinated biphenyls (PCBs)
	Biological detoxification of agroindustrial wastes	Coffee pulp, cassava peels, canola meal, coffee husk.

(Guerra *et al*., 2003; Mienda *et al*., 2011)

Steps involved in SSF process of substrates

- Microbial culture made into suspension.
- Nutrient enrichment of substrates.
- Moisture optimization
- Autoclaving and cooling of substrates.
- Inoculation with microbial suspension.
- Incubation of inoculated substrates.
- Oven drying of fermented substrates.
- Milling and storage of fermented substrates.

Table 4: Microorganisms used in SSF

Microorganisms	Substrate/Solid supports	Source
Bacteria		
Amycolatopsis Mediterranean MTCC 14	GOC and COC	Vastrad and Neelagund (2011)
Pseudomonas spp. BUP6	GOC, COC, SOC, and CSC	Faisal *et al.* (2014)
Bacillus licheniformis MTCC 1483	Wheat straw, sugarcane baggase, maize straw, and paddy straw	Kaur *et al.* (2015)
Fungi		
Aspergillus niger	Rice bran, wheat bran, black gram bran, GOC, and COC	Suganthi *et al.* (2011)
Aspergillus oryzae	Soyabean meal (waste)	Thakur *et al.* (2015)
Rhizopus arrhizus and Mucors ubtillissimus	Corn cob, cassava peel, soyabean, wheat bran, and citrus pulp	Nascimento *et al.* (2015)
Aspergillus niger	Rice bran, wheat bran, black gram bran, GOC, and COC	Mahalakshmi and Jayalakshmi. (2016)
Aspergillus terreus	Palm oil cake	Rahman *et al.* (2016)

(Sadh *et al.*, 2018)

Table 5: Substrates used for SSF

Enzymes	Microorganisms	Substrates/Solid support	Source
Lipase	*Candida rugosa*	Groundnut oil cake (GOC)	Rekha *et al.* (2012)
Pectin methyl Esterase	*Pseudomonas notatum*	Wheat bran and orange peel	Gayen and Gosh (2011)
α-Amylase	*Pseudomonas aeruginosa*	Linseed oil cake (LOC)	Dharmendra (2012)
α-Amylase	*Aspergillus niger*	Orange peel	Sindiri *et al.* (2013)
α-Amylase	*Aspergillus oryzae*	Coconut oil cake (COC)	Ramachandran *et al.* (2004)
α-Amylase	*Bacillus sp.*	Rice bran	Sodhi *et al.* (2005)
α-Amylase	*Bacillus sp.*	Corn bran	Sodhi *et al.* (2005)
α-Amylase	*Aspergillus niger*	Rice bran, wheat bran, black gram bran, and soyabean	Akpan *et al.* (1999)
Invertase	*Aspergillus niger*	Fruit peel waste	Mehta & Duhan (2014)

Monogastric nutrition and use of SSF

Monogastric animals, such as swine, horse and poultry eat rations high in concentrates. Monogastric animals require a good source of protein in their diet and are limited in their capacity to ferment fiber for the provision of energy. The horse however can obtain most of its energy through the fermentation of fibre or complex carbohydrates in the hindgut, while pigs and poultry obtain energy from the digestion of simple carbohydrates in the small intestines. Monogastric animal feeding is more challenged by feedstuff in the diets, immune traits, and meat quality. At present, numerous studies focus on feedstuffs from agricultural by-products on pigs and poultry. Moreover, over the last decade, there has been an interest in entirely natural, plant-derived antioxidants. Many agro-industry by-products as feeds have shown to improve the feed conversion ratio, body weight, antioxidant capacity, immunity, gut morphology and intestinal microflora of pigs and poultry after suitable treatments.

Pigs and poultry require a good source of protein and amino acids. Best source of protein for all these species are the oil seed meals such as soyabean meal, canola meal, as well as legumes. For energy, poultry and pigs are best fed with cereals such as wheat and corn.

Protein sources are second most important components of monogastric diets. Due to fluctuation in the price of feed sources like Corn-SBM diet which is the most commonly used feed for monogastric animal production and persistent increase in prices of these ingridents, nutritionists have been exploring alternate feed sources. This could reduce human-livestock competition for feed sources like soyabean, corn and support production of more animal protein. However, the use of these alternate feed sources is limited due to presence of anti-nutritional factors such as glucosinolates (Rapeseed meal), gossypol (Cottonseed meal), non-starch polysaccharides in lupin flour, total phenolic contents and phytic acid (Canola meal), high fiber (Palm kernel cake) which are known to impair animal performance, nutrient digestibility and feed utilization and have negative health effects on the monogastric animal. As processing technique, SSF has been researched for long in food industry. An important objective of this technique is the production of enzymes, organic acids, and other metabolites of economic importance. In recent times the technique of SSF has been employed to enhance nutrient bioavailability, inhibition of gut pathogenic bacteria and reduction of anti-nutritional factors in different feed sources. It has resulted in improved digestibility, thereby improving performance and gut health in poultry. The use of fermented feed products does not have any negative effect on performance and nutrient digestibility in growing-finishing pigs, and a reduction in the levels of dust in swine barns. Solid-state fermentation has resulted in high counts of lactic acid bacteria and low counts of enterobacteria in the substrate. Moreover, feeding a diet containing solid-state fermented feed, free of antibiotics, can result in similar performance and nutrient digestibility in growing-finishing pigs to a regular diet with antibiotics. The possible mechanism responsible for solid-state fermented feed in replacing antibiotics may be due to the following characteristics gained from solid-state fermentation:

- Increased counts of lactic acid bacteria and bacillus and low counts of enterobacteria.
- Increased concentration of organic acids and low pH.
- Increased water soluble protein to crude protein ratio (WSP/CP).

Corn, the main energy feed while Soybean meal (SBM) is the principal source of protein for the feed industry worldwide and is used in large proportions in the diets of monogastric animals. Soybean protein contains unsaturated, essential fatty acids such as linoleic acid and linolenic acid. Efforts have been made to increase soybean protein products acceptance in animal feed for the low cost and high nutritive value with a good amino acid balance. But SBM contains various anti- nutritional factors that limit its application in animal feed. Anti- nutritional factors of SBM include trypsin inhibitors, protease inhibitors, lectins, phytoestrogens, stachyose and raffinose, phytates, allergens etc. Phytate of plant origin is present as phytate- phosphorus in feedstuffs which is only partially utilized by monogastrics that is reflected in the poor bioavailability of total phosphorus (P) in monogastric animals. Two- third of phosphorus in soybean is in bound form as phytate. Soybean antigenic proteins in the diets of weaned pigs have shown to provoke a transient hypersensitivity associated with the abnormal morphology of the small intestine. These morphological changes in intestines can cause malabsorption syndrome, growth depression, and diarrhea. Presence of Phytate may reduce mineral bioavailability and protein digestibility when it is fed to pigs. Furthermore, high levels of soy oligosaccharides particularly stachyose and raffinose, have been reported to cause intestinal disorder in weaning piglets. The various soybean products are therefore processed by different fermentation and non- fermentation methods which have been applied to improve the nutrient bioavailability of feed and reduce the wastage. Fermentation process offers new fermented products that can enhance the production of growth promoting factors. From enormous traditional fermentation methods, solid state fermentation (SSF) offers numerous advantages over submerged fermentation (SmF). Subunits of soybean antigenic proteins, including β-conglycinin of α, α′ and β, and acidic and basic glycinin in soybean protein are separated on fermentation. First-stage fermentation with B. subtilis significantly affects the characteristics of proteins in feed. The α and α′ subunits of β-conglycinin and the acidic subunits of glycinin in the feed are almost completely degraded during SSF. In contrast, fermentation led to increase in the number of small peptides (<25 kDa) compared with the fermented uninoculated substrate. However, no effect on the protein profile during the second-stage of fermentation with E. faecium compared with the first-stage fermented feed is observed. The SSF systems have been reported to be an effective way to enhance phytase production. Phytase production increases progressively with different incubation times compared to unfermented SBM. Similarly phytase production of fermented canola meal using SSF by A. ficuum was noticed. Phytase activity of fermented SBM by *A. niger* increased with increasing fermentation time. Solid state fermentation has also been used to increase bioavailability of nutrients and reduce the level of antinutritional factors in rapeseed meal and canola meal.

Table 6: The effect of solid-state fermented rapeseed meal and canola meal on performance, intestinal microflora and intestinal morphology of broiler chickens.

Substrate	Microorganism	Result	Reference
Rapeseed meal	*Lactobavillus fermentum, Enterococcus faecium, Saccharomyces cerevisiae, Bacillus subtilis*	Improved BWG and FCR compared to broilers fed unfermented rapeseed mea but did not differ from soyabean meal control, Increased LAB counts in the colon and caecal digesta. Improved villus height and VH:CD ratio in ileum and jujenum.	Chiang *et al.* (2010)
	Lactobacillus fermentum, Bacillus subtilis	Had no negative effect on performance of broilers at 10% inclusion in place of SBM, but BWG decreased at 15% inclusion. Upto 10% inclusion improved VH:CD ratio in jujenum of broilers.	Xu *et al.* (2012)
	Bacillus subtilis, Candida utilis, Enterococcus faecalis	Increased villus height and VH:CD ratio, decreased crypt depth and intestinal wall thickness in duodenum, jujenum, ileum and caecum in broilers	Hu *et al.* (2016)
Canola meal	*Lactobacillus salivarius*	Inclusion rates higher than 10% reduced performance during 1 to 28 d, but no detrimental effect was observed when used upto 30% during 29 to 35 d under heated and unheated conditions.	Aljuobori *et al.* (2014)

FCR: feed conversion ratio; LAB: Lactic acid bacteria; VH:CD ratio: villus height to crypt depth; SBM: Soyabean meal.

Two-stage fermentation of corn-SBM with *B. subtilis* followed by *E. faecium* effectively reduces the ANFs (soy-antigenic protein, NDF, and phytic acid) in corn-SBM mixed feed and increased the TCA-SP (consist of small molecular peptides (2–20 amino acid residues) and free AAs and CP content of the diet.

Cottonseed meal which is a byproduct of oil extraction from cottonseeds has a crude protein content of 22.2 to 56.5%, but is used in limited amounts in poultry diets due to its gossypol and low lysine levels compared to soyabean meal. Free gossypol in cottonseed meal binds to lysine and inhibits its availability in cottonseed meal. Free gossypol could reduce growth performance and cause increased mortality in broiler chickens.

Bacillus strains have been predominantly used for the SSF of cottonseed meal. *Bacillus subtulis* produces highly active protease, lipase and amylase to degrade complex carbohydrates in plant and lead to increased nutritional digestibility thus providing more nutrition to animals. The use of SSF in CSM resulted in decreased DM content which can be attributed to the consumption of carbohydrates by microorganisms. There is increase in CP content due to decrease in DM. Crude fat content is reduced which may be attributed to the lipase producing ability of *Bacillus subtulis.* Crude fiber content is also reduced which may be attributed to the fiber degrading enzymes secreted by the microorganisms. The concentration of free gossypol is reduced.

Solid-state fermented CSM increases lactic acid bacteria (LAB) population in cecal digesta of broiler chicken. Coliform bacteria counts in caeca also showed a decline. Increased villus height in duodenum and linearly elevated villus height and the villus height to crypts depth ratio in jejunum is seen. There is comparable improvement in jejunal villus height.

Palm kernel cake is by-product of oil extraction from the kernels of oil palm. Palm kernel cake has been used as an energy source in ruminant and non-ruminant diets because of its palatability. The limitations in using palm kernel cake in monogastric animal feeding esp. poultry is due to poor amino acid balance, high indigestible fibre content, coarse texture, grittiness, possible deterioration under unhygienic conditions and high concentrations of NSP such as mannan, xylan and cellulose which leads to reduced feed intake and indigestion in poultry. Thus the dietary inclusion of palm kernel meal in poultry diets does not exceed 40%.

Different strains like *Aspergillus niger, A wentii, Sclerotium rolfsii, Trichoderma spp*. etc. have been in SSF of palm kernel cake. The use of SSF has resulted in improved nutritive value, performance, digestibility, intestinal microflora and intestinal morphology of broiler chicken.

Lupin flour which is obtained by grounding lupin (leguminous crop) seeds contains NSP, tannins and protease inhibitors which has a daunting effect on its use. Fermented lupin however is gaining more attention as a diet component in monogastric feeding. Fermentation contributes to the improvement of nutritional value of lupin by increasing the nutrient availability and causing effective degradation of ANFs. Various bacterial and yeast species have been used in the fermentation process of lupin viz. *S. cerevisiae, E. faecium, L. plantarum, L buchneri* and *L casei.*

Interest in the use of fermented feed for improving the health of pigs increased dramatically after the European Union banned the use of antibiotics as antimicrobial growth promoters for swine.

Generally available literature confirms the feasibility of improving the nutrient composition of alternative feed sources with SSF. Fermentation enhanced the crude protein concentration and other nutriment but led to reduction of many anti-nutritional factors, crude fiber content and toxic ingredients. Organic acid, several amino acids and other metabolites are increased by fermentation In particular no decline in nutritional profile has been reported. Similar or even better nutrient composition in solid-state fermented feed sources compared to their unfermented or conventional forms has been reported.

Conclusion

Due to the increase in the population of humans, there is scarcity of food grains (Maize & Soybean) for feeding poultry. Hence, utilization of agricultural byproducts has generated an interest of nutritionist for utilizing them in efficient ways in order to improve the production of animals. In this concern, solid state fermentation (SSF) is a promising and novel technique, which has a huge impact on nutritive composition of feed, performance, hemobiochemical status, gut morphology, gut microbiota, carcass attributes and rumen fermentation along with the reduction in enteric methane emission of animals and poultry birds.

References

Akpan, I., Bankole, M.O., Adesemowo, A.M. and Latunde-Dada, G.O. 1999. Production of amylase by A. niger in a cheap solid medium using rice bran and agricultural materials. Tropical science, 39: 77-79.

Aljubori, A., Idrus, Z., Soleimani, A.F., Abdullah, N. and Juan Boo, L. 2017. Response of broiler chickens to dietary inclusion of fermented canola meal under heat stress condition. Italian Journal of Animal Science, 16(4): 546-551.

Canibe, N. and Jensen, B.B. 2003. Fermented and non-fermented liquid feed to growing pigs: effect on aspects of gastrointestinal ecology and growth performance. Journal of Animal Science, 81(8): 2019-2031.

Chiang, G., Lu, W.Q., Piao, X.S., Hu, J.K., Gong, L.M. and Thacker, P.A. 2009. Effects of feeding solid-state fermented rapeseed meal on performance, nutrient digestibility, intestinal ecology and intestinal morphology of broiler chickens. Asian-Australasian Journal of Animal Sciences, 23(2): 263-271.

Dharminder, P.K. 2012. Production of lipase utilizing linseed oilcake as fermentation substrate. International Journal of Environmental Science and Technology 1(3): 135-143.

Faisal, P.A., Hareesh, E.S., Priji, P., Unni, K.N., Sajith, S., Sreedevi, S., Josh, M.S. and Benjamin, S. 2014. Optimization of parameters for the production of lipase from Pseudomonas sp. BUP6 by solid state fermentation. Advances in Enzyme Research, 2(04), p.125.

Gayen, S. and Ghosh, U. 2013. Purification and characterization of tannin acyl hydrolase produced by mixed solid state fermentation of wheat bran and marigold flower by Penicillium notatum NCIM 923. BioMed Research International, 2013.

Hu, Y., Wang, Y., Li, A., Wang, Z., Zhang, X., Yun, T., Qiu, L. and Yin, Y. 2016. Effects of fermented rapeseed meal on antioxidant functions, serum biochemical parameters and intestinal morphology in broilers. Food and Agricultural Immunology, 27(2): 182-193.

Kaur, P.S., Kaur, S., Kaur, H., Sharma, A., Raj, P. and Panwar, S. 2015. Solid substrate fermentation using agro industrial waste: new approach for amylase production by Bacillus licheniformis. International Journal of Current Microbiology and Applied Science, 4: 712-717.

Koyani, R.D. and Rajput, K.S. 2015. Solid state fermentation: comprehensive tool for utilization of lignocellulosic through biotechnology. Journal of Bioprocessing & Biotechniques, 5:258. doi:10.4172/2155- 9821.1000258

Mehta, K. and Duhan, J.S. 2014. Production of invertase from Aspergillus niger using fruit peel waste as a substrate. International Journal of Pharmacology and Biological Science, 5(2), pp.B353-B360.

Mienda, B.S., Idi, A. and Umar, A. 2011. Microbiological features of solid state fermentation and its applications-An overview. Research in Biotechnology, 2(6).

Parmar, A.B., Patel, V.R., Usadadia, S.V., Rathwa, S.D. and Prajapati, D.R. 2019. A solid state fermentation, its role in animal nutrition: A review. International Journal of Chemical Studies, 7(3): 4626-4633.

Pérez-Guerra, N., Torrado-Agrasar, A., López-Macias, C. and Pastrana, L. 2003. Main characteristics and applications of solid substrate fermentation. Electronic Journal of Environmental, Agricultural and Food Chemistry, 2(3).

Prabhakar, A., Krishnaiah, K., Janaun, J. and Bono, A. 2005. An overview of engineering aspects of solid state fermentation. Malaysian Journal of Microbiology, 1(2): 10-16.

Rahman, K.H.A., Yusof, S.J.H.M. and Zakaria, Z. 2016. Bioproteins production from palm oil agro-industrial wastes by Aspergillus terreus UniMAP AA-1.

Ramachandran, S., Patel, A.K., Nampoothiri, K.M., Francis, F., Nagy, V., Szakacs, G. and Pandey, A. 2004. Coconut oil cake flf flfa potential raw material for the production of á-amylase. Bioresource technology, 93(2): 169-174.

Rekha, K.S.S., Lakshmi, M.V.C., Devi, V.S. and Siddartha Kumar, M. 2012. Production and optimization of lipase from Candida rugosa using groundnut oilcake under solid state fermentation. biosensors, 27, p.31.

Sadh, P.K., Duhan, S. and Duhan, J.S. 2018. Agro-industrial wastes and their utilization using solid state fermentation: a review. Bioresources and Bioprocessing, 5(1): 1-15.

Sindiri, M.K., Machavarapu, M. and Vangalapati, M. 2013. Alfa-amylase production and purification using fermented orange peel in solid state fermentation by Aspergillus niger. Indian Journal of Applied Research, 8: 49-51.

Singh nee' Nigam, P., Gupta, N. and Anthwal, A. 2009. Pre-treatment of agro-industrial residues. biotechnology for agro-industrial residues utilisation: Utilisation of agro-residues, pp.13-33.

Sodhi, H.K., Sharma, K., Gupta, J.K. and Soni, S.K. 2005. Production of a thermostable α-amylase from Bacillus sp. PS-7 by solid state fermentation and its synergistic use in the hydrolysis of malt starch for alcohol production. Process Biochemistry, 40(2): 525-534.

Suganthi, R., Benazir, J.F., Santhi, R., Ramesh Kumar, V., Hari, A., Meenakshi, N., Nidhiya, K.A., Kavitha, G. and Lakshmi, R. 2011. Amylase production by Aspergillus niger under solid state fermentation using agroindustrial wastes. International Journal of Engineering Science and Technology, 3(2): 1756-1763.

Thakur, A.K., Thakur, D.S., Patel, R.K., Pradhan, A. and Kumar, P. 2015. Effect of Different Plant Geometry and Nitrogen Levels, in relation to Growth Characters, Yield and Economics on Sweet Corn (Zea Mays Sachharata L.) At Bastar Plateau Zone. The Bioscan, 10(3): 1223-1226.

Vastrad, B.M. and Neelagund, S.E. 2011. Optimization and production of neomycin from different agro industrial wastes in solid state fermentation. International Journal of Pharmaceutical Sciences and Drug Research, 3(2): 104-111.

Xu, F.Z., Zeng, X.G. and Ding, X.L. 2012. Effects of replacing soybean meal with fermented rapeseed meal on performance, serum biochemical variables and intestinal morphology of broilers. Asian-Australasian Journal of Animal Sciences, 25(12): 1734-1741.

18

Alternative Feed Resources for Poultry Rations

Y.A. Beigh, A.M. Ganai, M.T. Banday, Haidar Ali Ahmad and S. Adil

Faculty of Veterinary Science and Animal Husbandry, Sher-e-Kashmir University of Agricultural Sciences and Technology of Kashmir, Srinagar-190 006 Jammu and Kashmir, India

Introduction

Limited feed supply and poor quality of the available feeds are the major constraints for optimal livestock and poultry productivity in all developing nations like India. Most of the regions in India are characterized by irregular rainfall and thus livestock have to survive on persistent shortage of feed resources of low nutritive value for most part of the year. The poultry industry is an important livestock sub-sector in India with a potential to solve the problem of malnutrition, unemployment and augmenting rural economy. However, high feed cost decreases animal production which contributes to lower animal protein availability for human consumption. This vicious cycle of low productivity and intake of animal protein has been maintained and sustained by the scarcity of feedstuff.

A major gap exists between the demand and supply of conventional feed resources for feeding livestock in the world. To manage this problem, it is essential to increase the availability of feed resources for optimum livestock production. But most poultry feeds have very similar characteristics being low in fiber and essentially cereal based, as such often comprise between 50 and 75% of the diet. Maize and soybean meal form the major source of energy and protein sources in the diet of poultry. Thus feeding of poultry presents a challenge to farmers as poultry shares the feed similarity with humans in terms of the fact that ingredients used in formulating poultry rations are equally consumed by humans. Also, the production level of these feeds has not been adequate to meet the growing needs of the poultry industry. In the coming times, poultry sector has definitely to look beyond maize and soybean meal based diets because of their availability; cost and also maize-soybean production cannot keep pace with the ever-increasing poultry production. So there is a scope for inclusion of alternate feed ingredients in poultry diets for curtailing the production cost.

As feed constitutes 60-70% of the total cost of production, any attempt to reduce the feed cost may lead to a significant reduction in the total cost of production. So there is need to improve the scientific knowledge for utilizing low cost locally available agro-industrial by-products in poultry feed in order to reduce the feed cost. Attempts to utilize locally available cheap by-products may benefit the end users in reducing the feed cost which in turn can reduce the total cost of production of meat and egg and making them easily available at a cheaper cost. The traditional sources of proteins used in poultry rations such as fish meal, meat and bone meal, soybean meal, groundnut cake, etc. are becoming expensive in developed countries. The availability of such feed ingredients is not adequate because of the spiraling cost of raw materials and ever-increasing competition with human beings for the same food items. Hence, the search for alternative feed sources has become inevitable to reduce feed cost. There is an opportunity to utilize locally available AFR for economic production of poultry. Although, there has been a lot of work done in India in the area of alternate feed ingredients; however, still a lot more needs to be done in this direction.

Alternative feed resources (AFR)

AFR generally refer to all those feeds that have not been traditionally used for feeding livestock and are not commercially used in the production of livestock feeds. Several known examples include leaf meals, spent brewer's grains, rubber seed meal and some aquatic plants. The term AFR has been frequently used to describe sources such as oil palm by-products, single-cell proteins and feed materials derived from agro-industrial by-products of plant and animal origin, and other agro-industrial by-products such as slaughter-house by-products and those from the processing of sugar, cereal grains, citrus fruits and vegetables from the processing of food for human consumption also comes under category of AFR.

Need for alternative feed resources

With an increasing demand for livestock products as a result of rapid growth in the world economies and shrinking land area causing serious shortages of conventional animal feed, future hopes of feeding the animals and safeguarding their food security will depend on the better utilization of AFR which do not compete with human food. Alternative feeds could partly fill the gap in the feed supply, decrease competition for food between humans and animals, reduce feed cost, and contribute to self-sufficiency in nutrients from locally available feed sources.

Generation of alternative feed resources

The generation of AFR is essentially from agriculture and various agro-based industries and is a function of many factors. Such factors include the quantity and quality of the materials produced which is dependent on the prevailing agro-climatic conditions and cropping patterns, the type of raw materials, the production process, the production rate, the type of inputs used, the regulations affecting product quality use and the constraints imposed upon effluent discharge (Devendra, 1985). Most AFR are usually regarded as waste so, they can be used to supplement the existing limited feed resources. Recycling, reprocessing and utilization of all or a portion of the wastes, offers the possibility of returning these materials to beneficial use as opposed to the traditional methods of disposal and relocation of the same residues. The demonstration of potential value can thus make any of these waste products new feeds of value and importance.

Characteristics of alternative feed resources

- They are mainly organic and can be in a solid, slurry or liquid form
- Their economic value is less than that the cost of collection and transportation for use thus referred to as wastes
- Some feeds contain toxic factors and have a deleterious effect e.g castor bean meal, neem seed cake
- These are by-products of food production systems that have not been used, recycled or salvaged.
- They have considerable potential as feed materials. In the case of feeds, they can be subjected to value addition if processing techniques are employed.
- Most of AFR feed resources are low in energy, protein, minerals

Constraints in the utilization of alternative feed resources

A. Nutritional aspects

- Limited knowledge of the chemical composition and feeding values of alternative feeds.
- Variability in nutrient level and quality (soil, temperature, humidity, variety, harvest method, processing)
- Presence of naturally occurring anti-nutritional and/or toxic factors (alkaloids, non-starch polysaccharides, glycosides, tartrates, heavy metals) in some resources like sal seed meal, neem seed cake and mahua

seed cake, rendering them non-suitable for use in animal feed, and little knowledge about their characterization, quantification in ingredient, and their long-range effects on animal health and productivity.

- Presence of pathogenic micro-organisms (Salmonellae; present if waste is not processed/ sterilized properly).
- Need for supplementation (minerals, most limiting essential amino acids)

B. Technical aspects

- Seasonal and unreliable supply (need for storage) (wine, apple, dates; duration of transport) Bulkiness, wetness and/or powdery texture impose difficulties in collection, handling, transportation, and processing of these feeds (need for pelleting) (Brewers' spent grains; poultry manure, sludge; potato starch)
- Processing requirements (drying, detoxification) (availability of machinery; knowledge of processing; energy source)
- Lack of research and development efforts (feed industries) (cooperation developed/developing countries; transfer of knowledge).
- Non-availability of AFR in large quantities.
- Production is scattered in definite areas.

Benefits derived from the use of non-conventional feed resources

1. Environmental sanitation: The sanitary disposal of offal, such as the by-products of the slaughterhouse, presents great difficulties. Not only does this offal attract vermin and present danger of spreading disease, but it also tends to decompose, rapidly forming an ideal substrate for microorganisms and leads to objectionable odors. Burning or burying of inedible offal, or its use as fertilizer leads to a total loss of potential by-products and, unless properly carried out, it may also lead to spread in disease (El Boushy, 1990). The effluents from slaughterhouses and from the processing of fruits and vegetables can be used to produce a sludge that in dry form can be utilized for livestock and poultry feeding purposes. The sludge can also be activated by means of micro-organisms through solid state fermentation process to produce a higher nutritional value in comparison with the original sludge.
2. Livestock health and productive agriculture: Offal can be used either to manufacture fertilizers or livestock feedstuffs depending on the speed with which they are handled and the freshness of the raw materials.
3. Price structure: The use of by-products and recycling waste will influence the price of meat and eggs. Depending on local circumstances, the return

derived from the use of by-products (animal, vegetable and fruit wastes) may be used to decrease the prices of meat and eggs to the consumer or to give the livestock producers more gain for their product and by-products.

4. Creation of new employment: There is no doubt that the disposal of waste (inedible offal, fruit, and vegetables, tannery or municipal refuse) needs manpower in developing market economies. The conversion of offal, however, into valuable by-products creates new employment and skills at the place of production.
5. Reducing imports of feedstuffs (foreign currency) by upgrading local waste: If a local industry such as the poultry industry is able to transfer all the offals by rendering and produce poultry offal meal (blood, feet, heads, intestines, and feathers), a product will be created with high nutritive value. This application may lower the present imports of feedstuffs, fertilizers, cereals and soya, animal products and total agricultural products that require foreign currency.

Alternative poultry feeds

1. Energy sources

i. **Rice kani:** Rice kani (broken rice) a by-product obtained through milling of rough rice or paddy is a potential unconventional energy source for poultry feeding. There is tremendous scope for using rice kani as a substitute for high energy feed ingredient like maize in poultry feed in order to reduce the feed cost as well as the competition with human beings for conventional energy source. Besides, rice kani is not associated with aflatoxins, which pose threat to the survivability of poultry and other livestock. Its CP value ranges from 7.19-11.41%, and the apparent metabolizable energy content is comparable to that of maize (Swain *et al.*, 2006). Rice kani can be used at a level of 15 % in the diet of Vanaraja growing chickens in order to reduce the feed cost and economize the cost of production. In Japanese quails chicks, rice kani can replace maize up to a level of 20 % in the diet without any adverse effect on their performance with appreciable reduction in the feed cost.

ii. **De-oiled salseed-meal**: It is a byproduct from processing of Sal fruits for oil. The composition of meal resembles cereals. But its use is very much limited to poultry because of high tannin content.

iii. **Palm oil:** Palm oil (PAO) and palm kernel oil (PKO) are produced from the fruits of *Elaeis quineensis* tree. Palm oil is the second most common vegetable oil produced in the world following soybean oil. The oil palm a perennial crop, is harvested throughout the year. PAO contains no cholesterol and trans fatty acids.PAO can be used in the diet of laying hens up to a level of 5.5 % replacing maize in the diet without affecting the egg production performance. However, the yolk cholesterol content increased due to incorporation of palm oil in the laying hens' diet (Swain *et al.*, 2014).

iv. **Tapioca-meal**: It is obtained from the tubers of tapioca. The meal is a good source of energy. Certain varieties contain gynogenic substances. These can be removed during the processing of tapioca by sun drying or heating.

v. **Molasses:** May be used to replace cereal grains upto 45% of the ration. Higher percentage produces loose excreta because of high mineral content of molasses.

vi. **Small millets:** The demand for maize has increased tremendously for use as human and other industrial use making it less available for animal feed. Millets grossly resemble maize in proximate composition except variation in protein and minerals. Replacement of maize with coarse cereals, reduces feed cost and pressure on use of maize. Small millets such as *kodon* and *sawan* can be used in place of maize up to 20 per cent in the ration. *Ragi, kambu* and *cholam,* available in southern India, may also be satisfactorily used to replace maize to an extent of 50 per cent. Bajra is a satisfactory feed ingredient for laying hens that can be included in unground form at moderate levels as per the results of research work conducted by earlier workers (Rao *et al.*, 2000).

2. Vegetable protein sources

i. **Brewers' dried grains (BDG):** BDG is a valuable by-product of brewery which has a potential to be used as supplementary feed for livestock and poultry. These materials are considered to be good sources of un-degradable protein, energy and water-soluble vitamins. Brewer's grain is the materials that remain after grains have been fermented during the beer making process. These materials can be fed as wet brewer's grains or dried brewer's grains. BDG is a by-product of barley malt, corn or rice that is treated to remove most of the readily soluble carbohydrates, protein, fibre, linoleic acid, vitamins and minerals. Brewery waste protein can replace 20% soya protein in the diet of chickens without causing significant differences in the growth and feed intake. A study in Rhode Island Red chicks indicated that BDG could be incorporated at a level of 20% in RIR chick ration without any adverse effect on their growth and feed efficiency (Swain *et al.*, 2014).

ii. **Mustard-cake:** It is superior to groundnut-cake in lysine content. Its use in poultry ration is limited because of the presence of glycosides and goitrogens. Even after treatment its use should be limited to 5% in chick and 10% in laying hen diets.

iii. **Soybean-meal:** Soybean contains about 35 to 40% protein and 18 to 21 % fat. The oil may be removed in several ways. Expeller processing of the beans yielded a meal which contained 42% protein and 5% fat. Suitable heat treatment improves the protein quality of the meal. It is a high-quality vegetable protein rich in lysine, arginine, glycine, tryptophan and cystine. The limiting amino acid is methionine.

iv. **Sesame-meal:** It is a good source of protein supplement and a good source of arginine, methionine and tryptophan, but poor in lysine, cystine and glycine.

v. **Cluster bean:** It is a byproduct in the manufacture of vegetable gum from the seeds of cluster bean plants. It is rich in protein but its use is limited by residual cluster bean gum and due to the presence of trypsin inhibitor.

vi. **Sunflower seed meal:** It is superior to groundnut-meal in nutritive value. But because of high fibre content its use is restricted in poultry rations. Compared to soybean-meal it is richer in methionine and arginine but poor in lysine. It is an excellent source of pantothenic acid and niacin.

vii. **Safflower-meal:** It is a good substitute to groundnut-cake up to 25 per cent level in the ration. Lysine deficiency appears to be one of the main limitations in total utilization of this cake.

viii. **Ramtil-cake:** It can replace satisfactorily up to 50 and 100 per cent of groundnut-cake in chicks and layer rations respectively.

ix. **Cotton-cake:** High in protein content but deficient in lysine. It can be used up to 15 per cent as a substitute for groundnut-cake. Continuous use causes yolk mottling on stored eggs due to the presence of gossypol in the cake.

x. **Maize gluten-meal:** A byproduct of maize starch industry it is rich in protein and xanthophylls but deficient in lysine, tryptophan and arginine.

xi. **Penicillin mycelium waste:** It is a byproduct from the manufacture of penicillin. It is a good protein source and contains some residual antibiotic activity. It can be used at levels of 5 per cent in the ration.

xii. **Linseed-meal:** It is a good source of tryptophan but contains cyanogenic glycoside and antipyridoxial factor, cannot be used more than 5% if not processed. The meal can be rendered non-toxic by boiling.

xiii. **Green materials:** A wide range of materials are available including herbs, fodder leaves (e.g., leucaena, calliandra, sesbania), leaves from cultivated plants (e.g., cassava) and aquatic plants (e.g., azolla, water hyacinth, duckweed) for inclusion in the diet of poultry. These feeds can be harvested and fed directly to poultry in fresh form. Likewise, cowpea (*Vigna unguiculata* [L.] is an important grain and fodder legume crop grown in many parts of the world. Cowpea is used at all stages of its growth including as vegetables (Ofori and Stern, 1986). Cowpea leaves can be fed to vanaraja laying hens for more income generation due to significant reduction in feed cost (Swain *et al.*, 2014). Such feeds are not only good sources of protein, but they are also rich in pigments, vitamins and minerals.

3. Animal protein sources

i. **Blood-meal:** It contains 80 per cent protein and is rich in lysine, arginine, methionine, cystine and leucine, but deficient in isoleucine. The maximum dietary level of inclusion is not greater than 2 to 3 per cent due to unpalatability and low biological value of its protein.

ii. **Liver residue-meal:** It is a good source of lysine, methionine, cystine and tryptophan, and an excellent source of riboflavin, choline and vitamin B12.

iii. **Silkworm pupae-meal:** Deoiled silkworm pupae-meal is a good protein supplement. Because of high fibre content and poor protein digestibility its use is restricted in poultry rations.

iv. **Hatchery byproduct-meal:** The poultry hatchery waste (PHW) is the product left over in the poultry hatchery after the hatching process is completed. Poultry hatchery waste is primarily composed of dead chicks, infertile whole eggs and shells from hatched eggs (Hamm and Whitehead 1982). It contains approximately 25-34 per cent crude protein depending upon the material that goes into its making.

vi. **Feather-meal:** It contains 80-85 per cent of crude protein and may be used up to 5 per cent level in poultry rations.

vi. **Poultry byproduct-meal:** It is a product from poultry processing plants, and includes heads, feet and entrails. It must not contain more than 16 per cent ash and no more than traces of feathers. The meal may contain 55 to 60 per cent protein and 12 per cent fat if not extracted.

vii. **Meat and meat-cum-bone-meal:** Besides a good source of high quality protein, it is a good source of calcium and phosphorus. The quality of meal is variable depending upon the processing methods and the proportion of gelatin it contains. The variable quality and content of phosphorus limit the use of these meals to 5 to 10 per cent of the diet.

viii. **Insect meals:** Insects can be used to produce cheaper proteins from non-food animals. Insects are part of the natural diet of poultry, and scavenging poultry consume a wide variety, including grasshoppers, crickets, termites, aphids, scale insects, beetles, caterpillars, pupa, flies, fleas, bees, wasps and ants. Insects are rich in protein, with reported protein contents ranging from 40 to 75%. These novel protein sources can be collected from surrounding areas. There is also opportunity for the production of insects using waste materials.

ix. **Insect larva:** The biological digestion of animal wastes by the larval stage of flies (especially house and soldier flies), and the harvest and use of larvae and pupae is a cheap way of supplying high-protein materials to family poultry. Insect larva can be produced from kitchen and animal wastes. The materials are left to decompose in a protected area, where insects come and lay their eggs. In medium- to large-scale production of fly pupae using animal wastes, light is used to induce the migration of larvae out of the waste through a screen into a lower compartment, where they pupate and are harvested.

x. **Termites**: Termites are not only collected from nature, but can also be grown near the family unit and harvested. Termites have a unique ability to digest fibre, and the production of termites should be linked to the recycling of wood and paper wastes. A simple method of rearing termites on crop residues for family poultry supplementation is practiced in some African countries. This involves the use of inverted clay pots containing termites and filled with moistened fibrous material. The pots must be protected against excessive heat and desiccation, and the termite larvae can be harvested after three to four weeks.

Conclusion

Shortage of feedstuffs in the future is an alarming issue at present in the poultry industry. A distinctive gap exists between the requirements and supplies of nutrients, the non- conventional feeds could partly fill this gap. Presently these by-products are not exploited to the full extent for inclusion in the poultry feed. These feed resources have good nutrient composition and reported to contribute to the productive value for egg and meat with reduction in cost of production. Hence, based on chemical compositions and potential feeding value, these by-products can be incorporated in the poultry feed formulations to economise the feed cost and to increase the profit margin for the poultry farmers. Adoption of these feed resources in poultry nutrition will be a sure way to achieve the strategic plans on suitable animal production for national food security and poverty alleviation.

References

Devendra, C. 1985. Non-conventional feed resources In Asia and the Pacific. 2nd Ed. Food and Agriculture Organization of the United Nations, Regional Animal Production and Health Commission for Asia, the Far East and the South-West Pacifie (APHCA), Bangkok.

El Boushy, A.R. 1990. Using non-traditional feed as a feedstuff will reduce the competition for food between human kind and poultry. Third International Symposium on Feed Manufacturing and Quality Control, 7-9 may 1990, Cairo, Egypt, pp. 305-320.

Hamm, D. and Whitehead, W. K. 1982. Holding techniques for hatchery wastes. Poultry Science 61: 1025-1028.

Ofori, F. and Stern, W. R. 1986. Maize/cowpea intercrop system. Effect of nitrogen fertilizer on productivity and efficiency. Field crops Research 14: 247-261.

Rao, S. V. R., Reddy, M. R., Praharaj, N. K. and Sundar, G. S. 2000. Laying performance of broiler breeder chickens fed various millets or broken rice as a source of energy at a constant nutrient intake. Tropical Animal Health and Production, 32: 329-338.

Swain, B. K., Naik, P. K. and Singh, N. P. 2014. Unconventional feed resources for efficient poultry production. Technical Bulletin No. 47, ICAR-ICAR Research Complex for Goa, Old Goa 403 402, Goa, India, pp. 39-41.

Swain, B. K., Sundaram, R.N.S., Chakurkar, E.B. and Barbuddhe, S. B. 2006 Feeding value of broken rice for Japanese quail layers. Indian Journal of Animal Nutrition 23: 193-195.

19

Low Protein Diets with Supplemental Amino Acids for Economical & Eco-friendly Broiler Production

T.M. Prabhu, B.N. Suresh and C. Basavanta Kumar

Department of Animal Nutrition, Veterinary College, Hebbal, Bengaluru-560 024
Karnataka Veterinary, Animal and Fisheries Sciences University, Bidar

Introduction

Feed is the main contributor to economic and environmental costs of poultry production. This applies in particular to the protein fraction of the diet as the protein constitutes the second abundant and the most expensive nutrient in the broiler diets. Quantitatively, protein rich feed sources constitute 25 to 40 per cent of the diets, next to cereal grains as energy sources accounting for 60 to 70 per cent. In terms of input cost, protein sources account for 40 to 50 per cent of feed cost as these ingredients are highly expensive and play a major role in determining the cost of broiler production.

Proteins are made up of amino acids and it is universally accepted that birds as such do not have need for crude protein (CP) rather there is a need for amino acids (AA). The AA are essential primarily for biosynthesis of muscle mass apart from serving various biochemical functions inside the body. The modern broiler genotypes which are bred for higher body weight gain and feed efficiency, require high amount of protein with optimal AA profiles in their diet. Hence, practical broiler diets are formulated with higher CP levels in order to ensure supply of all essential AA excepting commercially available crystalline AA such as methionine, lysine and threonine. The surplus dietary CP excreted in the excreta which emits ammonia and also contributing to poor litter quality and health status of birds.

Reduction of protein is one of the easiest methods to reduce the feed cost as well as to reduce impact of nitrogen pollution on the environment. For protein reduction, locally available feed ingredients such as sunflower cake, rapeseed meal, de-oiled rice bran and other alternative ingredients can be used to partially replace soybean meal, the conventional protein source in broiler diets.

However, reduction of protein in commercial broiler diets invariably reduce the broiler performance since, in such formulations although the first three limiting AA are supplemented, the second line of limiting AA namely valine, isoleucine and occasionally tryptophan become limiting (Basavanta Kumar *et al*., 2016). It is a challenging situation and the extent to which protein can be decreased without compromising with the bird's performance. Lowering the dietary CP levels and use of synthetic AA perhaps can reduce the feed cost and also reduce the environmental pollution of nitrogen (Corzo *et al.*, 2009). Further, Szczurek (2010) suggested to formulate the diets on digestible or ileal digestible AA basis to prevent AA deficiency and to improve environmental stewardship.

Protein and amino acid requirement of broilers

The requirement of energy, CP and various AA during different phases of broiler production is presented in Table 1. In view of the faster growth observed in the present-day broilers, the nutrient levels recommended are higher than the previous values. Current practice in the field is to supply nutrients somewhat excess of the recommended requirements.

Table 1: Recommended amino acids (%) levels in broiler diets by various agencies

Phase (Feeding period, days)	AMEn Kcal/kg	Crude protein	Dig Lys	Dig Met	Dig. Met +Cys	Dig Try	Dig Thr	Dig Arg	Dig Val	Dig Ile
NRC (1994)[1]										
Starter (0-21 days)	3200	23.0	0.99	0.45	0.81	0.18	0.67	1.15	0.78	0.70
Grower (22-42 days)	3200	20.0	0.90	0.34	0.65	0.16	0.62	1.01	0.71	0.64
Finisher (43-56 days)	3200	18.0	0.77	0.29	0.54	0.15	0.57	0.92	0.61	0.55
ICAR (2013)										
Starter (0-14 days)	3000	22.0	1.08	0.47	0.80	0.18	0.80	1.24	-	0.80
Grower (15-21days)	3050	21.5	0.96	0.43	0.75	0.18	0.78	1.12	-	0.78
Finisher (22-42 days)	3100	19.5	0.84	0.37	0.62	0.15	0.67	0.95	-	0.69
Cobb 500 (2018)										
Starter (1-8 days)	2975	21-22	1.22	0.46	0.91	0.20	0.83	1.28	0.89	0.77
Grower (9-18 days)	3025	19-20	1.12	0.45	0.85	0.18	0.73	1.18	0.85	0.72

Finisher 1 (19-28 days)	3100	18-19	1.02	0.42	0.80	0.18	0.66	1.07	0.76	0.67
Finisher 2 (>29 days)	3150	17-18	0.97	0.40	0.76	0.17	0.63	1.02	0.73	0.64
Ross 308 (2019)										
Starter (0-10 days)	3000	23.0	1.28	0.51	0.95	0.20	0.86	1.37	0.96	0.86
Grower (11-24 days)	3100	21.5	1.15	0.47	0.87	0.18	0.77	1.23	0.87	0.78
Finisher (>25 days)	3200	20.0	1.03	0.43	0.80	0.16	0.69	1.10	0.78	0.71

AMEn = Apparent metabolizable energy corrected by nitrogen

[1]Values derived by multiplying individual amino acid with its digestibility co-efficient

Amino acid profile and their digestibility values in feed ingredients

Various ingredients and crystalline AAs are used in broiler diets to supply the required AA. However, the digestibility co-efficient of AA in different feed ingredients differs depending on several factors. The quantum of AA digested and absorbed is more important than the AA intake. Thus, expression of the ideal amino acid ratios and the feed formulation on digestible amino acid basis or standardized ileal AA basis (SIDAA) is preferred than total AA basis. The AA profile and its standardized ileal digestibility coefficients of commonly used ingredients in poultry diets is presented in Table 2.

Table 2: Amino acid profile and its standardized ileal digestibility coefficients of feed ingredients used in poultry diets

Ingredient	**Lys**	**Met**	**Met+ Cys**	**Thr**	**Val**	**Ile**	**Trp**	**Leu**	**Arg**	**Phe**	**Gly+ Ser**	**His**
Total amino acid composition (%, as is)												
Maize	0.255	0.173	0.357	0.306	0.408	0.296	0.061	1.050	0.408	0.418	0.745	0.255
Soybean meal	2.727	0.577	1.214	1.712	2.080	2.000	0.577	3.364	3.334	2.279	4.656	1.184
Rapeseed meal	1.741	0.690	1.641	1.481	1.801	1.421	0.510	2.482	2.352	1.471	3.239	1.021
De-oiled rice bran	0.732	0.321	0.631	0.621	0.892	0.571	0.200	1.162	1.223	0.732	1.620	0.451
Meat and bone meal	2.121	0.523	0.898	1.292	1.815	1.115	0.207	2.457	3.187	1.391	8.320	0.681
Percentage standardized ileal digestibility coefficients[1]												
Maize	92	94	90	85	92	95	81	94	93	94	75/83	95
Soybean meal	90	91	86	85	88	89	89	89	93	89	80/84	92
Rapeseed meal	80	84	73	79	79	79	80	82	87	83	76/72	82
De-oiled rice bran	74	77	72	69	75	75	79	73	86	76	70/67	82
Meat and bone meal	69	72	62	32	70	69	53	71	77	70	69/52	71

[1]Adopted from Hoehler *et al.* (2006) and as apparent digestible coefficients for Gly+Ser from Bryden *et al.* (2009).

Limiting amino acids in low protein diets

The *de novo* protein synthesis requires all twenty-two AA (physiologically essential) to be present at the cellular level for mRNA translation (NRC, 1994). However, the broilers are able to synthesize twelve of them which are termed dispensable or non-essential AA and rest of the ten AA that can't be synthesized by birds to meet the requirement as indispensable or essential AA (D'Mello, 2003). The essential AA requirement must be met solely through dietary supply while non-essential AA need not be supplied in the diet. However, under certain circumstances, the non-essential AA also become essential depending on the demand at times of rapid growth or certain physiological conditions, which are categorised as conditionally essential AA which includes tyrosine, cysteine, proline and glycine (Leeson and Summers, 2008).

Limiting AA (LAA) refers to the AA which are deficit in a particular type of diet in relation to the requirement of the birds. Since it depends on the bird's requirement and the AA composition of the diet, the order of LAA keeps changing depending on the phase of growth as well as on the type of diet. In practical type of corn-soybean meal based broiler diets, methionine is the first limiting AA and lysine and threonine follows as second and third LAA, respectively. Further, any attempt to reduce the cost of the diet by reducing protein level would result in deficiency of subsequent LAA such as valine, isoleucine, arginine and tryptophan.

Table 3: Order of limiting amino acids in practical type of corn-soybean meal based broiler diets upon sequential protein reduction

Limiting Order	Amino acid	Function	Commercial sources
1	Methionine	Synthesis of muscle, keratin, feather protein and all enzymes systems, essential for expression of myogenic gene and initiation of protein synthesis, precursor for cysteine, methyl group donor in creatine synthesis, prevent fat accumulation in liver	DL-Methionine, DL-2-hydroxy-4-(methylthio)butanoic acid (DL-HMTBA) DL-methionine hydroxy analog-free acid (MHA-FA) Liquid Herbal extracts
2	Lysine	Synthesis of protein and carcass composition, synthesis of nucleotides, chromoproteins, formation of erythrocytes and deposition of calcium in bones and absorption of phosphorus	L-Lysine HCl L-Lysine Sulfate
3	Threonine	Breast meat yield, gut physiology	L-Threonine
4/5	Valine	Body protein accretion, feather protein synthesis, various physiological functions	L-Valine
5/4	Isoleucine	Muscle and feather protein synthesis, immune function	L-Isoleucine
6	Arginine	Muscle protein synthesis, immune and hormone function	L-Arginine
7	Tryptophan	Muscle protein synthesis, precursor for synthesis of neurotransmitters (serotonin, melatonin) and niacin	L-Tryptophan

Performance of broilers on low protein diets with supplemental amino acids

The results of recently conducted trials with reduced CP in broiler diets is presented in Figures 1 to 3. The comparable feed intake in low protein LAA supplemented diets was observed in most studies. In all such low protein diets, even though the protein was less yet they were formulated to contain same levels of LAA and hence the feed intake was homogenous between high protein and low protein AA supplemented diets as the feed ensured sufficient intake of AA. However, in some cases, depressed feed intake as the negative effect of low CP diets was noticed. The addition of non-essential AA like glycine has shown partially to alleviate the negative effect of low CP diets, though the dietary NEAA/EAA ratio is poorly understood, factor in defining the performance of broilers fed on low CP diets.

The protein reduction with supplementation of EAA resulted in equal or better body weight gain and feed conversion ratio than control (Kerr and Kidd, 1999; Kamran *et al.*, 2004; Si *et al.,* 2001; Waldroup *et al.*, 2005; Darsi *et al.*, 2012; Han, 2019). In these studies, the extent of protein reduction ranged between 0.6 to 2.7 percentage points with exception of one study with 4 per cent protein reduction. In contrary, the negative performance observed in few studies (Ferguson *et al.*, 1998a, b; Bregendahl *et al.*, 2002) was in fact noticed with relatively higher protein reduction (2.4 to 6.0 percentage points). In this context, a protein reduction beyond 2 percentage point appears to decrease the growth performance of broilers hence protein reduction within this limit perhaps be regarded as safe.

Liveability was not affected under low protein diets even with a steep protein reduction up to 6 percentage point regardless of amino acid supplementation (Kerr and Kidd, 1999, Si *et al.*, 2001; Waldroup *et al.*, 2005; Maksoud *et al.*, 2010). Hence, there is no impact of protein reduction with or without amino acid supplementation on increasing mortality and hence liveability was not affected with protein reduction.

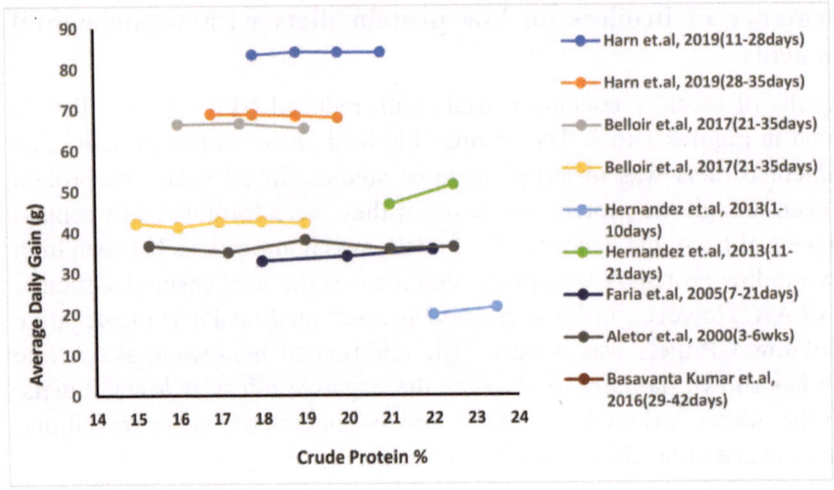
Average Daily Gain (g)
90
80
70
60
50
40
30
20
10
0
14 15 16 17 18 19 20 21 22 23 24
Crude Protein %
Harn et.al, 2019(11-28days)
Harn et.al, 2019(28-35days)
Belloir et.al, 2017(21-35days)
Belloir et.al, 2017(21-35days)
Hernandez et.al, 2013(1-10days)
Hernandez et.al, 2013(11-21days)
Faria et.al, 2005(7-21days)
Aletor et.al, 2000(3-6wks)
Basavanta Kumar et.al, 2016(29-42days)

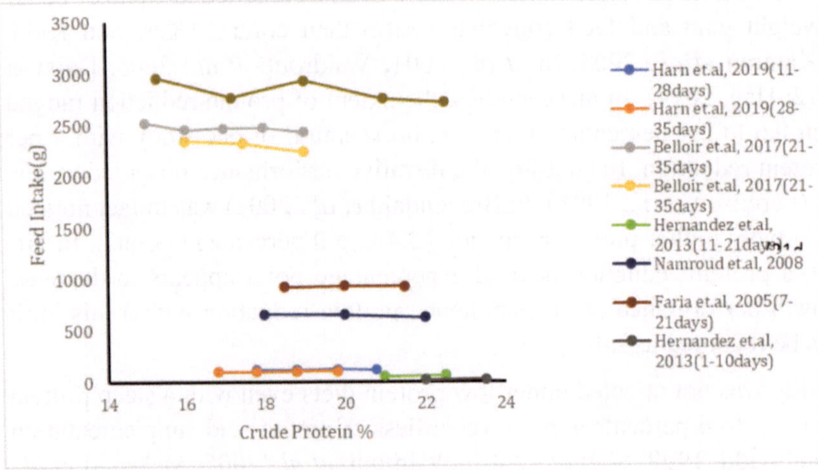
Feed Intake(g)
3500
3000
2500
2000
1500
1000
500
0
14 16 18 20 22 24
Crude Protein %
Harn et.al, 2019(11-28days)
Harn et.al, 2019(28-35days)
Belloir et.al, 2017(21-35days)
Belloir et.al, 2017(21-35days)
Hernandez et.al, 2013(11-21days)
Namroud et.al, 2008
Faria et.al, 2005(7-21days)
Hernandez et.al, 2013(1-10days)

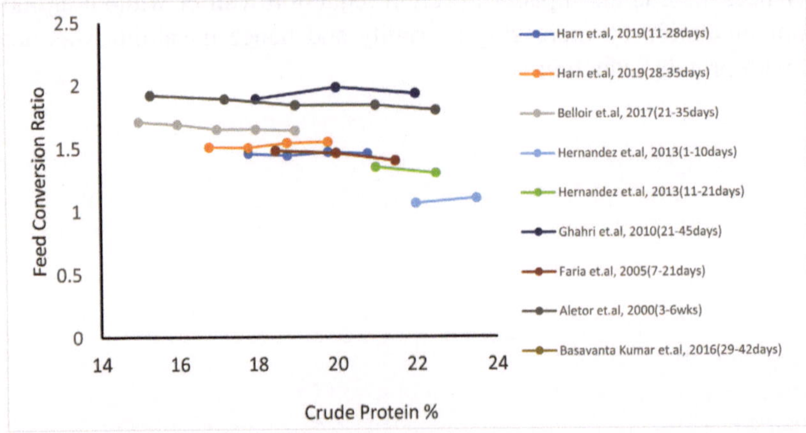
Feed Conversion Ratio
2.5
2
1.5
1
0.5
0
14 16 18 20 22 24
Crude Protein %
Harn et.al, 2019(11-28days)
Harn et.al, 2019(28-35days)
Belloir et.al, 2017(21-35days)
Hernandez et.al, 2013(1-10days)
Hernandez et.al, 2013(11-21days)
Ghahri et.al, 2010(21-45days)
Faria et.al, 2005(7-21days)
Aletor et.al, 2000(3-6wks)
Basavanta Kumar et.al, 2016(29-42days)

Carcass characteristics not affected by low protein diets with supplemental amino acids

The broilers fed with the amino acid balanced low-protein diets have shown similar breast meat yield (Rezaei *et al.*, 2004; Sterling *et al.*, 2005, 2006; Belloir *et al.*, 2017) and carcass yield (Harn *et al.*, 2019). The breast muscle yield was significantly decreased on protein reduction (4 percentage point) and with supplementation of LAA, the breast muscle yield was significantly (P<0.05) similar to control in broilers. With further protein reduction, the breast yield significantly (P<0.05) decreased not with standing the LAA supplementation (Kerr and Kidd, 1999). On the other hand the thigh, drumstick and wing yields were not affected by protein reduction either with or without amino acid supplementation. Similarly, no difference in thigh yield (Namroud *et al.*, 2008; Darsi *et al.*, 2012) was observed in broilers when the protein level was reduced and formulated to satisfy the LAA needs. It may be concluded that, if the essential AA particularly the lysine and methionine are in a good balance then decreasing the dietary protein does not decrease the breast meat yield because it is very sensitive to dietary lysine and methionine levels (Si *et al.*, 2001).

The most consistent problem of low protein diets is increased abdominal fat deposition which deteriorates the quality of carcass. This perhaps occurs as a consequence of increased lipogenesis, as the ratio between NE and protein in such diets is increased. Smith and Pesti (1998), Neto *et al.* (2002) and Sterling *et al.* (2005) found significantly P<0.05) increased abdominal fat content with low protein diets. However, when an amino acid balanced low protein diet is given, the birds fed such diets are expected to utilise the energy for protein accretion than for abdominal fat synthesis. In line with this, Kerr and Kidd (1999) reported supplementation of LAA with gluatamic acid in a 6 percentage point protein reduction resulted in a similar AF levels to that of control. Similarly, Si *et al.*, (2004) also reported no alteration of AF percentage with a protein reduction of 4.40 percentage points with supplementation of LAA in 0-21 day old broilers. In contrast, Namroud *et al.* (2008) were able to reduce protein only by 2.0 percentage points with supplementation of LAA, however, further protein reduction was found to significantly (P<0.05) increase the AF percentage. Similar observation was also made by Darsi *et al.* (2012).

The liver is the main lipogenic organ in chickens. As a consequence of enhanced lipogenesis in the liver of birds fed the low protein diets, the liver weights are expected to increase due to increase in ME:CP ratio (Rosebrough and Steele, 1985; Swennen *et al.*, 2006). However, Cheng *et al.* (1997) and Sterling *et al.* (2005) did not find any effect of dietary protein levels on liver weights. In contrast, Namroud *et al.* (2008) reported a significant (P<0.005) increase in relative liver weight, which in fact was noted only at high level of protein reduction (6 percentage points) but not at moderate reduction (2 and 4 percentage points). Since the weights of other two giblet organs were not anticipated to alter, were not illustrated in any low protein amino acid supplemented studies and hence due to lack of literature are not discussed.

Utilisation of alternative protein sources to reduce protein in broiler diets

In India, due to diversified crop production, many alternative protein sources are available for poultry feeding. Rapeseed meal (RSM), a by-product from oil industry is a good source of crude protein, lysine and methionine. However, RSM inclusion in boiler diets is limited due to the presence of glucosinolates (120μmol/g). The broilers can tolerate 10 μmol glucosinolates/g feed without any impact on growth performance and theoretically RSM can be included up to 8.0 per cent of their diets. Similarly, De-oiled rice bran (DORB), a by-product of rice milling industry which is available in plenty at a reasonably lower price and a moderate source of protein, can be incorporated in broiler rations up to 20%.

A preliminary study conducted with incorporation of RSM and DORB at 6 per cent of the diets to reduce protein revealed significant ($P<0.05$) decrease in growth performance of broilers due to deficiencies of second line limiting amino acids *viz*., valine, isoleucine and occasionally tryptophan (Basavanta Kumar *et al.,* 2015). Further trials (Table 3) with incorporation of 3 and 6 per cent of RSM or DORB (replacing soybean meal) to reduce protein with supplementation of LAA (Lys, Met, Thr, Val, Ile) showed similar feed intake, body weight gain and feed efficiency compared to control diets with recommended CP level. No impact of levels of DORB or RSM on carcass parameters is indicative of the supplemental amino acids in overcoming the deficiency of valine and isoleucine. Further, in both the trials, formulation of diets on SID amino acid found to perform better than TAA based formulation.

Table 3: Performance of broilers fed DORB and RSM based low protein diets with supplemental LAA

Attribute	**Trial 1: CP reduction by incorporating DORB**				**Trial2: CP reduction by incorporating RSM**			
DORB/RSM Level	**0**	**3**	**6**	**p-value**	**0**	**3**	**6**	**p-value**
CP reduction	**0**	**-0.75**	**-1.5**		**0**	**-0.75**	**-1.5**	
Supplemental AA	Lys, Met, Thr	Lys, Met, Thr, Val	Lys, Met, Thr, Val, Ile		Lys, Met, Thr	Lys, Met, Thr, Val	Lys, Met, Thr, Val, Ile	
Growth performance								
Feed intake (g)	3455	3426	3449	0.579	3455	3463	3499	0.647
Body weight gain (g)	2098[b]	2053[ab]	2034[a]	<0.001	2098	2088	2084	0.554
Feed conversion ratio	1.680[a]	1.705[b]	1.723[b]	<0.001	1.680	1.686	1.700	0.124
Carcass characterises (% of pre-slaughter weight)								
Carcass yield	71.96[b]	71.93[ab]	71.24[a]	0.040	71.28	71.83	72.38	0.280
Breast yield	21.94[b]	21.59[ab]	21.14[a]	0.044	21.70	21.60	22.09	0.466
Thigh yield	13.48[b]	13.14[ab]	12.68[a]	0.012	13.24	13.15	13.63	0.354
Drumstick yield	9.995	9.660	9.400	0.080	9.60	9.78	10.30	0.522
Liver	2.07	2.04	2.03	0.915	2.06	2.03	2.05	0.656
Heart	0.44	0.43	0.44	0.831	0.44	0.44	0.45	0.857
Gizzard	1.93	1.97	1.97	0.424	1.95	1.95	1.95	0.278
Abdominal fat	1.85	1.71	1.61	<0.001	1.80	1.67	1.56	0.172
Nitrogen balance								
N excretion (g/d)	1.794[b]	1.726[ab]	1.608[a]	0.004	-	-	-	-
N retention (g/d)	4.263	4.271	4.163	0.522	-	-	-	-
Serum uric acid (mg/dL)	10.45	10.28	9.85	0.098	10.40	10.05	10.50	0.806

DORB = De-oiled rice bran, RSM = Rape seed meal

Low protein diets decreased nitrogen excretion in birds

A large part of the dietary nitrogen intake is not retained by the bird, but excreted into the environment. The most nitrogen losses through excreta are due to the inability of dietary protein to meet the AA requirements and particularly the imbalances between different AA (Gous, 1998). Lowering the CP content of the diet could therefore be a tool to reduce the nitrogen excretion and ammonia emission from broiler houses. However, the balance of AA is important while reducing CP because birds need AA in certain ratios to ensure optimum performance. The dietary protein level has significantly ($p<0.05$) minimized nitrogen excretion at 1.5% protein reduction compared to normal protein diet (Table 3). The serum uric acid level was also significantly reduced in 1.5% low protein diet compared to normal protein diets.

Further, if the available EAA content of the diet is closer to the amino acid requirement of birds for growth and maintenance, a minimum amino acid degradation and excretion will occur (Gous, 1998). As a result, efficiency of protein utilisation in broilers would be better under low protein amino acid supplemented diets as compared to high protein diets (Maksoud *et al*., 2010). On the other hand, reduction of protein reduces the N level in excreta and litter and therefore, decreases the disposal problems and pollution potential of the litter (Moran *et al*., 1996). It is most efficient and possibly the cheapest method of controlling ammonia production. By this method, nitrogen excretion can be reduced up to 21 per cent with a 2.5 percentage point reduction in dietary protein (Jacob *et al*., 1994). It is, therefore, reduced protein degradation/AA oxidation leads to more efficient retention of dietary protein as a compensatory mechanism for a reduced protein intake. As a general rule, one percentage point reduction in dietary protein will lead to reductions of 10% nitrogen in manure, 10% ammonia emissions into the air, 3 % water consumption and 5% manure volume.

Low protein diets reduces wet litter and footpad lesions

A reduced CP content in broiler diets can reduce water intake, because there is a reduced need to excrete the surplus of nitrogen. A lower water intake might reduce the risk of wet litter, and thus the risk of impaired welfare, since wet litter is the main reason for skin dermatitis such as footpad lesions, hock burns and breast blisters (Martland, 1985). The normal or higher CP diets are prepared with inclusion of soybean meal at higher levels. As a result, the potassium content and the electrolyte balance (dEB) also increases. The water intake increases with the increase of both dEB and potassium (Mushtaq *et al*., 2013). This also result in deteriorated litter quality and the higher footpad score of the broilers.

Harn *et al.,* (2019) reported that, the incidence of footpad lesions decreased linearly with the reduction of the dietary CP content. The most important factor causing footpad lesions is considered to be wet litter (Shepherd and Fairchild, 2010). Broilers fed with the control feeding program had the lowest scores for litter quality and the highest footpad scores.

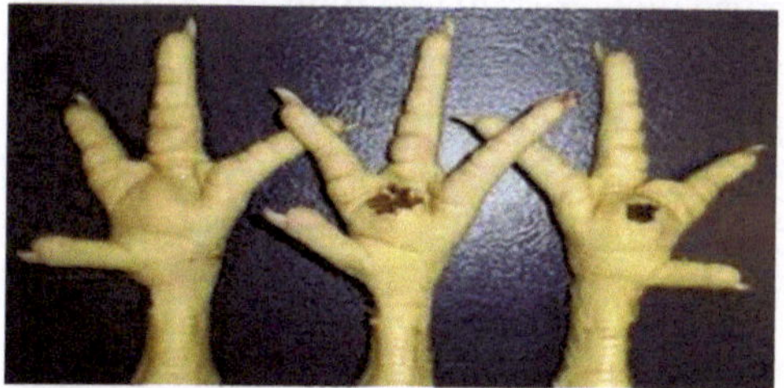

Footpad lesion

Effect of feeding low-protein diets on gut health of broilers

Feeding low crude protein diets reduces the *Clostridium perfringens* counts in the intestine. *C. perfringens* is the gram-positive and obligate bacteria associated with necrotic enteritis in poultry. Toxins produced by the bacteria cause damage to the small intestine, liver lesions, and mortality. Most often the only sign of necrotic enteritis in a flock is a sudden increase in mortality. However, birds with depression, ruffled feathers, and diarrhoea may also be seen. The gross lesions are primarily found in the small intestine (jejunum/ileum), which may be ballooned, friable, and contain a foul-smelling, brown fluid. The mucosa is usually covered with a tan to yellow pseudo membrane often referred to as a "Turkish towel" in appearance. This pseudo membrane may extend throughout the small intestine or be localized. The disease usually persists in a flock for 5–10 days, and mortality is 2%–50%. Feeding high CP diets has a negative impact on gut health. It causes increased flow of indigestible protein to the large intestine, thus increasing metabolite production in the caecum.

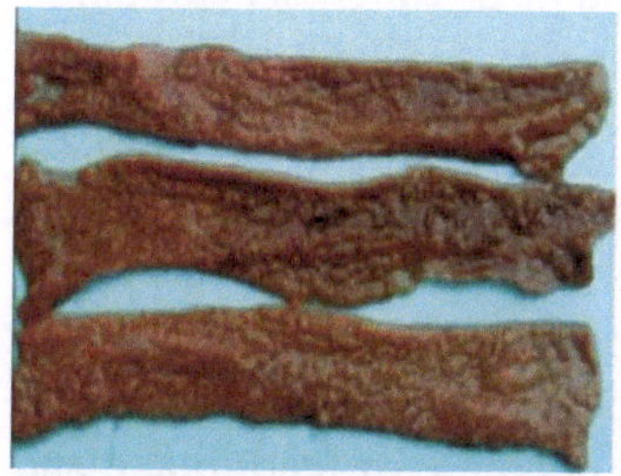

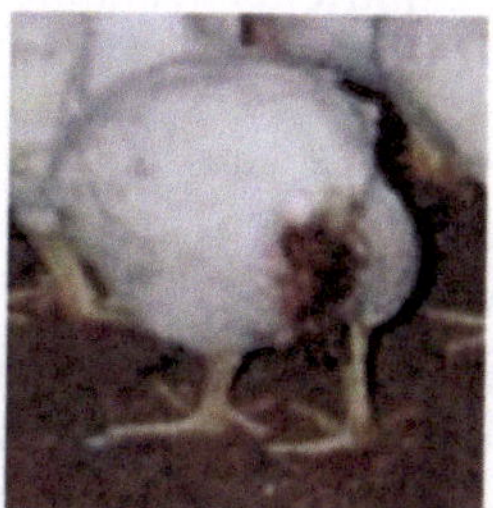

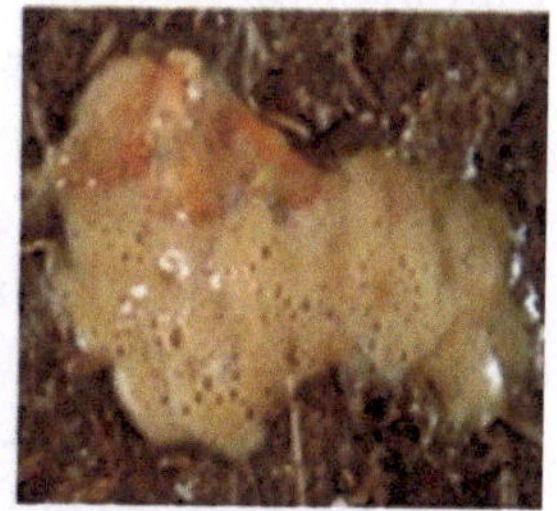

Intestinal lesion Diarrhoea due to Necrotic Enteritis
(*Courtesy*: Engormix)

Low protein diets in hot climates and during heat stress

In the hot and humid tropics, irrespective of the level of inputs, the full genetic potential of the commercial meat-type chickens may not be able to be expressed because of environmental constraints. The concept of maximising growth performance of broiler chickens should be matched with economic considerations. Thus, it is possible to use diets formulated with lower nutrient specifications under such conditions. The nutrient requirement of poultry is profoundly affected by ambient temperature and relative humidity. According to Awad *et al* (2016), crude protein of broilers starter (1-21 days) diet can be reduced upto 19.2% with EAA fortification and without any adverse effects on growth performance under the hot, humid tropics.

The main reason behind the low protein diets apart from cost reduction is that, with supplementation of LAA one can reduce overindulgence of essential amino acids, which will have a bearing on minimising the bird's energy expenditure for excreting excess of amino acids as the energy cost of excretion is more than the energy cost of amino acid incorporation for protein synthesis as described previously. In tropical countries like India, where the ambient temperature is expected to be more than thermo neutral comfort zone for broilers, the impact of high protein or excess of EAA would indeed reduce feed intake to avoid heat increment which consequently might reflect on the bird's growth performance.

Effect of protease supplementation in low-protein diets in broilers

Apart from using crystalline amino acids, addition of exogenous protease enzyme to the low-protein diets is another strategy to maintain the performance of broilers. Sometimes, depending on the local contexts of the feedstuff production and markets, and consumer's demand, broiler producers consider incorporating alternative protein sources, with a lesser digestibility of the nitrogen fraction and suboptimal amino acid availability (Ajayi, 2015), which may reduce the performances. In this direction, supplementation of exogenous enzymes help to make more nutrients available and also reduce the amount of nutrients voided in faeces (Oxenboll *et al*., 2011).

The use of exogenous proteases can help in the reduction of the protein contents of a given feed by improving the digestibility and availability of the protein thereby reducing the cost of feed contributed by the protein feedstuff. According to Ajayi *et al* (2015), performance of birds on the lower CP diets were enhanced by the supplementation with protease; there was significant increase in the body weight gain and decrease in feed intake and feed conversion ratio of birds fed the 15.5/12.5% CP and the 17.5/14.4%CP diets with added protease. Further, there was no negative effect on carcass characteristics of same birds. Recent findings also support the addition of protease to low protein diets for broilers to enhance growth performance and increase production efficiency (Ndazigaruye *et al.*, 2019; Law *et al.*, 2019) and to decrease abdominal fat deposition and increase the profit margin (Law *et al.*, 2019). The CP in broiler chicken diets can be reduced by about 5.6% without deleterious effect on performance if the protease is used in a tropical environment similar to the one in this study.

Practical Utility

- Formulation of low protein poultry diets is essential for combating rising feed and production costs, as well as animal welfare and environmental concerns.
- Formulation of poultry diet with supplemental amino acids increases flexibility and efficiency in the use of locally available diverse protein rich feedstuffs in India, including reducing dependency on soybean.
- Increased accuracy of poultry diet formulation based on amino acid digestibility in comparison to total amino acids lead to more feed efficiency and productivity of birds.

Conclusion

- CP level in the broiler diets can be reduced by at least two percentage points without affecting performance and carcass quality when balanced for essential AAs.
- Low CP diets using supplemental AA is cost effective and environment-friendly. On an average, one percentage point dietary CP reduction result in 10 % decrease in nitrogen excretion.
- Exogenous protease helps in better utilization of dietary protein sources of low quality.
- Amino acid balanced low protein diets under high temperature are advantageous in terms of sustaining production and health status of broilers.

References

Ajayi, H. L. 2015. Effect of protease supplementation on performance and carcass weights of broiler chickens fed low protein diets, Nigerian Journal of Agriculture, Food and Environment, 11(1):29-32.

Aletor, V. A., Hamid. I.I., Nies. E. and Pfeffer, E. 2000. Low-protein amino acid supplemented diets in broilers chickens: effects on performance, carcass characteristics, whole-body composition and efficiencies of nutrient utilization. Poultry Science, 80: 243–253.

Awad, E. A. 2016. Effects of feeding low-protein diets fortified with amino acids on broiler chickens under high environmental temperatures. PhD Thesis, Universiti Putra Malaysia.

Basavanta Kumar, C., Gloridoss, D.G., Singh, K.C., Prabhu, T.M. and Suresh, B.N. 2016. Performance of broiler chickens fed low protein, limiting amino acid supplemented diets formulated either on total or standardised ileal digestibile amino acid basis. Asian Australasian Journal of Animal Science, 29: 1616-1624.

Basavanta Kumar, C., Gloridoss, D.G., Singh, K.C., Prabhu, T.M., Siddaramanna, Suresh, B.N. and Anand, M.G. 2015. Impact of second line limiting amino acids deficiency in broilers fed low protein diets with rape seed meal and de-oiled rice bran. Veterinary World, 8: 350-357.

Basavanta Kumar, C., Gloridoss, D.G., Singh. K.C., Venkata Reddy, K., Prabhu, T.M., Siddaramanna, Suresh, B.N. and Anand, M.G. 2015. Performance of broiler chickens fed rapeseed meal based low protein, amino acid supplemented diets formulated either on total or standardised ileal digestible amino acid basis. Mysore Journal of Agricultural Science, 49(1): 79-88.

Belloir, P., M′Eda. B., Lambert. W., Corrent. E., Juin. H., Lessire, M. and Tesseraud, S. 2017. Reducing the CP content in broiler feeds: impact on animal performance, meat quality and nitrogen utilization. Animal, 11: 1881–1889

Bregendahl, K., Sell. J.L. and Zimmerman, D. L. 2002. Effect of low-protein diets on growth performance and body composition of broiler chicks. Poultry Science, 81: 1156-1167.

Cheng T.K., Hamre M.L. and Coon, C.N. 1997. Responses of broilers to dietary protein levels and amino acid supplementation to low protein diets at various environmental temperatures. Journal of Applied Poultry Research, 6: 18-33

Corzo, A., Loar, R.E and Kidd, M.T. 2009. Limitations of deficiency isoleucine and valine in broiler chick diets. Poultry Science, 88: 1934-1938.

D'mello, J.P.F. 2003, Amino acids in animal nutrition, 2nd edition, CABI publishing, Wallingford, UK.

Darsi, E., Shivazad, M., Zaghari, M., Namroud, N. F. and Mohammadi, R. 2012. Effect of reduced dietary crude protein levels on growth performance, plasma uric acid and electrolyte concentration of male broiler chicks. Journal of Agricultural Science and Technology, 14: 789-797.

Ferguson, N. S., Gates. R.S., Taraba. J.L., Cantor. A.H., Pescatore, A.J., Ford, M.J. and Burnham, D.J. 1998. The effect of dietary crude protein on growth, ammonia concentration, and litter composition in broilers. Poultry Science, 77: 1481–1487.

Ghahri, H., Gaykani, R. and Toloie, T. 2010. Effect of dietary crude protein level on performance and lyine requirements of male broiler chickens. African Journal of Agricultural Research, 5:1228-1234.

Gous, R.M. 1998. Lysine: Making progress in the nutrition of broilers. Poultry Science, 77(1): 111-7

Harn, J.V., Dijkslag, M.A. and Van Krimpen, M.M. 2019. Effects of low-protein diets supplemented with free amino acids on growth performance, slaughter yield, litter quality and footpad lesions of male broilers. Poultry Science, 98: 4868-4977.

Hernandez, F., Megias. M.D., Orengo. J., Martinez. S., Lopez. M.J. and Madrid, J. 2013. Effect of dietary protein level on retention of nutrients, growth performance, litter composition and NH_3 emission using a multi-phase feeding programme in broilers. Span. Journal of Agricultural Research, 11: 736–746.

Kamran, Z., Sarwar, M., Nisa, M.U., Nadeem, M.A. and Mahmood, S. 2010. Effect of low levels of dietary crude protein with constant metabolizable energy on nitrogen excretion, litter composition and blood parameters of broilers. International Journal of Agricultural Biololgy, 12: 401–405.

Kerr, B.J. and Kidd, M.T. 1999. Amino acid supplementation of low-protein broiler diets: 1. Glutamic acid and indispensable amino acid supplementation. Journal of Applied Poultry Research, 8: 298–309.

Law, F.L., Idrus, Z., Farjam, A.S., Boo, L.J. and Awad, E.A 2019. Effects of protease supplementation of low protein and/or energy diets on growth performance and blood parameters in broiler chickens under heat stress condition, Italian Journal of Animal Science, 18(1): 679-689.

Leeson, S. and Summers, J.D. 2008. Commercial Poultry Nutrition, Third Edition. University Books, Guelph, Canada

Maksoud, A. A., Yan, F., Cerrate, S., Coto, C., Wang, Z. and Waldroup, P. W. 2010. Effect of dietary crude protein, lysine level and amino acid balance on performance of broilers 0 to 18 days of age. International Journal of Poultry Science, 9: 21–27.

Martland, M. F. 1985. Ulcerative dermatitis in broiler chickens – The effect of wet litter. Avian Pathology, 14: 353–364.

Moran, E.T. and Stilborn, B. 1996. Effect of glutamic acid on broiler given sub-marginal crude protein with adequate essential amino acids using feeds high and low in potassium. Poultry Science, 75: 120-129

Mushtaq, M., Pasha, T., Mushtaq, T. and Parvin, R. 2013. Electrolytes, dietary electrolyte balance and salts in broilers: An updated review on growth performance, water intake and litter quality. World's Poultry Science Journal, 69: 789–802.

Namroud, N. F., Shivazad, M. and Zaghari, M. 2008. Effects of fortifying low crude protein diet with crystalline amino acids on performance, blood ammonia level, and excreta characteristics of broiler chicks. Poultry Science, 87: 2250–2258.

Ndazigaruye, G., Kim, D.H., Kang, C.W., Kang, K.R., Joo, Y.J., Lee, S.R. and LEE, K.W. 2019. Effects of low-protein diets and exogenous protease on growth performance, carcass traits, intestinal morphology, caecal volatile fatty acids and serum parameters in broilers. Animals, 9: 226

Neto, M.G., Pesti, G.M. and Bakalli, R.I. 2002. Influence of dietary protein level on the broiler chicken's response to methionine and betaine supplements. Poultry Science, 79:1478-1484.

NRC (National Research Council). 1994. Nutrient Requirements of Poultry. 9th revised edition, National Academic Press, Washington, DC.

Oxenboll, K. M., Pontoppidan, K. and Fru-Nji, F. 2011. Use of a protease in poultry feed offers promising environmental benefits. International Journal of Poultry Science, 10(11): 842-848.

Rezaei, M., Moghaddam, H. N., Reza, J. P. and Kermanshahi, H. 2004. The effects of dietary protein and lysine levels on broiler performance, carcass characteristics and N excretion. International Journal of Poultry Science, 3: 148–52.

Rosebrough, R.W. and Steele, N. C. 1985. Energy and protein relationships in the broiler. 1. Effect of protein levels and feeding regimens on growth, body composition, and in vitro lipogenesis of broiler chicks. Poultry Science, 64: 119–126.

Shepherd, E. M. and Fairchild, B.D. 2010. Footpad dermatitis in poultry. Poultry Science, 89: 2043–2051.

Si, J., Fritts, C.A., Burnham, D.J. and Waldroup, P.W. 2001. Relationship of dietary lysine level to the concentration of all essential amino acids in broiler diets Poultry Science, 80: 1472-1479

Si, J., Fritts, C.A., Burnham, D.J. and Waldroup, P.W. 2004. Extent to which crude protein may be reduced in corn-soybean meal broiler diets through amino acid supplementation. International Journal of Poultry Science, 3: 46–50.

Smith, E. R. and Pesti. G.M. 1998. Influence of broiler strain cross and dietary protein on the performance of broilers. Poultry Science, 77: 276-281.

Sterling, K.G., Vedenov, D.V., Pesti, G.M. and Bakalli, R.I. 2005. Economically optimal crude protein and lysine levels for starting broiler chicks. Poultry Science, 84: 29-36.

Swennen Q., Janssens, G.P.J., Collin, A., Bihanduval, E.L., Verbeke, K., Decuypere, E. and Buyse, J. 2006. Diet-induced thermogenesis and glucose oxidation in broiler chickens: Influence of genotype and diet composition. Poultry Science, 85: 731-742.

Szczurek, W. 2010. Practical validation of efficiency of the standardised ileal digestible amino acid values in diet formulation for broiler chickens. Journal of Animal Feed Science, 19: 592-598.

Waldroup, P. W., Jiang, Q. and Fritts, C.A. 2005. Effect of supplementing broiler diets low in crude protein with essential and nonessential amino acids. International Journal of Poultry Science, 4: 425-431.

20

Functional Feed Ingredients and Supplements in Poultry Nutrition

B.N. Suresh, M.C. Shivakumar and G.P. Hombegowda

Department of Livestock Farm Complex, Veterinary College, Hassan-560 024 Karnataka, Karnataka Veterinary, Animal and Fisheries Sciences University, Bidar

Introduction

Nutrients are essential substances present in different types of foods which perform various life-sustaining functions in the body. They are required for growth, maintenance and the reproductive process. Poultry require more than 40 such nutrients, which are classified into six major groups - water, carbohydrates, protein (amino acids), fats, minerals and vitamins. Poultry diets must be formulated to provide all these essential nutrients as per the bird's requirement to achieve optimum growth and production. Several ingredients including cereal grains, cereal by-products, fats, plant protein sources, animal by-products, vitamin and mineral supplements, crystalline amino acids and feed additives are commonly used to prepare poultry diets. Further, specialist areas such as immuno-nutrition are rapidly gaining attention due to continued advancement in the field of poultry nutrition (Beski *et al*., 2015). Hence, besides supplying essential nutrients, present day feed formulation necessitates choosing ingredients to maximize nutrient availability, better gut functioning and to enhance immune system (Ravindran, 2005) and to increase tolerance to stress (Campbell *et al*., 2003; Campbell *et al*., 2006b) and disease challenges in birds (Campbell *et al*., 2006a).

Functional feed ingredients are those which have a potentially positive effect on health of the birds beyond the basic nutrition. Such ingredients or products should be typically high in important nutrients or contains biologically active components, besides being highly digestible and devoid of anti-nutritional factors. Inclusion of such functional ingredients in broiler diets, especially at an earlier age of birds, can assist early gut development and digestive physiology, support immune system and improve their growth performance (Beski *et al*., 2015). Some of these ingredients can also increases the birds' tolerance to diseases (Campbell *et al*., 2006a) and stress in a wide variety

(Campbell *et al*., 2006b; Gonzalez-Esquerra *et al*., 2020). Hence, the poultry feed industry always scouting for sustainable and high-quality alternatives for diet formulations. Single cell proteins (SCP), spray-dried plasma (SDP), yeast extracted nucleotides (YEN) and other specialized protein products are some examples for such unique ingredients.

Single cell proteins

Single cell proteins (SCP) are broad range of very diverse products produced from microorganisms as fungi, algae (*Spirulina, Chlorella*), yeasts (*Saccharomyces cerevisiae*) or bacteria (*Methylococuus, Cyanobacteria)*. SCP is produced by a fermentation process. The high growth rates of micro-organisms, their high efficiency of substrate conversion and protein synthesis forms the basis for the production of SCP (Ritala *et al*., 2017). The possibility of large-scale production from high-tech bioreactors using inexpensive raw materials and a continuous harvest are other advantages of SCP production (Ritala *et al*., 2017; Linder, 2019). The methods of SCP production are also standardized to maintain consistency of the product and also can enable traceability. This is a huge advantage compared to existing sources of protein that are plagued by safety and contamination challenges. SCPs contains ~ 65 % crude protein and has an amino acid profile similar to fishmeal (Hombegowda, 2019). Studies indicated that SCPs can be included up to 5% level or to meet 30-40 % of total crude protein in broiler diets with improved weight gain, feed conversion ratio and economic efficiency in broilers (Ayed and Ghaoui, 2011; Saied *et al*., 2011; El-Nagha, 2012).

Our study showed that SCP can be included up to 5% in the commercial broiler diets as a protein source replacing soybean meal or fish meal without any adverse effect on the growth performance of broiler birds (Hombegowda, 2019). Further, the livability was significantly improved upon inclusion of SCP up to 10%. The effect of dietary inclusion of SCP at different levels on the gut development and its morphometry is presented in Table 1. The relative length of the different segments of small intestine viz., duodenum, jejunum and ileum of broiler birds were significantly ($P<0.01$) increased with incremental level of SCP in diets. The duodenal villi length, crypt depth and length to depth ratio were higher ($P<0.01$) in groups fed 5% SCP diets compared to control. The incorporation of SCP at 5% in diets showed beneficial effect on the gut health of jejunum of broiler birds while no adverse effect on ileal health was observed.

Table 1: Effect of single cell protein (SCP) on intestinal development and morphology of broilers at 42nd day

SCP Level %	Intestinal Length (cm/100g body weight)			Intestinal morphometry (µm)								
				Duodenum			Jejunum			Ileum		
	Duodenum	Ileum	Jejunum	Villi Length	Crypt Depth	Villi: Crypt	Villi Length	Crypt Depth	Villi: Crypt	Villi Length	Crypt Depth	Villi: Crypt
0	1.13^{a}	3.43^{a}	3.40^{a}	2205.8^{b}	246.0^{a}	9.1^{a}	1180.6^{bc}	151.1^{b}	7.9	841.0^{b}	135.4	6.2
2.5	1.18^{ab}	3.38^{a}	3.36^{a}	2188.5^{ab}	232.2^{a}	9.5^{ab}	1184.7^{bc}	149.7^{b}	8.0	835.8^{b}	131.6	6.4
5	1.12^{a}	3.38^{a}	3.39^{a}	2942.2^{c}	288.5^{b}	10.3^{b}	1232.7^{c}	150.3^{b}	8.2	848.9^{b}	129.3	6.6
7.5	1.22^{ab}	3.61^{ab}	3.61^{ab}	2094.9^{ab}	233.0^{a}	9.1^{a}	1111.8^{b}	144.9^{ab}	7.7	784.6^{ab}	129.4	6.1
10	1.28^{b}	3.76^{b}	3.76^{b}	2031.6^{a}	228.8^{a}	8.9^{a}	1017.7^{a}	134.2^{a}	7.7	768.6^{a}	130.6	5.9
SEM	0.016	0.003	0.008	<0.001	0.001	0.047	<0.001	0.029	0.778	0.036	0.567	0.208
P-value[1]	0.02	0.08	0.06	34.08	6.54	0.21	17.98	2.56	0.21	13.67	1.83	0.14

[1]An effect with a probability of less than 0.05 is considered significant

[a-d] Means column bearing different superscripts differ significantly

(Hombegowda, 2019)

Similarly, supplementation of *Bacillus subtilis* SCP at 0, 0.2, 0.5 and 1% levels to the basal mash diet up to 28 days showed significantly (P<0.05) higher villus length of the duodenum in 0.2% SCP group compared to control (Samanya *et al.*, 2002). The improvement in villi length in the duodenum, jejunum and ileum upon incorporation of SCP could be due to an elevated production of short chain fatty acids by lactic acid bacteria in the intestinal lumen and also production of antimicrobial and antioxidant compounds with a reduction of substrates available in the intestinal lumen which could diminish the bacterial population of Gram-negative and anaerobic bacteria, therefore decreasing the level of intestinal inflammation and enhancing epithelial integrity, nutrient absorption and bone strength and composition.

Spray-dried plasma protein

Spray-dried blood products such as spray dried plasma (SDP), serum, or globulin concentrate are a combination of bioactive compounds such as peptides, albumin, immunoglobulins, fibrinogen, lipids, growth factors, enzymes, and other components that exert specific biological activities. Such protein products are commonly derived from bovine or porcine origins and are highly digestible protein sources with good amino acid profiles (Torrallardona, 2010). SDP improves early intestinal health and supports an efficient immune system response both locally at the intestine and systemically, thereby benefiting growth, feed efficiency, and survival of broilers in conventional commercial production and under challenging conditions such as disease or environmental stressors.

SDP is produced from the fresh blood collected at abattoir and treated with an anticoagulant. The plasma and blood cell fractions are separated by centrifugation. The plasma is then heated and spray-dried, with the final product being a fine granulated powder (Cole and Sprent, 2001). The spray-drying technique is a mild dehydration process that maintains the functional physicochemical and biological properties of the product. These products may be further processed to standardize the immunoglobulin concentration. This step facilitates its handling at manufacturing plant, or makes it to be in the form of water-soluble product (Pettigrew, 2006). SDP has excellent water-holding capacity, foaming and emulsifying properties and gel strength when heated above 80^{0}C (Polo *et al.*, 2005).

SDP is commonly used as a functional protein ingredient in diets of farm animals to improve performance and health conditions (Torrallardona, 2010; Boyer *et al.*, 2015). It plays a multifaceted mode of action. Modulation of the immune system, antibody functions, inflammatory response, and modification in the intestinal morphology as responses to dietary SDP have been confirmed in numerous studies in young pigs (Campbell *et al*., 2009; Owusu-Asiedu *et al*., 2002). Mobilization of the mucosa membrane and the expression of the activation of immunological areas have been observed after inclusion of SDP in broiler diets (Jamroz *et al*., 2011; Jamroz *et al*., 2012). The recommended level of inclusion of SDP in broiler diets ranged from 0.25 to 4% in broiler diets.

The SDP has beneficial effect on the intestinal integrity of animals and birds. The tendency of SDP to improve the absorptive capacity by increasing villus height and the villus height/crypt depth ratio has been reported in pigs (King *et al*., 2008; Zhao *et al*., 2007). The longer intestinal villi have been observed after inclusion of spray-dried porcine plasma in broiler diets (Jamroz *et al*., 2011, 2012).

Studies also indicated that SDP have antibacterial action, both the external benefits on the microbial community of the intestine as well as the internal effects on pigs (Edwards *et al*., 2010). This is essentially due to the immunoglobulins and glycoproteins exist in plasma products which has potential to bind with pathogenic bacteria receptors and thus reduce their adhesion to the mucosal wall in the gastrointestinal tract (Bosi *et al*., 2001; Garriga *et al*., 2005; Pierce *et al*., 2005). Furthermore, antibodies that exist in SDP also have the ability to inhibit or reduce pathogenic colonization in the GIT (Owusu-Asiedu *et al*., 2002). These theories could explain the greater efficiency of plasma in high-pathogen environments than in clean environments. An improvement in the health and growth efficiency has been observed in animals fed on diets containing SDP and challenged with *Escherichia coli* (Bosi *et al*., 2001; Quigley and Drew, 2000) and necrotic enteritis by *Eimeria* and *Clostridia* (Campbell *et al*., 2006a).

The inclusion of SDP in diets, particularly in the starter phase has also improved the performance of broilers raised under challenge conditions (Henn *et al*., 2013). SDP contains a diversity of functional proteins that are more efficient during animal exposure to environmental or immunological challenges. Good responses to spray-dried serum have also been observed in broilers housed in different environments (Campbell *et al*., 2003).

Yeast extracted nucleotides

The advancement of biotechnology has opened the door to the possibility of utilizing yeast extract, the cell contents of yeast, in animal and poultry feeding to fill the void left by the loss of animal proteins. Yeast extract, rich in nucleotides, is a functional nutrient which upon supplementation in poultry diets provides a range of benefits when compared to standard commercial formulations.

Yeast extracted nucleotides (YEN) are extracted from specific strain of yeast *Saccharomyces cerevisae*. The seed yeast is added to the fermenters to start industrial fermentation. The growth conditions are continuously adjusted to ensure consistency of the final product. The biomass is harvested by separating live yeasts from the culture medium and washed by centrifugation to obtain yeast cream. It is subjected for further processing depending on the desired product. Under controlled conditions yeast's own enzymes disrupt live yeast cells. Then the product is subjected for centrifugation to separate the yeast cell walls and yeast extract.

Presence of nucleotides, glutamic acid, inositol, amino acids and peptides in the yeast extract offers a significant advantage particularly in young chicks. The amino acids and short chain peptides present in yeast extract are in a highly digestible form. Hence, its dietary inclusion improves growth (Dozier *et al.,* 2000), nutrient utilization (Santos *et al.*, 2007), gastrointestinal tract development and immune system function particularly in young chicks (Rutz *et al.,* 2007).

A study was conducted to ascertain the effect of incorporating YEN @ 2% in the broiler diets for a period 0-7, 0-14 and 0-42 days of age. YEN used in the trial was obtained from *Saccharomyces cerevisiae*[1026] which is a rich source of nucleotides, highly digestible peptides, glutamic acid and inositol. The birds fed YEN from 0-14 days recorded significantly ($P<0.05$) longer intestinal length and weight than all other groups on 14th day. This could be due to that the nucleotides supply essential nutrients needed for gut development and repair, as also expressed by Grimble and Westwood (2000).

There was no significant ($P\geq0.05$) differences in the length of villi and depth of crypt measured at all the three regions of the intestine. However, numerically increase in length of villi and crypt depth observed in test groups is due to the fact that feeding of nucleotide hastens the villi maturation and maintains the gut health. Mateo (2004) reported that the villus height and crypt depth were higher in glutamine fed group than the control group in pigs. Bohorquez *et al.* (2008) who fed turkey poults with Nupro yeast extract for 21 days and noticed enhanced intestinal morphology and development. Further, they reported that significant increase in length and crypt depth at the age of 7 days in poults.

The feeding of YEN significantly ($P\leq0.05$) decreased *E.coli* and increased *Lactobacillus* counts in all the intestinal samples studied at different periods. Thus feeding of YEN is expected to provide a better environment for the birds to digest the feed consumed and also to assimilate the same in order to convert it into meat. Feeding two per cent YEN also resulted in non-significant ($P\geq0.05$) difference in gut pH from first to six weeks of age irrespective of the period for which the particular group was fed with nucleotides. It can be concluded that the feeding nucleotides from 0 to 14 days of age can improve the intestinal development and its microbial establishment.

Table 2: Effect of feeding yeast extracted nucleotides (YEN) on intestinal development and morphometry of broilers

	Attribute	Control	YEN 0-7 days	YEN 0-14 days	YEN 0-42 days	SEM
Intestinal length (cm)	Day 7	105.7	107.9	107	106.7	3.18
	Day 14	113.9[a]	114.2[a]	121.0[b]	115.1[a]	1.92
	Day 42	191.6	196.2	200.4	202.2	3.09
Intestinal thickness (mm)	Day 7	0.731	0.721	0.724	0.719	0.021
	Day 14	0.818	0.739	0.778	0.757	0.021
	Day 42	1.060[a]	1.264[ab]	1.157[ab]	1.410[b]	0.038
Intestinal weights (gm)	Day 7	12.84	14.44	13.31	13.39	0.29
	Day 14	9.145[a]	9.557[ab]	10.327[b]	9.207[a]	0.138
	Day 42	5.00	5.71	5.11	5.73	0.103
Duodenum	Villi height	155.68	164.84	205.63	209.79	1.28
	Crypt depth	74.93	84.15	101.57	123.21	0.90
Jejunum	Villi height	245.59	268.07	268.07	273.06	2.10
	Crypt depth	99.9	87.41	109.89	129.87	1.20
Ileocaecocolic junction	Villi height	99.9	108.23	131.54	113.22	0.93
	Crypt depth	52.45	65.77	84.92	51.62	0.87
***E coli* count, *log*$_{10}$CFU/g**	Day 7	1.60 X10^{4} [a]	1.40 X10^{4} [ab]	1.35 X10^{4} [ab]	1.30 X10^{4} [b]	0.039
	Day 14	25.5 X10^{4} [a]	2.60 X10^{4} [b]	2.40 X10^{4} [b]	3.01 X10^{4} [b]	0.196
	Day 42	20.20 X10^{4} [a]	1.89 X10^{4} [b]	1.81 X10^{4} [b]	2.02 X10^{4} [b]	0.525
***Lactobacillus*, *log*$_{10}$ CFU/g**	Day 7	1.80 X10^{3} [a]	2.71 X10^{3} [b]	2.03 X10^{3} [a]	2.10 X10^{3} [a]	0.073
	Day 14	1.16 X10^{3} [a]	1.25 X10^{3} [a]	1.28 X10^{3} [a]	2.41 X10^{3} [b]	0.063
	Day 42	*2.29 X10^{2} [a]*	*2.72 X10^{2} [a]*	*12.90 X10^{2} [b]*	*26.89 X10^{2} [c]*	*1.218*

[1]An effect with a probability of less than 0.05 is considered significant

[a-d] Means column bearing different superscripts differ significantly

(Shivakumar, 2009)

Conclusions

It has become apparent that gut health (intestinal morphometry and microbial community), immune function and tolerance to stress and diseases incidence are critical contributing factors to poultry performance. Some feed ingredients and supplements having such properties have been identified. Among these, single cell proteins, spray dried plasm and yeast extracted nucleotides have received recent attention as candidates for commercial application in poultry.

References

Ayed, M.H. and Ghaoui, F. 2011. Efficiency of supplementing Sacharomyes cerevissiae var. ellipsoideus for improved growth performance and carcass yield in broiler. Research Opinions in Animal and Veterinary Science, 1: 371-374.

Beski, S.S.M., Swick, R.A. and Iji, P.A. 2015. Specialized protein products in broiler chicken nutrition: A review. Animal Nutrition, 1: 47-53

Bohorquez, D.V., Santos, Jr. A.A., Nanneey, R.L. and Ferket, P.R. 2008. Small intestine development and growth performance of turkey poults is enhanced by dietary supplementation of Nupro yeast extract. In: Proc. XXIII World Poultry Congress, Brisbane, Australia.

Bosi, P., Han, I.K., Jung, H., Heo, K., Perini, S., Castellazzi, A. 2001. Effect of different spray dried plasmas on growth, ileal digestibility, nutrient deposition, immunity and health of early-weaned pigs challenged with E. coli K88. Asian Australasian Journal of Animal Science, 4: 1138-43.

Boyer, P.E., D'Costa, S., Edwards, L.L., Milloway, M., Susick, E., Borst, L.B., Thakur, S., Campbell, J.M., Crenshaw, J.D., Polo, J. and Moeser, A.J. 2015. Early-life dietary spray-dried plasma influences immunological and intestinal injury responses to later-life Salmonella typhimurium challenge. British Journal of Nutrition, 113(5): 783–793.

Campbell, J.M., Crenshaw, J.D., Russel, L.E., Hayes, S.K. 2009. Management of the inflammatory response using plasma as an immune modulator and its impact on swine production. In: Proceeding of 16th International Conference, Krmiva, Opatija, Croatia. p. 43.

Campbell, J.M., Le Russell, Crenshaw, J.D. and Koehnk, H.J. 2006a. Effect of spray-dried plasma form and duration of feeding on broiler performance during natural necrotic enteritis exposure. Journal of Applied Poultry Research, 15: 584-591.

Campbell, J.M., Le Russell, Crenshaw, J.D., Behnke, K.C. and Clark, P.M. 2006b.Growth response of broilers to spray-dried plasma in pelleted or expanded feed processed at high temperature. Journal of Animal Science, 84: 2501-2508.

Campbell, J.M., Quigley III, J.D., Le Russell and Kidd, M.T. 2003. Effect of spray-dried bovine serum on intake, health and growth of broilers housed in different environments. Journal of Animal Science, 81: 2776-2782.

Cole, M. and Sprent, M. 2001. Protein and amino acid requirements of weaner pigs. In: Varley MA, Wiseman J, editors. The weaner pig: nutrition and management. Wallingford, UK: CAB Int. p. 45-64

Dozier, B., Edwin Moran and James Pierce. 2000. Responses of male broilers to biopeptide protein from placement until 17 days of age. Alltech Technical Update.

Edwards, M., Campbell, R., Mikkelsen, L. and Choct, M. 2010. Nutritional strategies to limit the post-weaning growth check in young pigs [PhD thesis]. University of New England; p. 26.

EL-Naga, M.K.A. 2012. Effect of dietary yeast supplementation on broiler performance. Egyptian Poultry Science Journal, 32(1): 95-106.

Garriga, C., Perez-Bosque, A., Amat, C., Campbell, J.M., Russell, L., Polo, J. 2005. Spray-dried porcine plasma reduces the effects of staphylococcal enterotoxin B on glucose transport in rat intestine. Journal of Nutrition, 135: 1653-8.

Gonzalez-Esquerra, R., Campbell, J. and Javier Polo. 2020. Using spray-dried plasma in broilers –lessons learned. Asian Poultry Magazine, May 2020: 28-30.

Grimble, G.K. and Westwood, M.R. 2000. Nucleotides. In: Nutrition and Immunology: Principles and practice (M.E. Gershwin, J.B. German ad C.L. Keen, Eds), Humana press, Totowa, NJ, USA, pp. 135-144.

Henn, J.D., Bockor, L., Vieira, M.S., Ribeiro, A.M.L., Kessler, A.M., Albino, L., Rostagno, H., Crenshaw, J.D., Campbell, J.M. and Rangel, L.P.S. 2013. Inclusion of porcine spray-dried plasma in broiler diets. Journal of Applied Poultry Research, 22: 229-237.

Hombegowda, G.P. 2019. Nutritional evaluation of single cell protein in broilers. MVSc Thesis, Karnataka Veterinary, Animal and Fisheries Sciences University, Bidar, India

Jamroz, D., Wiliczkiewicz, A., Orda, J., Kuryszko, J., Stefaniak, T. 2012. Use of spray-dried porcine blood by-products in diets for young chickens. Journal of Animal Physiology and Animal Nutrition, 96: 319-33.

Jamroz, D., Wiliczkiewicz, A., Orda, J., Skorupi_Nska, J, S³upczy_Nska, M. and Kuryszko, J. 2011. Chemical composition and biological value of spray dried porcine blood by-products and bone protein hydrolysate for young chickens. British Poultry Science, 52: 589-605.

King, M., Morel, P., Pluske, J. and Hendriks, W. 2008. A comparison of the effects of dietary spray dried bovine colostrum and animal plasma on growth and intestinal histology in weaner pigs. Livestock Science, 119: 167-73.

Linder, T. 2019. Making the case for edible microorganisms as an integral part of a more sustainable and resilient food production system. Food Security, 11: 265–278.

Owusu-Asiedu, A., Baidoo, S., Nyachoti, C. and Marquardt, R. 2002. Response of early-weaned pigs to spray-dried porcine or animal plasma-based diets supplemented with egg yolk antibodies against enterotoxigenic Escherichia coli. Journal of Animal Science, 80: 2895-903.

Pettigrew, J.E. 2006. Critical review of functional animal proteins. Des Moines, Iowa USA.

Pierce, J., Cromwell, G., Lindemann, M., Russell, L. and Weaver, E. 2005. Effects of spray-dried animal plasma and immunoglobulins on performance of early weaned pigs. Journal of Animal Science, 83: 2876-85.

Polo, J., Rodríguez, C., Saborido, N. and Ródenas, J. 2005. Functional properties of spray-dried animal plasma in canned petfood. Animal Feed Science and Technology, 122: 331–343.

Quigley, J. and Drew, M. 2000. Effects of oral antibiotics or bovine plasma on survival, health and growth in dairy calves challenged with Escherichia coli. Food Agricultural Immunology, 12: 311-8.

Ravindran, R. 2005. Perspectives on early nutrition e development of digestive function and possible physiological limitations in neonatal poultry. Poultry beyond 2010. Auckland, New Zealand.

Ritala, A., Hakkinen, S.T., Toivari, M. and Wiebe, M. G., 2017. Single cell protein-state of the art, industrial landscape and patents 2001-2016.Frontiers in Microbiology, 8: 1-18.

Rutz, F., Xavier, E.G., Anciuti, M.A., Victor Fernando B Roll and Patricia Rossi. 2007. The role of nucleotides in improving broiler prestarter diets: The Brazilian experience. Proceedings of 23rd Alltech' s Annual Symposium: 175-181.

Saied, J.M., Al-Jabary, Q.H. and Thalij, K.M. 2011. Effect of dietary supplement yeast culture on production performance and hematological parameters in broiler chicks. International Journal of Poultry Science, 10: 376-380.

Samanya, M. and Yamauchi, K.E. 2002. Histological alterations of intestinal villi in chickens fed dried Bacillus subtilis var. natto. Comparative Biochemistry Physiology A. Molecular Integrative Physiology, 133: 95–104.

Santos Jr., A.A., Bohoquez, D.V., Nanney, R.L. and Ferket, P.R. 2007. Nutrient digestibility value of a yeast extract, Nupro in broiler male chicks. International Poultry Scientific Forum, Georgia World Congress Center, Atlanta, USA, p 10.

Shivakumar, M.C. 2009. Role of yeast cell extracted nucleotides in improving performance of broiler chickens. PhD Thesis, Karnataka Veterinary, Animal and Fisheries Sciences University, Bidar, India

Torrallardona, D. 2010. Spray dried animal plasma as an alternative to antibiotics in weanling pigs: a review. Asian-Australasian Journal of Animal Science, 23:131e48.

Zhao, J., Harper, A., Estienne, M., Webb, K., Mcelroy A and Denbow, D. 2007. Growth performance and intestinal morphology responses in early weaned pigs to supplementation of antibiotic-free diets with an organic copper complex and spray-dried plasma protein in sanitary and non-sanitary environments. Journal of Animal Science, 85: 1302e10.

Index

D

E.

F

R

S

T

V

W

X

Y

Z

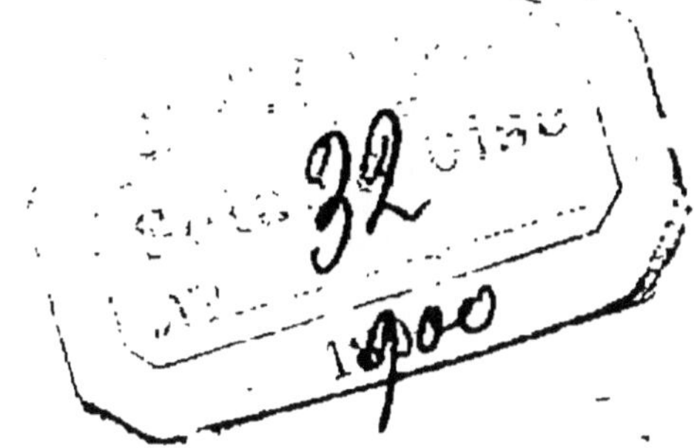